Speech–Language Pathology Assistants

A Resource Manual

Second Edition

Speech–Language Pathology Assistants

A Resource Manual

Second Edition

Jennifer A. Ostergren, PhD, CCC-SLP

PLURAL
PUBLISHING
INC.

PLURAL PUBLISHING
INC.

5521 Ruffin Road
San Diego, CA 92123

e-mail: information@pluralpublishing.com
Website: https://www.pluralpublishing.com

Typeset in 10.5/13 Palatino by Flanagan's Publishing Services, Inc.
Printed in the United States of America by McNaughton & Gunn, Inc
22 21 20 19   2 3 4 5

For permission to use material from this text, contact us by
Telephone: (866) 758-7251
Fax: (888) 758-7255
e-mail: permissions@pluralpublishing.com

*Every attempt has been made to contact the copyright holders for material originally printed
in another source. If any have been inadvertently overlooked, the publishers will gladly make
the necessary arrangements at the first opportunity.*

Library of Congress Cataloging-in-Publication Data:

Names: Ostergren, Jennifer A., author.
Title: Speech-language pathology assistants : a resource manual / Jennifer A.
   Ostergren.
Description: Second edition. | San Diego, CA : Plural, [2020] | Includes
   bibliographical references and index.
Identifiers: LCCN 2018045684 | ISBN 9781944883263 (alk. paper) | ISBN
   1944883266 (alk. paper)
Subjects: | MESH: Speech-Language Pathology--methods | Allied Health
   Personnel | Language Disorders--therapy
Classification: LCC RC424.7 | NLM WL 21 | DDC 616.85/5--dc23
LC record available at https://lccn.loc.gov/2018045684

Contents

Preface

Speech-language pathology assistants (SLPAs) are "support personnel who, following academic and/or on-the-job training, perform tasks prescribed, directed, and supervised by American Speech-Language-Hearing Association (ASHA)-certified speech-language pathologists (SLPs) (ASHA, n.d.-a., para. 2). The use of SLPAs and support personnel is not new. As early as the 1970s, support personnel in the field of speech-language pathology were being used and regulated by different states in the United States (ASHA, n.d.-a.). ASHA has had guidelines for the use of support personnel since 1969. According to ASHA, attention to the use of SLPAs has increased as professionals in the field look for ways to contain costs and expand clinical services (ASHA, n.d.-a.). ASHA maintains and periodically updates formal policy and guidelines on the training, use, and supervision of SLPAs. Recognizing national inconsistency in SLPA use and training, ASHA also created an optional associates program in 2011 (Robinson, 2010). The program extends ASHA affiliation to qualified support personnel who agree to follow all ASHA policies and guidelines pertaining to the use and supervision of support personnel (McNeilly, 2010). In 2017, ASHA's Board of Directors also voted in favor of approving funding and implementation of new Assistants Certification Programs for audiology assistants and SLPAs (ASHA, n.d.-b.). This new program is scheduled to launch sometime in 2020.

CONTENT

This book is written specifically for SLPAs, addressing their unique needs. It is intended to be a practical resource on a wide range of topics that SLPAs may find of value. It does not cover normal processes of communication or communicative disorders in-depth. Rather, it is intended as a "what now" or real-world perspective offering technical and clinical procedure suggestions for SLPAs, including SLPA professional issues and ethics, and instruction in workplace behaviors, such as implementing treatment and collecting and summarizing data. Specialized topics applicable to SLPAs, such as augmentative and alternative communication, cultural and linguistic diversity, play and literacy in therapy, speech sound remediation, and autism spectrum disorder are also included to extend SLPAs' foundational knowledge to real-world applications. This book is written for individuals with a variety of SLPA experience and training. It is my hope that SLPAs with all levels of experience and background will find tools and resources of value to them in this book. If you are an SLPA who has been in the field for many years, this book may offer you a fresh perspective on your role and ideas for continuing to refine your skills. If you are an SLPA just starting your career, this book offers you important information to take with you on your journey. If you are an SLPA in training, the book provides you with information relevant for your training, particularly to your clinical practicum and future employment as an SLPA.

ORGANIZATION

The first six chapters cover broad topics, including an overview of the roles and responsibilities of SLPAs and their supervisors. The initial chapters also cover professional conduct, ethics, cultural and linguistic diversity, and topics important to the health and safety of SLPAs and the individuals they serve. Within these sections, ASHA documents are a cornerstone when referencing policies, procedures, rules, and regulations applicable to SLPA practice. At present, there is considerable variability between states' regulations applicable to SLPAs. As such, ASHA, as the sole national organization for the profession in the United States, serves as an important and primary resource on the topic. That is not to say that SLPAs should ignore state regulations. Rather, as will be discussed, SLPAs must be cognizant of both ASHA and individual state regulations. References and suggestions for accessing state-specific information are provided. Furthermore, given the dynamic nature of policies and procedures, readers should view the information in this book as an overview of regulations and policies in place at the time of publication. The reader is referred to ASHA's website, at https://www.asha.org, for the most recent information.

The next six chapters of the book are organized as "skill development" chapters. These chapters cover a specific set of skills needed by SLPAs across a wide variety of settings. They include the important topics of data collection, note writing, therapy implementation techniques for individual and group sessions, and a newly added chapter on the use of behavioral principles. Throughout each skill development chapter, helpful tips and applicable references and resources are provided, with the major emphasis on providing information that will be of value in actual clinical work as an SLPA.

The remaining seven chapters include treatment foundations and suggestions for specific populations, including newly added chapters on early intervention, language interventions for children, and foundational knowledge for working with adults with acquired neurologic disorders. This is not an exhaustive list of all the populations and disorders SLPAs may encounter in their clinical work. Rather, these chapters serve as additional considerations for common populations and disorders SLPAs might encounter.

COMPANION WEBSITE

This book has a companion website with important forms SLPAs can use in their clinical work. These forms can be freely modified and copied. Explanations about the content on the companion website are embedded within the chapters of the book. The following symbol denotes where the content of the companion website is referenced.

REFERENCES

American Speech-Language-Hearing Association (ASHA). (n.d.-a.). *Frequently asked questions: Speech-language pathology assistants (SLPAs).* Retrieved from https://www.asha.org/associates/SLPA-FAQs/

American Speech-Language-Hearing Association. (n.d.-b.). *Assistants certification program.* Retrieved on June 6, 2018 from https://www.asha.org/associates/Assistants-Certification-Program/

McNeilly, L. (2010, November). ASHA will roll out associates program in 2011. *ASHA Leader, 15,* 7. doi: 10.1044/leader.AN1.15142010.7

Robinson, T. L., Jr. (2010). Associates in ASHA: A new initiative. *ASHA Leader, 15,* 17. doi:10.1044/leader.FTP.15092010.17

Acknowledgments

Foremost, I would like to acknowledge and thank my husband and daughter for their patience and unwavering support. Without your words of encouragement and gifts of time to focus on my writing, this book would not have been possible. I would also like to thank my colleagues who contributed chapters to this book. Their names and accomplishments follow. Your expertise has added greatly to the depth of information available to speech-language pathology assistants (SLPAs) on very important topics. I would also like to thank all the students who completed their clinical practicum within my (SLPA) course at California State University, Long Beach. You have positively shaped the content of this book through your experiences as SLPAs in training. A special thank you, as well, to Ben, for his wonderful illustrations, which add additional insight and detail to each chapter. I would also like to acknowledge Plural Publishing and my publishing team for their commitment to excellence and constant support from start to finish. Thank you as well to Carley, my research assistant. Carley, your help and attention to detail has been invaluable in the process of revising for this second edition.

Contributors

Sara M. Aguilar, MA, CCC-SLP
Chapter 16
Sara M. Aguilar is a school-based speech language pathologist in Southern California. Her professional areas of interest include augmentative and alternative communication, early literacy intervention, and supervision and training of support personnel. She has published and presented research on the training, supervision, and use of SLPAs in California. Sara was a recipient of the Contemporary Issues in Communication Sciences and Disorders Editor's Award at the 2012 American Speech Language Hearing Association Conference.

Carolyn Conway Madding, PhD, CCC-SLP
Chapter 5
Carolyn Conway Madding, Professor Emerita, formerly Chair of the Department of Speech-Language Pathology at California State University, Long Beach, is a fellow of the ASHA and ASHA Minority Champion. She received the Diversity Award from the California Speech-Language-Hearing Association (CSHA) and has published and presented nationally and internationally on bilingualism and linguistic and cultural diversity within the profession of speech-language pathology.

Sarah Guzzino-Herrick, MA, CCC-SLP
Chapter 12
Sarah Guzzino-Herrick is a speech-language pathologist in Southern California working in an elementary school and private practice. She co-authored the first edition of Chapter 11, titled Group Ther-

apy, while in graduate school and working as a licensed speech-language pathology assistant at an elementary school. She received her BA and MA in Communicative Disorders from California State University, Long Beach.

Pei-Fang Hung, PhD, CCC-SLP
Chapter 6
Pei-Fang Hung is an assistant professor in the Department of Speech-Language Pathology at the California State University, Long Beach. Her research interests are aphasia assessment and intervention, neurogenic cognitive-communication disorders, and language changes related to normal aging and early dementia. She is a bilingual speech-language pathologist who holds certificates and licenses in both the United States and Taiwan.

Jodi Robledo, PhD, BCBA
Chapter 17
Jodi Robledo is an associate professor in Special Education at California State University, San Marcos and serves as the program coordinator of the Education Specialist Credential Programs and Master's Degree option. In addition, she is the program director for the Applied Behavior Analysis Certificate of Advanced Study and the Autism Spectrum Disorder Added Authorization. She also teaches courses in the Speech and Language Pathology Department. Prior to this appointment, she was a K–12 autism specialist and education specialist in an urban multicultural school district. Dr. Robledo currently teaches courses with a focus on autism spectrum disorder, supporting individu-

als with moderate to severe disabilities, and inclusive education. She has journal publications, several book chapters, and numerous national conference presentations on these and other topics. Recently, one of her studies received Tier 2 distinction in *Frontiers in Integrative Neuroscience*. Her research interests focus on autism spectrum disorder, supportive relationships, sensory and movement differences, and inclusive education.

Lei Sun, PhD, CCC-SLP
Chapter 13
Lei Sun is an associate professor in the Department of Speech-Language Pathology at the California State University Long Beach. She served as an SLP in preschools and elementary schools. She has expertise in preschool and school-age language development and disorders, theory of mind and language, parent training/coaching, and speech sound disorders.

Margaret Vento-Wilson, MA, CCC-SLP
Chapters 14, 15, and 18
Margaret Vento-Wilson is a speech-language pathologist working at an elementary school in Southern California. She is also an adjunct instructor at California State University, Long Beach in the department of Speech-Language Pathology. Her primary areas of interest include augmentative and alternative communication and language acquisition. She has published on motor speech disorders, fluency, congenital aglossia, and AAC. She has presented the topics of AAC in the acute care setting, AAC and literacy, and interdisciplinary collaboration in the school setting.

ILLUSTRATIONS

Ben Philpott
Chapter illustrations were provided by Ben Philpott. Ben Philpott lives in Tucson, Arizona, and earned his BA in communicative disorders from California State University, Long Beach. He has worked as an SLPA in school, clinic and home settings. He currently works for Scientific Learning, where he trains teachers on how to implement reading intervention software.

PART I

Defining Roles: Speech–Language Pathology Assistants (SLPAs)

CHAPTER 1

Defining Roles: SLPAs

Confidence, like art, never comes from having all the answers;
it comes from being open to all the questions.

—Earl Gray Stevens

The American Speech-Language-Hearing Association (ASHA) defines SLPAs as "support personnel who perform tasks as prescribed, directed, and supervised by an ASHA-certified speech-language pathologist (SLP)" (ASHA, 2013, Executive Summary, para. 1). SLPAs are not independent practitioners, but rather work specifically under the direction and guidance of a qualified SLP to increase the availability, frequency, and efficiency of services provided by the SLP. SLPAs provide services in a wide variety of settings. These settings include, but are not limited to the following (ASHA, 2013, Executive Summary, para. 1)[1]:

- Public, private, and charter elementary and secondary schools,
- Early intervention settings, preschools, and day care settings,
- Hospitals (in- and outpatient),

- Residential health care settings (e.g., long-term care and skilled nursing facilities),
- Nonresidential health care settings (e.g., home health agencies, adult day care settings, clinics),
- Private practice settings,
- University and college clinics,
- Research facilities,
- Corporate and industrial settings, and
- Student's patient's and client's residence.

SLPAs differ from other support personnel, such as speech and language aides, instructional aides, and communication aides both in the level of training and in the amount of supervision and oversight they receive. According to ASHA (n.d.-a.), "aides, for example, have a different, usually narrower, training base and more limited responsibilities than speech-language pathology assistants" (Defining Speech-Language Pathology Assistants, para 2).

The use of SLPAs is not new in the field of speech-language pathology. ASHA has had documents addressing support personnel since as early as the 1960s. The role of the SLPA in the field of speech-language pathology continues to evolve, however, given changes in health and educational service delivery models, increases in the number of individuals with communication disorders, expansion in the scope of services provided by SLPs, and the rising costs of providing these services.

ASHA (2013) outlines that "some tasks, procedures, or activities used to treat individuals with communication and related disorders can be performed successfully by individuals other than an SLP, if the persons conducting the activity are properly trained and supervised by ASHA-certified or licensed SLPs" (Executive Summary, para. 1). This chapter outlines recommendations for the training and use of SLPAs. Recommendations for the supervision of SLPAs are summarized in Chapter 2.

ASHA is the national professional organization in the United States in the field of speech-language pathology. For the purpose of this book, recommendations and standards reviewed are applicable to SLPAs in the United States, using ASHA recommendations and practice guidelines. At the writing of this book, ASHA's primary policy document on the training, use, and supervision of SLPAs was *Speech-Language Pathology Assistant Scope of Practice* (ASHA, 2013), which is available as Appendix 1–A and can also be retrieved from http://www.asha.org/

Internationally, there is variability in professional classification, services provided, and the use of assistants in the field of speech-language pathology. For individuals interested in obtaining information about SLPAs outside of the United States, Appendix 1–B contains a summary of international SLP professional organizations (this information is also available at http://www.asha.org/). These organizations are a good starting point for discovering if SLPAs exist at similar levels in other parts of the world. The International Association of Logopedics and Phoniatrics is also a source of information on this topic (http://www.ialp.info/).

In the United States, regulations for the training, use, and supervision of support personnel vary from state to state. The governing bodies that regulate or oversee the use of SLPAs also vary from state to state. In some locations, a state's department of education (or similar educational body) establishes and oversees specific requirements for SLPA training, use, and supervision in school settings. In some locations, state licensing boards regulate SLPA training, use, and supervision in nonschool settings. And in some cases, educational setting-specific requirements overlap with those of noneducation requirements, but in others they differ.

Figure 1–1 depicts a map highlighting states with official designation or regulation of SLPAs (ASHA, n.d.-b.). States not highlighted in gray either: (a) do not have an official regulating mechanism specifically for SLPAs (although they may recognize that SLPs use assistants, aides, or other types of paraprofessionals), or (b) use paraprofessional designations other than SLPA, such as communication aides, communication technicians, SLP apprentices, or SLP paraprofessionals.

As an SLPA, if you are working in a setting that requires formal licensure, certification, or registration for support personnel, it is imperative that you adhere to any applicable laws, regulations, and procedures. Not doing so could compromise the care of the individuals you serve and place you and your supervisor in legal jeopardy for actions outside your state's standards. SLPAs should familiarize themselves with the most recent regulations in their locations. Realize as well that state standards may change annually or without notice. Hence, it is your responsibility as an SLPA to be familiar with, and stay abreast of, the most recent regulations in your location.

ASHA's State Advocacy Team maintains a page on ASHA's website that summarizes each state's requirements, including requirements for support personnel (http://www.asha.org/advocacy/state/). This is an invaluable resource for SLPAs. SLPAs should also go directly to the website of their state's regulating body for information regarding SLPA regulations, laws, and procedures. An Internet search using terms such as the name of your state plus *speech-language pathology assistant*, *support personnel*, *registration*, *certification*, or *licensure*, will likely yield the contact information you need.

Lastly, before we begin a detailed discussion about SLPA training and use, it is helpful to understand what documents and guidelines ASHA has available on this and related topics. Appendix 1–C contains a description of cardinal sources from ASHA relative to SLPAs. ASHA also maintains a "Frequently Asked Questions" section on its website with current and helpful information about SLPAs. ASHA also has "practice portals" for professionals to access ASHA resources and policies on specific topics. The practice portal on the subject of SLPAs is highly valuable for current information on topics related to support personnel. It can be accessed via http://www.asha.org/ Practice-Portal/Professional-Issues/ Speech-Language-Pathology-Assistants/ or by searching *practice portal* and *SLPA* on ASHA's website.

The information discussed in this book applies to documents published by ASHA at the time this book was written. As an SLPA, you should make ASHA's website a favorite on your home page for ready access. Similar to state regulations, ASHA policies and documents change over time. As such, it is critical that you keep abreast of recent information from ASHA applicable to SLPAs. Following a description of SLPA use and training, the final section of this chapter describes ASHA affiliation for SLPAs, which is an additional avenue for keeping connected with ASHA's professional community.

Figure 1–1. States with formal SLPA designations (ASHA, n.d.-b). *Note.* States highlighted in gray formally recognize SLPAs, through registration, certification, licensure, or some other formal mechanism. Asterisks denote states with formal designations in the field of speech-language pathology other than SLPA, such as communication aide, technician, and speech-language pathology paraprofessional.

U.S. Territories with SLPA Designation
Guam
Puerto Rico

SLPA MINIMUM QUALIFICATIONS

As noted earlier, required training and education will vary by state, but ASHA recommends the following minimum qualifications for SLPAs (2013, Minimal Qualifications of an SLPA, para. 1)[1]:

- An associate's degree from an SLPA program, or a bachelor's degree in a speech-language pathology or communication disorders program;
- Successful completion of a minimum of one hundred (100) hours of supervised field work experience or equivalent clinical experience; and
- Demonstration of competency in the skills required of an SLPA.

SLPA DUTIES AND RESPONSIBILITIES

ASHA expectations for SLPAs working in the field of speech-language pathology include performing only those tasks that are prescribed by an SLP and adhering to all applicable guidelines and regulations, including state licensure and related rules regarding SLPAs in specific settings. Specifically, ASHA states that SLPAs are expected to do the following (ASHA, 2013, Expectations of an SLPA, para. 1)[1]:

- Seek employment only in settings in which direct and indirect supervision are provided on a regular and systematic basis by an ASHA-certified or licensed SLP.
- Adhere to the responsibilities for SLPAs and refrain from

performing tasks or activities that are the sole responsibility of the SLP.
- Perform only those tasks prescribed by the supervising SLP.
- Adhere to all applicable state licensure laws and rules regulating the practice of speech-language pathology, such as those requiring licensure or registration of support personnel.
- Conduct oneself ethically within the scope of practice and responsibilities for an SLPA.
- Actively participate with the SLP in the supervisory process.
- Consider securing liability insurance.
- Actively pursue continuing education and professional development activities.

ASHA's (2013) document makes a specific point of highlighting those activities SLPAs should not engage in, as they are specifically outside an SLPA's scope of service (Box 1–1). If you find yourself in a situation during your training or at any point during the course of your employment as an SLPA where you engage in (or are asked to perform) any of these activities, this is a clear warning sign that you should seek immediate assistance in addressing the issue. Chapter 3 discusses ethical dilemmas such as this and recommendations for resolving ethical conflict.

Now that you know what an SLPA must not do, ASHA's 2013 scope-of-practice document also outlines activities that are within the scope of responsibilities of an SLPA, including duties in the areas of service delivery, administrative support, and prevention and advocacy.

Box 1–1. Activities Outside an SLPA's Scope of Practice
(ASHA, 2013, Responsibilities Outside the Scope of SLPAs, para. 1)[1]

An SLPA must *not*

- Represent himself or herself as an SLP;
- Perform standardized or nonstandardized diagnostic tests, formal or informal evaluations, or swallowing screenings and checklists;
- Perform procedures that require a high level of clinical acumen and technical skill (e.g., vocal tract prosthesis shaping or fitting, vocal tract imaging and oral pharyngeal swallow therapy with bolus material);
- Tabulate or interpret results and observations of feeding and swallowing evaluations performed by SLPs;
- Participate in formal parent conferences, case conferences, or any interdisciplinary team without the presence of the supervising SLP or other designated SLP;
- Provide interpretative information to the student, patient, client, family, or others regarding the patient or client status or service;
- Write, develop, or modify a student's, patient's, or client's treatment plan in any way;
- Assist with students, patients, or clients without following the individualized treatment plan prepared by the certified SLP or without access to supervision;
- Sign any formal documents (e.g., treatment plans, reimbursement forms, or reports);
- Select students, patients, or clients for service;
- Discharge a student, patient, or client from services;
- Make referrals for additional service;
- Disclose clinical or confidential information either orally or in writing to anyone other than the supervising SLP;
- Develop or determine the swallowing strategies or precautions for patients, family, or staff;
- Treat medically fragile students, patients, and clients without supervision; or
- Design or select augmentative and alternative communication systems or devices.

Service Delivery

In the area of service delivery, ASHA recommends that SLPAs identify them-selves to clients, clients' families, and fellow service providers, both verbally and in writing, and wear a name badge (ASHA, 2013). Furthermore, as discussed in Chapter 3, SLPAs are expected to conduct themselves ethically, maintain client confidentiality, and adhere to all federal and state regulations in the provision of services in schools and medical settings. Provided SLPAs are under the direction of a qualified SLP and given adequate training and supervision, Box 1–2 outlines ASHA's recommendations for activities within the scope of an SLPA related to service delivery. SLPAs "may not perform tasks when a supervising SLP cannot be reached by personal contact, phone, pager, or other immediate or electronic means" (ASHA, 2013, Minimum Requirements in Frequency and Amount of Supervision, para. 1).[1] Furthermore, the purpose of an SLPA is to support the SLP in the provision of services, not to increase the caseload numbers of the SLP. ASHA recommends that SLPAs have liability insurance as protection for malpractice during service provision. Your employer may provide this insurance for you or

---

Box 1–2. SLPA Scope of Responsibility: Service Delivery
(ASHA, 2013, Service Delivery, para. 1)[1]

- Assist the SLP with speech, language, and hearing screenings **without** clinical interpretation.
- Assist the SLP during assessment of students, patients, and clients, exclusive of administration and interpretation.
- Assist the SLP with bilingual translation during screening and assessment activities exclusive of interpretation.*
- Follow documented treatment plans or protocols developed by the supervising SLP.
- Provide guidance and treatment via telepractice to students, patients, and clients who are selected by the supervising SLP as appropriate for this service delivery model.
- Document student, patient, and client performance (e.g., tally data for the SLP to use; prepare charts, records, and graphs) and report this information to the supervising SLP.
- Program and provide instruction in the use of augmentative and alternative communication devices.
- Demonstrate or share information with patients, families, and staff regarding feeding strategies developed and directed by the SLP.
- Serve as interpreter for patients, clients, students, and families who do not speak English.*
- Provide services under SLP supervision in another language for individuals who do not speak English and for English-language learners.*

Note: Chapter 5 contains a discussion of the use of SLPAs as interpreters and translators, including ASHA (2004) recommendations for training in this function.

you may be expected to independently acquire liability insurance. This should be done prior to providing services to clients. ASHA offers discounts on this insurance for SLPAs who are affiliated associates.

Administrative Support

In addition to providing clinical services, SLPAs may provide administrative support to their supervisors, including the activities listed in Box 1–3.

Prevention and Advocacy

SLPAs may also assist their supervisors in activities related to the prevention of communicative disorders and advocacy for individuals with communicative disorders and their families. Box 1–4 highlights activities within the scope of responsibilities of an SLPA in this area.

SLPA JOB DESCRIPTION: A DAY IN THE LIFE OF AN SLPA

After reading lists of duties and responsibilities, many SLPAs in training often still ask, "What will my job be like as an SLPA?" This is a valid question to ask but a difficult one to answer. The settings in which SLPAs work are highly variable, as are the populations of individuals for which SLPAs provide services. Equally variable is the nature of tasks SLPAs perform in these different settings. Appendix 1–D recounts several stories, collected from SLPAs throughout the United States, which tell of a "Day in the Life" of a specific SLPA. Lastly, Appendices 1–E and 1–F contain sample job descriptions for SLPAs in medical and educational settings, respectively. Each of these documents sheds a light on different roles of an SLPA. Ultimately, learning firsthand by meeting and speaking directly with SLPAs and SLPs themselves is one of the best ways to explore the field of speech-language pathology and the roles of SLPAs.

COMPETENCY ASSESSMENT

Webster's dictionary defines *competent* as "having requisite or adequate ability or qualities" or "having the capacity to function or develop in a particular way" (Merriam-Webster, 2003). Being a competent SLPA requires knowledge and the practical application of this knowledge in the execution of specific tasks (i.e., skill). In

---

Box 1–3. SLPA Scope of Responsibility: Administrative Support
(ASHA, 2013, Administrative Support, para. 1)[1]

- Assist with clerical duties, such as preparing materials and scheduling activities, as directed by the SLP.
- Perform checks and maintenance of equipment.
- Assist with departmental operations (e.g., scheduling, recordkeeping, maintaining supplies and equipment, monitoring equipment safety).

> ## Box 1–4. SLPA Scope of Responsibility: Prevention and Advocacy (ASHA, 2013, Prevention and Advocacy, para. 1)[1]
>
> ■ Present primary prevention information to individuals and groups known to be at risk for communication disorders and other appropriate groups; promote early identification and early intervention activities.
> ■ Advocate for individuals and families through community awareness, health literacy, education, and training programs to promote and facilitate access to full participation in communication, including the elimination of societal, cultural, and linguistic barriers.
> ■ Provide information to emergency response agencies for individuals who have communication or swallowing disorders.
> ■ Advocate at local, state, and national levels for improved public policies affecting access to services and research funding.
> ■ Support the supervising SLP in research projects, in-service training, public relations programs, and marketing programs.
> ■ Participate actively in professional organizations.

all settings, on-the-job-training is required to develop your knowledge and skills as an SLPA. To be competent in the performance of your duties in a specific work environment, you need additional knowledge and skills beyond what you learned in a training program to become an SLPA.

In the field of speech-language pathology, assessment based on competency is often used. As discussed in Chapter 2, it is your supervisor's responsibility to outline what specific competencies are required for you to operate effectively as an SLPA in your unique setting (ASHA, 2013). Your supervisor is also responsible for creating a mechanism for assessing your competency in these areas and for developing ways to improve your knowledge and skills to required levels. As an SLPA, it is your responsibility to be aware of the knowledge and skills required of you and to strive for competency in all areas.

Appendix 1–G (and the companion website of this book) contains an example of a competency-based measurement, given the responsibilities within the scope of an SLPA (ASHA, 2013). Note that it uses a continuum to rate competency in the responsibilities of an SLPA on a scale from *does not meet* (1) to *far exceeds requirements* (5). Table 1–1 contains a description of performance levels for this scale. It is important to remember, however, when descriptions of competency indicate the word *independent*, this does not mean SLPAs are performing any activity without the supervision of an SLP (e.g., operating as an independent clinician). Rather, this designation means that, under a supervising SLP's guidance, an SLPA has obtained a level of competency that allows her or him to operate with proficiency in the task described. Appendices 1–H to 1–K contain additional evaluation

Table 1–1. Examples of Competency-Based Assessment Levels (ASHA, 2013)

Does not meet	Requires education and training at the introductory level
Needs improvement	Requires input from supervisor or other resource for routine cases.
Meets requirements	Demonstrates proficiency independently in most cases: independently seeks resources for additional support
Exceeds requirements	Independently demonstrates proficiency for routine to complex cases
Far exceeds requirements	Demonstrates proficiency at all levels of complexity; able to serve as a role model to other staff

tools and forms recommended by ASHA for documenting the presence and degree of core proficiency levels for SLPAs.

These competency-based assessments illustrate an important point to consider throughout your career as an SLPA. Competency reflects your level of performance at any given point in time, for a specific set of circumstances (e.g., a specific task, client, and setting). You will likely not be equally competent across everything you do as an SLPA. That is completely normal. In fact, to expect that you will be perfect and exceed competencies in everything you do misses the potential of this type of assessment.

In each setting, additional, more specific competencies will be required, beyond the basic framework of SLPA responsibilities and job duties outlined by ASHA. For example, there are specific knowledge and skills needed to work with young children with autism spectrum disorder (ASD). These may be similar in some respects but different from the knowledge and skills needed to work with adults with aphasia. Similarly, if you are working in a school setting, there may be specific competencies needed that differ from those of a medical or private practice setting. As an SLPA, when you

enter a training or employment setting, it is critical that you review all competency assessment tools applicable to you and ask your supervisor about the range of specific knowledge and skills required of you in that unique setting.

Beyond minimal competency, as an SLPA, you should always strive for higher levels of performance in all areas of knowledge and skill applicable to your role. Your goal should be to continue to improve and enhance your knowledge and skills throughout your career. SLPAs who recognize there is always room for improvement and who seek ways to improve their performance are those who reach the highest levels of performance as an SLPA. ASHA also stipulates that SLPAs must "actively pursue continuing education and professional development activities" (ASHA 2013, Expectations of an SLPA, para. 1). Furthermore, many state regulating bodies specifically outline the amount and nature of continuing education required for SLPAs to maintain licensure, certification, or registration in that state. You should be familiar with what is required in your state.

It is your responsibility to seek out appropriate continuing education opportunities. You can work with your supervising SLP to identify these opportunities, but ultimately you are responsible for initiating them. Chapter 4 offers suggestions for self-assessment and reflection to evaluate your own skills and abilities and then, importantly, identify avenues for improvement and formal continuing education.

ASHA AFFILIATION

In 2011, ASHA initiated a new program that offered affiliation status to SLPAs, audiology assistants, and other support personnel in the field of communication sciences and disorders (Robinson, 2010). According to ASHA's president at the time, this new program was created to improve patient care by: (a) providing leadership in reconciling national inconsistencies regarding the training, use, and supervision of support personnel across the United States and (b) offering resources for support personnel and their supervisors (Robinson, 2010). However, this program is not a certification program. SLPA affiliates are referred to as ASHA associates. They are not full members of ASHA and are not eligible to vote or hold elected positions. In addition, ASHA does not provide direct oversight or regulation of certification for ASHA associates. This responsibility remains with the applicable state educational, statutory, and regulatory bodies. ASHA associates do however, have access to many ASHA member benefits, including the following ("Welcome!" 2011, para. 5):

■ Networking opportunities with other assistants,
■ Affinity benefits,
■ Consultation with ASHA professional practices staff,

■ Listing and search capabilities on ASHA's online member and affiliate directory,
■ Opportunities to participate in advocacy efforts,
■ Participation in mentoring programs,
■ Reduced registration fees for education programs and products,
■ Access to the online Career Center,
■ Subscription to *The ASHA Leader* and access to *The ASHA Leader Online* (ALO),
■ Access to four online scholarly journals,
■ Subscription to an e-newsletter for assistants,
■ Access to an assistants' e-group (i.e., e-mail discussion list, forum, social network), and
■ Opportunities to earn professional development hours (PDHs) in training, specifically designed for SLPAs and audiology assistants.

You are eligible to apply for ASHA affiliation if

1. You are employed as an SLPA and are supervised by an ASHA-certified SLP, or
2. You have completed your training as an SLPA, but are not currently employed as an SLPA.

If you are employed as an SLPA, your supervisor must sign your application, attesting that she or he is supervising you in accordance with ASHA policies and procedures on support personnel and that you are qualified to perform the tasks of an SLPA. If you have completed your

SLPA training but are not employed, the director for your SLPA training program must sign your application, attesting that you have received training and are qualified to perform the tasks of an SLPA.

ASHA associates must agree to the following (ASHA, 2011):

- Adhere to all applicable policies pertaining to the use and supervision of support personnel, including performing only those tasks assigned by a supervising SLP or audiologist.
- Work only under the supervision of an ASHA-certified SLP or audiologist.
- Adhere to all applicable state (or province) laws and rules regulating the professions listed above.
- Pay annual fees to maintain affiliation.

Additional information about becoming an ASHA associate, including frequently asked questions about the associate program (McNeilly, 2010), can be found on ASHA's website (http://www.asha.org/ associates/).

In 2017, ASHA's Board of Directors also voted in favor of approving funding and implementation of new Assistants Certification Programs for audiology assistants and SLPAs (ASHA, n.d.-c.). This was based on feasibility studies conducted by ASHA in 2016. This analysis revealed the following relative to certification for SLPAs (ASHA, n.d.-c., History):

- The majority of respondents believed a national credential for SLPAs would have a positive impact on client service delivery.

- The advantages to SLPs of working with assistants outweigh the challenges.
- A national SLPA credential could have multiple benefits for supervisors and employers.
- The vast majority of respondents believe ASHA is an appropriate entity to provide assistant certification.
- The inconsistency in SLPA qualifications and ability levels poses a challenge to the use (and credentialing) of assistants.
- There remains a need for resources to help supervisors and assistants to work together effectively to provide client services.

ASHA's Board of Directors tasked its Council for Clinical Certification (CFCC) with creating this new program At the writing of this book, ASHA's anticipated launch of the new certification for SLPAs was expected by the end of 2020 (ASHA, n.d.-c., Timeline).

REFERENCES

American Speech-Language-Hearing Association. (n.d.-a.). *Frequently asked questions: Speech-language pathology assistants (SLPAs).* Retrieved from http://www.asha.org/asso ciates/SLPA-FAQs/

American Speech-Language-Hearing Association. (n.d.-b.). *ASHA state-by-state.* Retrieved from http://www.asha.org/advocacy/state/

American Speech-Language-Hearing Association. (n.d.-c.). *Assistants certification program.* Retrieved from http://www.asha.org/asso ciates/assistants-certification-program/

American Speech-Language-Hearing Association. (n.d.-d.). *Audiology and speech-language pathology associations outside of the United States.*

Retrieved from http://www.asha.org/members/international/intl_assoc.htm

American Speech-Language-Hearing Association (ASHA). (2013). *Speech-language pathology assistant scope of practice*. Retrieved from http://www.asha.org/policy

McNeilly, L. (2010, November). ASHA will roll out associates program in 2011. *ASHA Leader*. Retrieved from http://www.asha.org/Publications/leader/2010/101123/ASHAWill-Roll-Out-Associates-Program-in-2011.htm

Merriam-Webster. (2003). *Merriam-Webster's collegiate dictionary* (11th ed.). Springfield, MA: Author.

Robinson, T. L., Jr. (2010). Associates in ASHA: A new initiative. *ASHA Leader*. Retrieved from http://www.asha.org/Publications/leader/2010/100803/From-President-100803.htm

CHAPTER ENDNOTE

1. American Speech-Language-Hearing Association (2013). *Speech-language pathology assistant scope of practice*. Available from http://www.asha.org/policy. Copyright 2013 American Speech-Language-Hearing Association. All rights reserved. Reprinted with permission.

APPENDIX 1–A
ASHA Speech–Language Pathology Assistant Scope of Practice (ASHA, 2013)

TABLE OF CONTENTS

ABOUT THIS DOCUMENT

This scope of practice for the speech-language pathology assistant (SLPA) was developed by the American Speech-Language-Hearing Association (ASHA) Speech-Language Pathology Assistant Scope of Practice ad hoc committee. It was approved by ASHA's Board of Directors (January 2013). Members of the committee were DeAnne Wellman Owre (chair), Diane L. Eger, Ashley Northam, Mary Jo Schill, Rosemary Scott, Monica Marruffo, and Lemmietta McNeilly (ex officio). Gail J. Richard, Vice President for Speech-Language Pathology Practice, served as the monitoring vice president. The composition of the ad hoc committee included

ASHA-certified speech-language pathologists with specific knowledge and experience working with support personnel in clinical practice in schools, health care, and/or private practice, as well as two members who have served on the ASHA Board of Ethics (Diane L. Eger and Mary Jo Schill).

The document is intended to provide guidance for SLPAs and their supervisors regarding ethical considerations related to the SLPA practice parameters. The document addresses how SLPAs should be utilized and what specific responsibilities are within and outside their roles of clinical practice. Given that standards, licensure, and practice issues vary from state to state, this document delineates ASHA's policy for the use of SLPAs.

DEDICATION

In loving memory of Lisa Cabiale O'Connor (1937–2012), whose dedication, commitment, and perseverance contributed to ensuring integrity and quality in addressing the topic of SLPAs within the ASHA structure.

EXECUTIVE SUMMARY

This scope of practice presents a model for the training, use, and supervision of support personnel in speech-language pathology. Support personnel in speech-language pathology, or speech-language pathology assistants (SLPAs), perform tasks as prescribed, directed, and supervised by ASHA-certified speech-language pathologists (SLPs). Support personnel

can be used to increase the availability, frequency, and efficiency of services.

Some tasks, procedures, or activities used to treat individuals with communication and related disorders can be performed successfully by individuals other than SLPs if the persons conducting the activity are properly trained and supervised by ASHA-certified and/or licensed SLPs. The decision to shift responsibility for implementation of the more repetitive, mechanical, or routine clinical activities to SLPAs should be made only by qualified professionals and only when the quality of care and level of professionalism will not be compromised. The utilization of evidence and ethical and professional judgment should be at the heart of the selection, management, training, supervision, and use of support personnel.

This scope of practice specifies the qualifications and responsibilities for an SLPA and indicates the tasks that are the exclusive responsibilities of the SLP. Additionally, the document provides guidance regarding ethical considerations when support personnel provide clinical services and outlines the supervisory responsibilities of the supervising SLP.

INTRODUCTION

The SLPA Scope of Practice provides information regarding the training, use, and supervision of assistants in speech-language pathology that was established by the American-Speech-Language-Hearing Association to be applicable in a variety of work settings. Training for SLPAs should be based on the type of tasks specified in their scope of responsibility. Specific education and on-the-job training may be necessary to prepare assistants for unique roles in professional settings (e.g., hospitals and schools).

ASHA has established an associate affiliation program for support personnel in speech-language pathology and audiology. Individuals who are working in this capacity under the direct supervision of ASHA-certified SLPs or audiologists are eligible for this category of affiliation with ASHA.

ASHA has addressed the topic of support personnel in speech-language pathology since the 1960s. In 1967, the Executive Board of ASHA established the Committee on Supportive Personnel and in 1969 the document *Guidelines on the Role, Training and Supervision of the Communicative Aide* was approved by the Legislative Council (LC). In the 1990s, several entities—including committees, a task force, and a consensus panel—were established, and the LC passed a position statement, technical report, guidelines, and curriculum content for support personnel. In 2002, ASHA developed an approval process for SLPA programs, and in 2003, a registration process for SLPAs was established. Both were discontinued by vote of the LC because of fiscal concerns. In 2004, a position statement on the training, use, and supervision of support personnel in speech-language pathology was passed by the LC. Since then, the number of SLPAs has increased, primarily in schools and private practice settings. Specific guidance from ASHA continues to be requested by ASHA members in many states.

This document does not supersede federal legislation and regulation requirements or any existing state licensure laws, nor does it affect the interpretation or implementation of such laws. The document may serve, however, as a guide for the development of new laws or, at the appropriate time, for revising existing licensure laws.

STATEMENT OF PURPOSE

The purpose of this document is to define what is within and outside the scope of responsibilities for SLPAs who work under the supervision of properly credentialed SLPs. The following aspects are addressed:

a. parameters for education and professional development for SLPAs;
b. SLPAs' responsibilities within and outside the scope of practice;
c. examples of practice settings;
d. information for others (e.g., special educators, parents, consumers, health professionals, payers, regulators, members of the general public) regarding services SLPAs perform;
e. information regarding the ethical and liability considerations for the supervising SLP and the SLPA; and
f. supervisory requirements for the SLP and the SLPA.

QUALIFICATIONS FOR A SPEECH–LANGUAGE PATHOLOGY ASSISTANT

Minimum Recommended Qualifications for a Speech–Language Pathology Assistant

An SLPA must complete an approved course of academic study, field work under the supervision of an ASHA-certified and/or licensed SLP, and on-the-job training specific to SLPA responsibilities and workplace behaviors.

The academic course of study must include or be equivalent to

a. an associate's degree from an SLPA program,
or
a bachelor's degree in a speech-language pathology or communication disorders program,
and
b. successful completion of a minimum of one hundred (100) hours of supervised field work experience or its clinical experience equivalent,
and
c. demonstration of competency in the skills required of an SLPA.

Expectations of a Speech-Language Pathology Assistant

a. Seek employment only in settings in which direct and indirect supervision are provided on a regular and systematic basis by an ASHA-certified and/or licensed SLP.
b. Adhere to the responsibilities for SLPAs specified in this document and refrain from performing tasks or activities that are the sole responsibility of the SLP.
c. Perform only those tasks prescribed by the supervising SLP.
d. Adhere to all applicable state licensure laws and rules regulating the practice of speech-language pathology, such as those requiring licensure or registration of support personnel.

e. Conduct oneself ethically within the scope of practice and responsibilities for an SLPA.
f. Actively participate with the SLP in the supervisory process.
g. Consider securing liability insurance.
h. Actively pursue continuing education and professional development activities.

RESPONSIBILITIES WITHIN THE SCOPE FOR SPEECH–LANGUAGE PATHOLOGY ASSISTANTS

The supervising SLP retains full legal and ethical responsibility for the students, patients, and clients he or she serves but may delegate specific tasks to the SLPA. The SLPA may execute specific components of a speech and language program as specified in treatment plans developed by the SLP. Goals and objectives listed on the treatment plan and implemented by the SLPA are only those within their scope of responsibilities and are tasks the SLP has determined the SLPA has the training and skill to perform. The SLP must provide at least the minimum specified level of supervision to ensure quality of care to all persons served. The amount of supervision may vary and must depend on the complexity of the case and the experience of the assistant. Under no circumstances should use of the ASHA Code of Ethics or the quality of services provided be diluted or circumvented by the use of an SLPA. Again, the use of an SLPA is optional, and an SLPA should be used only when appropriate.

Provided that the training, supervision, and planning are appropriate, tasks in the following areas of focus may be delegated to an SLPA.

Service Delivery

a. Self-identify as SLPAs to families, students, patients, clients, staff, and others. This may be done verbally, in writing, and/or with titles on name badges.

b. Exhibit compliance with the Health Insurance Portability and Accountability Act (HIPAA) and Family Educational Rights and Privacy Act (FERPA) regulations, reimbursement requirements, and SLPAs' responsibilities.

c. Assist the SLP with speech, language, and hearing screenings **without** clinical interpretation.

d. Assist the SLP during assessment of students, patients, and clients exclusive of administration and/or interpretation.

e. Assist the SLP with bilingual translation during screening and assessment activities exclusive of interpretation; refer to *Knowledge and Skills Needed by Speech-Language Pathologists and Audiologists to Provide Culturally and Linguistically Appropriate Services* (ASHA, 2004).

f. Follow documented treatment plans or protocols developed by the supervising SLP.

g. Provide guidance and treatment via telepractice to students, patients, and clients who are selected by the supervising SLP as appropriate for this service delivery model.

h. Document student, patient, and client performance (e.g., tallying data for the SLP to use; preparing charts, records, and graphs) and report this information to the supervising SLP.

i. Program and provide instruction in the use of augmentative and alternative communication devices.

j. Demonstrate or share information with patients, families, and staff regarding feeding strategies developed and directed by the SLP.

k. Serve as interpreter for patients/clients/students and families who do not speak English.

l. Provide services under SLP supervision in another language for individuals who do not speak English and English-language learners.

Administrative Support

a. Assist with clerical duties, such as preparing materials and scheduling activities, as directed by the SLP.

b. Perform checks and maintenance of equipment.

c. Assist with departmental operations (scheduling, recordkeeping, safety/maintenance of supplies and equipment).

Prevention and Advocacy

a. Present primary prevention information to individuals and groups known to be at risk for communication disorders, and other appropriate groups; promote early identification and early intervention activities.

b. Advocate for individuals and families through community awareness, health literacy, education, and training programs to promote and facilitate access to full participation in communication, including the elimination of societal, cultural, and linguistic barriers.

c. Provide information to emergency response agencies for individuals who have communication and/or swallowing disorders.

d. Advocate at the local, state, and national levels for improved public policies affecting access to services and research funding.

e. Support the supervising SLP in research projects, in-service training, public relations programs, and marketing programs.

f. Participate actively in professional organizations.

RESPONSIBILITIES OUTSIDE THE SCOPE FOR SPEECH-LANGUAGE PATHOLOGY ASSISTANTS

There is potential for misuse of an SLPA, particularly when responsibilities are delegated by administrative or nonclinical staff without the approval of the supervising SLP. It is highly recommended that the ASHA Scope of Practice in Speech-Language Pathology (ASHA, 2007) and the ASHA Code of Ethics (ASHA, 2010) be reviewed with all personnel involved when employing an SLPA. It should be emphasized that an individual's communication or related disorder and/or other factors may preclude the use of services from anyone other than an ASHA-certified and/or licensed SLP. The SLPA should not perform any task without the approval of the supervising SLP. The student, patient, or client should be informed that he or she is receiving services from an SLPA under the supervision of an SLP.

The SLPA should *not* engage in the following:

a. represent himself or herself as an SLP;

b. perform standardized or nonstandardized diagnostic tests, formal or informal evaluations, or swallowing screenings/checklists;

c. perform procedures that require a high level of clinical acumen and technical skill (e.g., vocal tract prosthesis shaping or fitting, vocal tract imaging and oral pharyngeal swallow therapy with bolus material);

d. tabulate or interpret results and observations of feeding and swallowing evaluations performed by SLPs;

e. participate in formal parent conferences, case conferences, or any interdisciplinary team without the presence of the supervising SLP or other designated SLP;

f. provide interpretative information to the student/patient/client, family, or others regarding the student/patient/client status or service;

g. write, develop, or modify a student's, patient's, or client's treatment plan in any way;

h. assist with students, patients, or clients without following an individualized treatment plan prepared by the certified SLP and/or without access to supervision;

i. sign any formal documents (e.g., treatment plans, reimbursement forms, or reports; the SLPA **should** sign or initial informal treatment notes for review and cosign with the supervising SLP as requested);

j. select students, patients, or clients for service;

k. discharge a student, patient, or client from services;

l. make referrals for additional service;

m. disclose clinical or confidential information either orally or in writing to anyone other than the supervising SLP (the SLPA must comply with current HIPAA and FERPA guidelines) unless mandated by law;

n. develop or determine the swallowing strategies or precautions for patients, family, or staff;

o. treat medically fragile students/patients/clients independently; or

p. design or select augmentative and alternative communication systems or devices.

PRACTICE SETTINGS

Under the specified guidance and supervision of an ASHA-certified SLP, SLPAs may provide services in a wide variety of settings, which may include, but are not limited to, the following:

a. public, private, and charter elementary and secondary schools;

b. early intervention settings, preschools, and day care settings;

c. hospitals (in- and outpatient);

d. residential health care settings (e.g., long-term care and skilled nursing facilities);

e. nonresidential health care settings (e.g., home health agencies, adult day care settings, clinics);

f. private practice settings;

g. university/college clinics;

h. research facilities;

i. corporate and industrial settings; and

j. student/patient/client's residences.

ETHICAL CONSIDERATIONS*

ASHA strives to ensure that its members and certificate holders preserve the highest standards of integrity and ethical practice. The ASHA Code of Ethics (2010) sets forth the fundamental principles and rules considered essential to this purpose. The code applies to every individual who is: (a) a member of ASHA, whether certified or not, (b) a nonmember holding the ASHA Certificate of Clinical Competence, (c) an applicant for membership or certification, or (d) a clinical fellow seeking to fulfill standards for certification.

Although some SLPAs may choose to affiliate with ASHA as associates, the Code of Ethics does not directly apply to associates. However, any individual who is working in a support role (technician, aide, assistant) under the supervision of an SLP or speech scientist must be knowledgeable about the provisions of the code. It is imperative that the supervising professional and the assistant behave in a manner that is consistent with the principles and rules outlined in the ASHA Code of Ethics. Since the ethical responsibility for patient care or for subjects in research studies cannot be delegated, the SLP or speech scientist takes overall responsibility for the actions of the assistants when they are performing assigned duties. If the assistant engages in activities that violate the Code of Ethics, the supervising professional may be found in violation of the code if adequate oversight has not been provided.

The following principles and rules of the ASHA Code of Ethics specifically address issues that are pertinent when an SLP supervises support personnel in the provision of services or when conducting research.

Principle of Ethics I

Individuals shall honor their responsibility to hold paramount the welfare of persons they serve professionally or who are participants in research and scholarly activities and they shall treat animals involved in research in a humane manner.

Guidance

The supervising SLP remains responsible for the care and well-being of the client or research subject. If the supervisor fails to intervene when the assistant's behavior puts the client or subject at risk or when services or procedures are implemented inappropriately, the supervisor could be in violation of the Code of Ethics.

Principle of Ethics I, Rule A

Individuals shall provide all services competently.

Guidance

The supervising SLP must ensure that all services, including those provided directly by the assistant, meet practice standards and are administered competently. If the supervisor fails to intervene or correct the actions of the assistant as needed, this could be a violation of the Code of Ethics.

Principle of Ethics I, Rule D

Individuals shall not misrepresent the credentials of assistants, technicians, support personnel, students, clinical fellows, or any others under their supervision, and they shall inform those they serve professionally of the name and professional credentials of persons providing services.

Guidance

The supervising SLP must ensure that clients and subjects are informed of the title and qualifications of the assistant. This is not a passive responsibility; that is, the supervisor must make this information easily available and understandable to the clients or subjects and not rely on the individual to inquire about or ask directly for this information. Any misrepresentation of the assistant's qualifications or role could result in a violation of the Code of Ethics by the supervisor.

Principle of Ethics I, Rule E

Individuals who hold the Certificate of Clinical Competence shall not delegate tasks that require the unique skills, knowledge, and judgment that are within the scope of their profession to assistants, technicians, support personnel, or any nonprofessionals over whom they have supervisory responsibility.

Guidance

The supervising SLP is responsible for monitoring and limiting the role of the assistant as described in these guidelines and in accordance with applicable licensure laws.

Principle of Ethics I, Rule F

Individuals who hold the Certificate of Clinical Competence may delegate tasks related to provision of clinical services to assistants, technicians, support personnel, or any other persons only if those services are appropriately supervised, realizing that the responsibility for client welfare remains with the certified individual.

Guidance

The supervising SLP is responsible for providing appropriate and adequate direct and indirect supervision to ensure that the services provided are appropriate and meet practice standards. The SLP should document supervisory activities and adjust the amount and type of supervision to ensure that the Code of Ethics is not violated.

Principle of Ethics II, Rule B

Individuals shall engage in only those aspects of the profession that are within the scope of their professional practice and competence, considering their level of education, training, and experience.

Guidance

The supervising SLP is responsible for ensuring that he or she has the skills and competencies needed in order to provide appropriate supervision. This may include seeking continuing education in the area of supervision practice.

Principle of Ethics II, Rule D

Individuals shall not require or permit their professional staff to provide services or conduct research activities that exceed the staff member's competence, level of education, training, and experience.

Guidance

The supervising SLP must ensure that the assistant only performs those activities and duties that are defined as appropriate for the level of training and experience and in accordance with applicable licensure laws. If the assistant exceeds the practice role that has been defined for him or her, and the supervisor fails to correct this, the supervisor could be found in violation of the Code of Ethics.

Principle of Ethics IV, Rule B

Individuals shall prohibit anyone under their supervision from engaging in any practice that violates the Code of Ethics.

Guidance

Because the assistant provides services as "an extension" of those provided by the professional, the SLP is responsible for informing the assistant about the Code of Ethics and monitoring the performance of the assistant. Failure to do so could result in the SLP's being found in violation of the Code.

LIABILITY ISSUES

Individuals who engage in the delivery of services to persons with communication disorders are potentially vulnerable to accusations of engaging in unprofessional practices. Therefore, liability insurance is recommended as a protection for malpractice. SLPAs should consider the need for liability coverage. Some employers provide it for all employees. Other employers defer to the employee to independently acquire liability insurance. Some universities provide coverage for students involved in practicum/fieldwork. Checking for liability insurance coverage is the responsibility of the SLPA and needs to be done prior to providing services.

SPEECH-LANGUAGE PATHOLOGIST'S SUPERVISORY ROLE

Qualifications for a Supervising Speech-Language Pathologist

Minimum qualifications for an SLP who will supervise an SLPA include:

a. current ASHA certification and/or state licensure,
b. completion of at least 2 years of practice following ASHA certification,
c. completion of an academic course or at least 10 hours of continuing education units (CEUs) in the area of supervision, completed prior to or concurrent with the first SLPA supervision experience.

Additional Expectations of the Supervising Speech-Language Pathologist

a. Conduct ongoing competency evaluations of the SLPAs.
b. Provide and encourage ongoing education and training opportunities for the SLPA consistent with competency and skills and needs of the students, patients, or clients served.
c. Develop, review, and modify treatment plans for students, patients, and clients that SLPAs implement under the supervision of the SLP.
d. Make all case management decisions.
e. Adhere to the supervisory responsibilities for SLPs.

f. Retain the legal and ethical responsibility for all students, patients, and clients served.
g. Adhere to the principles and rules of the ASHA Code of Ethics.
h. Adhere to applicable licensure laws and rules regulating the practice of speech-language pathology.

GUIDELINES FOR SLP SUPERVISION OF SPEECH-LANGUAGE PATHOLOGY ASSISTANTS

It is the SLP's responsibility to design and implement a supervision system that protects the students', patients', and clients' care and maintains the highest possible standards of quality. The amount and type of supervision should meet the minimum requirements and be increased as needed based on the needs, competencies, skills, expectations, philosophies, and experience of the SLPA and the supervisor; the needs of students, patients, and clients served; the service setting; the tasks assigned; and other factors. More intense supervision, for example, would be required in such instances as the orientation of a new SLPA; initiation of a new program, equipment, or task; or a change in student, patient, or client status (e.g., medical complications). Functional assessment of the SLPA's skills with assigned tasks should be an ongoing, regular, and integral element of supervision. SLPs and SLPAs should treat each other with respect and interact in a professional manner.

As the supervisory responsibility of the SLP increases, overall responsibilities will change because the SLP is responsible for the students, patients, and clients as well as for supervision of the SLPA.

Therefore, adequate time for direct and indirect supervision of the SLPA(s) and caseload management must be allotted as a critical part of the SLP's workload. The purpose of the assistant level position is not to significantly increase the caseload size for SLPs. Assistants should be used to deliver services to individuals on the SLP's caseload. Under no circumstances should an assistant have his or her own caseload.

Diagnosis and treatment for the students, patients, and clients served remains the legal and ethical responsibility of the supervisor. Therefore, the level of supervision required is considered the minimum level necessary for the supervisor to retain direct contact with the students, patients, and clients. The supervising SLP is responsible for designing and implementing a supervisory plan that protects consumer care, maintains the highest quality of practice, and documents the supervisory activities.

The supervising SLP must

a. hold a Certificate of Clinical Competence in Speech-Language Pathology from ASHA and/or a state licensure (where applicable),
b. have an active interest in use of and desire to use support personnel,
c. have practiced speech-language pathology for at least 2 years following ASHA certification,
d. have completed or be currently enrolled in at least one course or workshop in supervision for at least 1.0 CEUs (10 clock hours).

The relationship between the supervising SLP and the SLPA is paramount to the welfare of the client. Because the clinical supervision process is a close, interpersonal experience, the supervising SLP should participate in the selection of the SLPA when possible.

SLP to SLPA Ratio

Although more than one SLP may provide supervision of an SLPA, an SLP should **not** supervise or be listed as a supervisor for more than two full-time equivalent (FTE) SLPAs in any setting or combination thereof. The supervising SLP should assist in determining the appropriate number of assistants who can be managed within his or her workload. When multiple supervisors are used, it is critical that the supervisors coordinate and communicate with each other so that minimum supervisory requirements are met and that the quality of services is maintained.

Minimum Requirements for the Frequency and Amount of Supervision

First 90 Workdays

A total of at least 30% supervision, including at least 20% direct and 10% indirect supervision, is required weekly. Direct supervision of student, patient, and client care should be no less than 20% of the actual student, patient, and client contact time weekly for each SLPA. This ensures that the supervisor will have direct contact time with the SLPA as well as with the student, patient, or client. During each week, data on every student, patient, and client seen by the SLPA should be reviewed by the supervisor. In addition, the direct supervision should be scheduled so that all students, patients, and clients seen by the assistant are directly supervised in a timely manner. Supervision days and time of day (morning/afternoon) may be alternated to ensure that all students, patients, and clients receive some direct contact with the SLP **at least once every 2 weeks**.

After First 90 Workdays

The amount of supervision can be adjusted if the supervising SLP determines the SLPA has met appropriate competencies and skill levels with a variety of communication and related disorders.

Minimum ongoing supervision must always include documentation of direct supervision provided by the SLP to each student, patient, or client **at least every 60 calendar days**.

A minimum of 1 hour of direct supervision weekly and as much indirect supervision as needed to facilitate the delivery of quality services must be maintained.

Documentation of all supervisory activities, both direct and indirect, must be accurately recorded.

Furthermore, 100% direct supervision of SLPAs for medically fragile students, patients, or clients is required.

The supervising SLP is responsible for designing and implementing a supervisory plan that ensures the highest standard of quality care can be maintained for students, patients, and clients. The amount and type of supervision required should be consistent with the skills and experience of the SLPA; the needs of the students, patients, and clients; the service setting; the tasks assigned; and the laws and regulations that govern SLPAs. Treatment of the student, patient, or client remains the responsibility of the supervisor.

Direct supervision means on-site, inview observation and guidance while a clinical activity is performed by the assistant. This can include the supervising SLP viewing and communicating with the SLPA via telecommunication technology as the SLPA provides clinical services, because this allows the SLP to provide ongoing immediate feedback. Direct supervision does not include reviewing a taped session at a later time.

Supervision feedback should provide information about the quality of the SLPA's performance of assigned tasks and should verify that clinical activity is limited to tasks specified in the SLPA's ASHA-approved responsibilities. Information obtained during direct supervision may include, but is not limited to, data relative to (a) agreement (reliability) between the assistant and the supervisor on correct/incorrect recording of target behavior, (b) accuracy in implementation of assigned treatment procedures, (c) accuracy in recording data, and (d) ability to interact effectively with the patient, client, or student during presentation and application of assigned therapeutic procedures or activities.

Indirect supervision does not require the SLP to be physically present or available via telecommunication in real time while the SLPA is providing services. Indirect supervisory activities may include demonstration tapes, record review, review and evaluation of audio- or videotaped sessions, and/or supervisory conferences that may be conducted by telephone and/or live, secure webcam via the Internet. The SLP will review each treatment plan as needed for timely implementation of modifications.

An SLPA may not perform tasks when a supervising SLP cannot be reached by personal contact, phone, pager, or other immediate or electronic means. If for any reason (i.e., maternity leave, illness, change of jobs) the supervisor is no longer available to provide the level of supervision stipulated, the SLPA may not perform assigned tasks until an ASHA-certified and/or state-licensed SLP with experience and training in supervision has been designated as the new supervising SLP.

Any supervising SLP who will not be able to supervise an SLPA for more than 1 week will need to (a) inform the SLPA of the planned absence and (b) make other arrangements for the SLPA's supervision of services while the SLP is unavailable or (c) inform the clients/student/patients that services will be rescheduled.

CONCLUSION

It is the intent of this document to provide guidance for the use of speech-language pathology assistants in appropriate settings, thereby increasing access to timely and efficient speech-language services. It is the responsibility of the supervising speech-language pathologists to stay abreast of current guidelines and to ensure the quality of services rendered.

DEFINITIONS

Accountability: Accountability refers to being legally responsible and answerable for actions and inactions of self or others during the performance of a task by the SLPA.

Direct Supervision: Direct supervision means on-site, in-view observation and guidance by an SLP while an assigned activity is performed by support personnel. Direct supervision performed by the supervising SLP may include, but is not limited to, the following: observation of a portion of the screening or treatment procedures performed by the SLPA, coaching the SLPA, and modeling for the SLPA. The supervising SLP must be physically present during all services provided to a medically fragile client by the SLPA (e.g., general and telesupervision). The SLP can view and communicate with the patient and SLPA live via real-time telecommunication technology to supervise the SLPA, giving the SLP the opportunity to provide immediate feedback. This does not include reviewing a taped session later.

Indirect Supervision: Indirect supervision means the supervising SLP is not at the same facility or in close proximity to the SLPA, but is available to provide supervision by electronic means. Indirect supervision activities performed by the supervising SLP may include, but are not limited to, demonstration, record review, review and evaluation of audio or video-taped sessions, and interactive television and supervisory conferences that may be conducted by telephone, e-mail, or live webcam.

Interpretation: Summarizing, integrating, and using data for the purpose of clinical decision making, which may only be done by SLPs. SLPAs may summarize objective data from a session to the family or team members.

Medically Fragile: A term used to describe an individual who is acutely ill and in an unstable condition. If such an individual is treated by an SLPA, 100% direct supervision by an SLP is required.

Screening: A pass-fail procedure to identify, without interpretation, clients who may require further assessment following specified screening protocols developed by and/or approved by the supervising SLP.

Speech-Language Pathology Aides/Technician: Aides or technicians are individuals who have completed on-the-job training, workshops, and so forth and work under the direct supervision of ASHA-certified SLPs.

Speech-Language Pathology Assistant: Individuals who, following academic coursework, clinical practicum, and credentialing, can perform tasks prescribed, directed, and supervised by ASHA-certified SLPs.

Supervising Speech-Language Pathologist: An SLP who is certified by ASHA and has been practicing for at least 2 years following ASHA certification, has completed not less than ten (10) hours of continuing professional development in supervision training prior to supervision of an SLPA, and who is licensed and/or credentialed by the state (where applicable).

Supervision: The provision of direction and evaluation of the tasks assigned to an SLPA. Methods for providing supervision include direct supervision, indirect supervision, and telesupervision.

Support Personnel: Support personnel in speech-language pathology perform tasks as prescribed, directed, and supervised by ASHA-certified SLPs. There are different levels of support personnel based on training and scope of responsibilities. Support personnel include SLPAs and speech-language pathology aides/technicians. ASHA is operationally defining these terms for ASHA resources. Some states use different terms and definitions for support personnel.

Telepractice: This refers to the application of telecommunications technology to delivery of professional services at a distance by linking clinician to client, or clinician to clinician, for assessment, intervention, and/or consultation.

Telesupervision: The SLP can view and communicate with the patient and SLPA in real time via Skype, webcam, and similar devices and services to supervise the SLPA, providing the opportunity for the SLP to give immediate feedback. This does not include reviewing a taped session later.

REFERENCES

American Speech-Language-Hearing Association. (2004). *Knowledge and skills needed by speech-language pathologists and audiologists to provide culturally and linguistically appropriate services*. Retrieved from http://www.asha.org/policy

American Speech-Language-Hearing Association. (2007). *Scope of practice in speech-language pathology*. Retrieved from http://www.asha.org/policy

American Speech-Language-Hearing Association. (2010). *Code of ethics*. Retrieved from http://www.asha.org/policy

Source: American Speech-Language-Hearing Association. (2013). *Speech-language pathology assistant scope of practice.* Available from http://www.asha.org/policy. Copyright 2013 American Speech-Language-Hearing Association. All rights reserved. Reprinted with permission.

*Note: The ASHA Code of Ethics referenced within this document was updated as of 2016. As such, readers are referred to Chapter 3, which contains the most recent ASHA Code of Ethics.

APPENDIX 1-B
Speech-Language Pathology Associations
Outside of the United States

Argentina

Asociación Argentina de Logopedia
    Foniatría y Audiología (ASALFA)
http://www.asalfa.org.ar/
E-mail: asalfa@ciudad.com.ar

Australia

Speech Pathology Australia
http://www.speechpathologyaustralia.
    org.au/
E-mail: office@
    speechpathologyaustralia.org.au

Austria

Öesterreichische Gesellschaft für
    Sprachheilpädagogik (OGS)
http://www.sprachheilpaedagogik.at
E-mail: office@sprachheilpaedagogik.at

Öesterreichische Gesellschaft für
    Logopadie, Phoniatrie und
    Pädaudiologie
http://www.hno.at/hauptnav/
    ueber-die-gesellschaft/aktuelles/
E-mail: gerhard.friedrich@meduni-graz
    .at

Belgium

International Bureau for
    Audiophonology (BIAP)
http://www.biap.org/fr/
E-mail: secretariat@biap.org

Vlaamse Vereniging voor Logopedisten
    Belgium (VVL)

https://www.vvl.be
E-mail: pol.demeyere@skynet.be

Brazil

Sociedade Brasileira de
    Fonoaudiologia
http://www.sbfa.org.br/portal2017/
E-mail: diretoria@sbfa.org.br

Canada

Speech-Language and Audiology
    Canada (SAC)
https://www.sac-oac.ca
E-mail: info@sac-oac.ca

Caribbean Region

Caribbean Speech-Language-Hearing
    Association
https://caribsha.wordpress.com/
    contact-us/
E-mail: caribsha.slpa@gmail.com

Chile

Colegio de Fonoaudiólogos de Chile
    A.G.
http://www.colfonochile.cl
E-mail: info@colfonochile.cl

China

The Hong Kong Association of Speech
    Therapists
https://www.speechtherapy.org.hk
E-mail: hkast@speechtherapy.org.hk

Columbia

The Columbian Association of
  Phonoaudiology
https://asofono.co
E-mail: infoasofono.co

Cyprus

Association of Registered Speech-
  Language Pathologists of Cyprus
E-mail: info@speechtherapy.org.cy

Denmark

Audiologopaedisk Forening (ALF)
https://www.alf.dk
E-mail: alf@alf.dk

Egypt

Egyptian Society for Phoniatrics and
  Logopedics
http://www.phoniatrics-uep.org
E-mail: nkotby@cng.com.eg

Germany

Deutsche Gesellschaft für Phoniatrie und
  Pädaudiologie e.V.
http://www.dgpp.de/cms/pages/de/
  willkommen.php
E-mail: martina.hoellrigl@uki.at

Deutsche Gesellschaft für
  Sprachheilpädagogik e.V.
https://www.dgs-ev.de
E-mail: info@dgs-ev.de

Deutscher Bundesverband für Logopadie
  e.V.
https://www.dbl-ev.de
E-mail: info@dbl-ev.de

Greece

Panhellenic Association of Logopedics
http://www.logopedists.gr/
  logopedists/

E-mail: info@logopedists.gr

Association of Scientists of Speech
  Pathology—Speech Therapy of
  Greece
https://www.selle.gr
E-mail: info@selle.gr

Iceland

The Icelandic Association of Speech
  Therapists
https://www.talmein.is
E-mail: talmein@talmein.is

India

Indian Speech and Hearing Association
http://www.ishaindia.org.in
E-mail: president@ishaindia.org.in

All India Institute of Speech and
  Hearing
http://www.aiishmysore.com/en/index
  .html
E-mail: director@aiishmysore.in

Ireland

The Irish Association of Speech and
  Language Therapists (IASLT)
http://www.iaslt.ie
E-mail: info@iaslt.com

Israel

The Israeli Speech, Hearing and
  Language Association (ISHLA)
http://ishla.org.il
E-mail: ishla@netvision.net

Italy

Società Italiana Foniatria e Logopedia
  (SIFEL)
https://www.sifel.it
E-mail: meet@meetandwork.com

Japan

Japan Society of Logopedics and
    Phoniatrics (JSLP)
http://www.jslp.org
E-mail: onsei@jslp.org

The Japanese Association of Speech-
    Language-Hearing Therapists (JAS)
https://www.jaslht.or.jp/e_top.html
E-mail: kaiingai@jaslht.gr.jp

Korea

The Korean Academy of Speech-
    Language Pathology and Audiology
    (KASA)
https://kasa1986.or.kr
E-mail: kasa1986@kasa1986.or.kr

Latvia

Latvian Association of Speech Therapists
http://logopedi.lv
E-mail: lla@e-apollo.lv

Luxembourg

Luxembourg Association of
    Orthophonists
https://www.alo.lu/index.php/en/
    contact
E-mail: info@aol.lu

Malaysia

Malaysian Association of Speech-
    Language & Hearing (MASH)
http://mash.org.my
E-mail: thesecretary@mash.org.my

Malta

Malta Association of Speech and
    Language Pathologists

http://aslpmalta.org
E-mail: info@aslpmalta.org

The Netherlands

Nederlandse Vereniging voor Logopedie
    en Foniatrie (NVLF)
https://www.nvlf.nl/home
E-mail: logopedie@nvlf.nl

Nederlandse Vereniging voor Stem-,
    Spraaken Taalpathologie (NVSST)
http://www.nvsst.org
E-mail: info@nvsst.org

New Zealand

New Zealand Speech-language
    Therapists' Association
https://speechtherapy.org.nz
E-mail: nzsta@speechtherapy.org.nz

Norway

Norsk Logopedlag
http://norsklogopedlag.no
E-mail: ellen-malm.ofte@norsk.

Paraguay

Sociedad Paraguaya de Fonoaudiología
    (SOPAFO)
https://www.facebook.com/Sociedad-
    Paraguaya-de-Fonoaudiologia-
E-mail: my_avalos@hotmail.com;
    gisselfono@gmail.com

Philippines

Philippine Association of Speech
    Pathologists (PASP)
http://pasp.org.ph
E-mail: pasp_secretariat@yahoo.com

Poland

Polish Logopaedic Society
http://www.logopedia.umcs.lublin.pl
E-mail: ptl@poczta.umcs.lulin.pl

Portugal

Associação Portuguesa de Terapeutas
da Fala
www.aptf.org/home
E-mail: geral@aptf.org

Romania

Romanian Society of Audiology and
Pathology of Communication
http://srapc.ro
E-mail: office@srapc.ro

Russia

The Russian Public Academy of Voice
http://www.voiceacademy.ru
E-mail: foncentr@mail.ru

South Africa

South African Speech-Language-Hearing
Association (SASLHA)
https://www.saslha.co.za/
E-mail: admin@saslha.co.za

Spain

Sociedad Médica Española de Foniatría
(SOMEF)
http://www.somef.es
E-mail: contacto@somef.net

Sweden

Swedish Association of Phoniatrics and
Logopedics (SFFL)
http://www.sffl.se
E-mail: astrid.frylmark@telia.com

Svenska Logopedförbundet (Swedish
Logopedics Association)
https://www.srat.se/Logopederna/
E-mail list: info@logopedforbundet.se

Switzerland

Association Romande des Logopédistes
Diplômés (ARLD)
http://arld.ch
E-mail: secretariat@arld.ch

Associazione Logopedisti della Svizzera
Italiana (ALOSI)
https://alosi.ch
E-mail: emanuela.dicampli@live.it

Deutschschweizer Logopädinnen- und
Logopädenverband (DLV)
http://www.logopaedie.ch
E-mail: info.logopaedie.ch

Taiwan

The Speech-Language-Hearing
Association
http://www.slh.org.tw
E-mail: slha@slh.org.tw

Thailand

Thai Speech-Language and Hearing
Association: Auditory and Speech
Therapy Association of Thailand
http://www.thaisha.or.th
E-mail: thaisha1802@gmail.com

Trinidad and Tobago

Speech-Language and Audiology
Association of Trinidad and Tobago
(SLAATT)
http://www.slaatt.com
E-mail: lyscaw@hotmail.com or
speechassociationtt@gmail.com

Turkey

United Kingdom

Association of Speech & Language
    Therapists in Independent Practice
    (ASLTIP)
https://beta.helpwithtalking.com

E-mail: office@helpwithtalking.com

The Royal College of Speech & Language
    Therapists (RCSLT)
https://www.rcslt.org
E-mail: info@rcslt.org

APPENDIX 1–C
Relevant ASHA Topics and Documents

Available from http://www.asha.org

SLPA Scope of Practice

American Speech-Language-Hearing Association. (2013). *Speech-language pathology assistant scope of practice.*

Code of Ethics (see Chapter 3)

American Speech-Language-Hearing Association. (2016). *Code of ethics.*

Confidentiality (see Chapter 3)

American Speech-Language-Hearing Association. (2013). *Confidentiality.*

Ethical Issues Concerning the Use of Support Personnel

American Speech-Language-Hearing Association. (2017). *Issues in ethics: Speech-language pathology assistants.*

SLP Scope of Practice

American Speech-Language-Hearing Association. (2016). *Scope of practice in speech-language pathology.*

Clinical Supervision in SLP (in General)

American Speech-Language-Hearing Association. (2008). *Clinical supervision in speech-language pathology* [Position statement].

APPENDIX 1–D
A Day in the Life of an SLPA:
Interviews and Advice from SLPAs

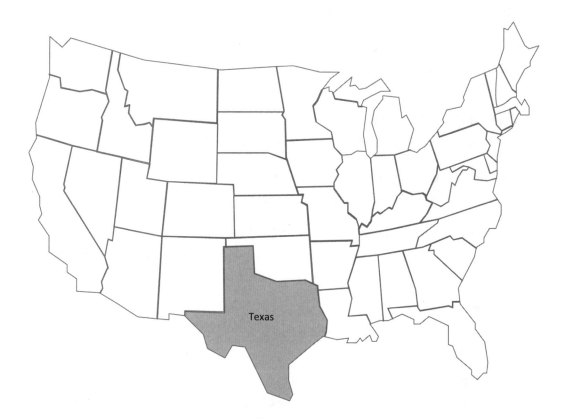

Texas

A DAY IN THE LIFE OF SARA

A Traveling SLPA

Sara is a licensed SLPA in the state of Texas. According to the ASHA (n.d., Statutory and Regulatory Requirements, para. 1), obtaining an SLPA license in Texas requires the following:

- a baccalaureate degree with an emphasis in communicative sciences and disorders,

- proof of completion of no fewer than 24 semester hours in speech-language pathology/audiology, and
- no fewer than 25 hours of clinical observation in the area of speech-language pathology *and* 25 hours of clinical assisting experience in speech-language pathology.

SLPAs in Texas must be supervised by a licensed SLP at least 2 hours per week, of which at least 1 hour must be face-to-face supervision at the location where the SLPA is employed.

Sara earned a bachelor's degree in communicative disorders. She feels fortunate to have attended a bachelor's program that also offered her the opportunity to obtain 100 hours of clinical practicum as an SLPA.

Sara is currently employed as an SLPA for a company that provides services to individuals in home settings, head start programs, and daycares. A typical day for Sara consists of traveling to these different locations to provide treatment services. Sara typically sees clients for 30-minute treatment sessions and makes about 125 to 200 visits per month. Her clients are very diverse, many of whom come from low-income households. They range in age from as young as 18 months to as old as 17 years. They have a wide spectrum of disorders, including a variety of speech and language impairments.

Rewards

Sara enjoys building rapport with her clients and their families. She finds the most rewarding aspect of her job the positive impact that she can make on her clients' lives and in seeing the joy of the children she works with when she travels to their homes to provide services. She reports that in some cases, her clients and their families tell her that her services are the highlight of their day/week.

Challenges

One of the challenges of Sara's job is moving from home to home, hauling her equipment in and out of her car. She feels though, that being in a client's home is also a big advantage, as she is able to get to know the parents and families of her clients.

Words of Wisdom

Sara reports that being an SLPA is "highly rewarding." To individuals interested in pursuing a career as an SLPA, Sara recommends attending a school that offers an opportunity to complete your degree in communicative disorders, as well as obtain the observation and clinical hours required to become an SLPA.

Reference

American Speech-Language-Hearing Association (ASHA). (n.d.). *ASHA state-by-state*. Retrieved from https://www.asha.org/Advocacy/state/info/TX/Texas-Support-Personnel-Requirements/

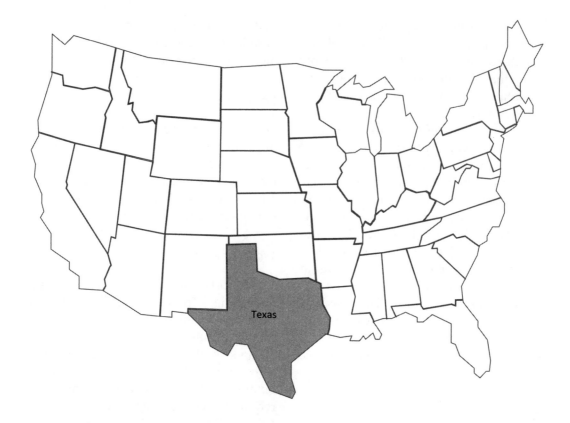

A DAY IN THE LIFE OF STEPHANIE

Never Give Up!

Stephanie is been a licensed SLPA in the state of Texas for 5 years. She has a bachelor's degree in communicative disorders and completed 50 hours of clinical practicum as part of her training to become an SLPA.

Stephanie currently works in a private practice, providing treatment services to individuals who range in age from 2 to 11 years, including individuals with ASD, speech sound disorder (SSD), stuttering, Down syndrome, and cleft lip/palate.

A typical day for Stephanie starts at 8:30 AM. First, she retrieves the speech folders for each client on her treatment schedule. These folders contain an initial evaluation, testing, monthly summary reports, a calendar, and speech notes (which include each client's individual goals). Next, Stephanie plans her sessions, writing out the goals developed by her supervising SLP and possible activities for each. She then decides which activities work best for each client's goals and collects her materials.

Stephanie sees three to five clients every morning and then an additional three to four clients in the afternoon. Treatment is provided on a one-to-one basis, although sometimes social skills are targeted in group sessions. During her sessions, she tallies the client's responses on a blank sheet of paper, where she has written each client's goals for that session. After each of her sessions, Stephanie writes a formal Subjective Objective Assessment and Plan (SOAP) note for each client. Her supervising SLP reviews these notes at the end of each day.

Stephanie is also charged with keeping the treatment rooms orderly, which includes cleaning and sanitizing materials. She assists with administrative duties, such as auditing therapy folders quarterly to ensure all needed information is present and up to date. Stephanie participates twice weekly in team meetings, one with the entire staff and the other with her fellow SLPAs and SLP supervisor.

Rewards

Stephanie's greatest reward as an SLPA is watching her clients make progress.

Challenges

Stephanie's biggest challenge is working with children who have behavioral issues, such as children who are not compliant with requests during the session. She also has clients who can exhibit aggressive behavior during treatment sessions when they become frustrated or are asked to complete nondesired tasks.

Words of Wisdom

Stephanie's words of wisdom to new SLPAs are: (a) take the time to do research about different diagnoses and disabilities and (b) "Don't give up!" When Stephanie first started working as an SLPA, she worked primarily with individuals with ASD. She recalls this was very challenging because many of her clients did not interact with her. As Stephanie put it, they seemed to be "in their own world." She also recalls they often cried, screamed, hit, or bit themselves.

In these early days of her career, Stephanie remembers sitting in her car during lunch one day, crying and thinking, "I can't do this. I don't know what I am doing!" Her supervising SLP told her that once she understands autism, working with these clients will not be so hard. For Stephanie, this advice was absolutely correct. With perseverance, research, and a knowledgeable supervising SLP, Stephanie now has the techniques needed to help her clients succeed (those with ASD and all her clients). Now, she remembers to take it one day at a time and she realizes, "I can do this!"

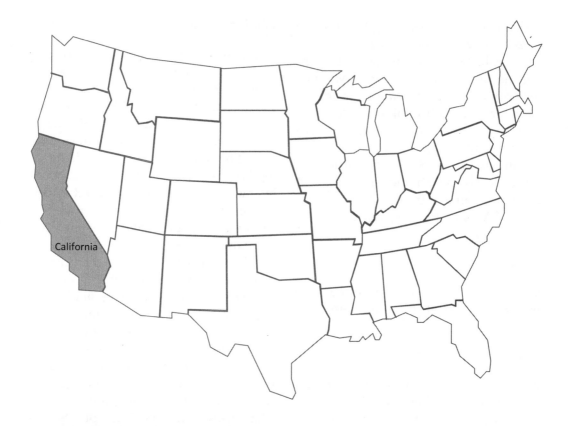

A DAY IN THE LIFE OF MIKA

Training To Be an SLP

Mika is a licensed SLPA in the state of California. According to ASHA (n.d., Statutory and Regulatory Requirements, para. 1), to obtain an SLPA license in California requires at least one of the following qualifications:

- an associate of arts or sciences degree from an SLPA-accredited and board-approved program, or
- a bachelor's degree in speech-language pathology or communicative disorders from an accredited and board-approved program, and

completion of 70 hours of fieldwork/clinical experience.

Mika has a bachelor's degree in communicative disorders and completed 100 hours of clinical practicum as an SLPA.

Mika currently works as an SLPA in a private practice, providing treatment services to children, mostly ages 2 to 5 years, who have a variety of impairments including expressive/receptive language delay and ASD. She also provides treatment to older children as part of a social skills group focused on pragmatic skills, such as problem solving, perspective taking, appropriate/inappropriate conversation topics, and understanding nonverbal cues. These groups comprise three to five children, with similar ages and abilities, all who have been diagnosed with ASD.

Mika's typical day is roughly 8 hours. She arrives 30 minutes early to review each client's file and any notes from her supervising SLP. In the mornings, she also gathers the toys and materials needed for each session. She carries out treatment goals, mostly through play-based intervention. Her treatment sessions occur throughout the course of her day and are generally 50-minute sessions, provided on a one-on-one basis with each client. In the afternoons, Mika prepares files and lesson plans for the next day. She also answers phones and helps with administrative duties as needed.

Mika is currently enrolled in a master's program in speech-language pathology. Her long-term goal is to become a fully licensed and ASHA-certified SLP. She plans to continue working as an SLPA while attending graduate school. She feels that her experience as an SLPA will allow her to incorporate what she has learned in the therapy room with what she learns in the classroom. She is very eager to learn more, including procedures for assessment and diagnosis and an expanded range of treatment procedures. She is particularly excited to participate in internships and clinical practica with individuals she has not yet worked with as an SLPA, such as individuals with swallowing disorders and aphasia.

Rewards

Mika feels extremely lucky to be working with a supervising SLP and fellow clinicians who view her as a full member of a team. Her greatest reward is in having an opportunity to provide services to clients on a one-on-one basis for 50-minute sessions. She believes this provides truly individualized treatment, which leads to dramatic progression over time. She says that "watching her clients inch closer and closer to their goals is an amazing feeling." As an SLPA, she has been able to make a connection with her clients and share in their feeling of excitement when they progress, make changes, and overcome challenges.

Challenges

Mika finds controlling the environment, addressing behavior, and building rapport among the most challenging aspects of her role as an SLPA. She believes that to be truly effective as an SLPA, she must be able to multitask, simultaneously implementing treatment goals (as developed by her supervising SLP), collecting data, and modifying the environment. This must be done while considering each client's behavior, performance, and needs, such as the following:

- Will this client cry?
- Is this the first time away from mom or dad?
- How do I keep the client on task while I take notes?
- What encourages good behavior?
- How do I make therapy fun but still task driven?

Words of Wisdom

First and foremost, Mika recommends that all SLPAs thoroughly understand their scope of practice. Mika also stresses that as an SLPA, you must be knowledgeable and passionate about what you do. Mika has learned that it is important to know pertinent information in the field, but it is equally important to deliver what you know in a motivating and fun environment that is geared to each client's individual needs. She recommends that SLPAs take advantage of their environment and be willing to learn. She has found it very helpful to observe other clinicians and brainstorm ways she can improve her performance as an SLPA.

Reference

American Speech-Language-Hearing Association (ASHA). (n.d.). *ASHA state-by-state*. Retrieved from https://www.asha.org/Advocacy/state/info/CA/California-Support-Personnel-Requirements/

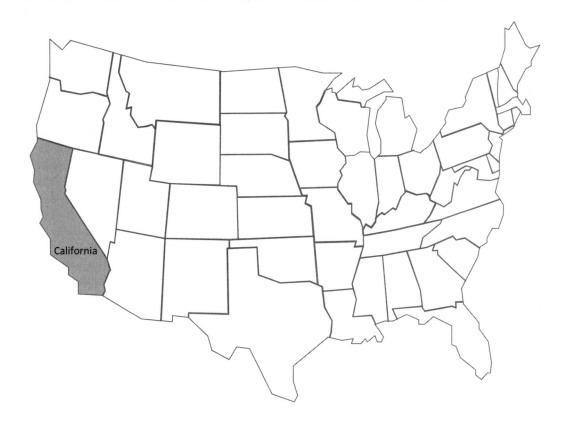

A DAY IN THE LIFE OF JACKIE

Set Yourself Apart

Jackie is a licensed SLPA in the state of California. Jackie became an SLPA by completing an associate's degree in speech-language pathology assisting. Jackie currently works in a public school setting, with children in kindergarten through eighth grade. She works at two separate elementary school campuses, providing treatment to students with a variety of impairments, including individuals with SSD and ASD. Between her two campuses, Jackie works in self-contained, functional skills classrooms and ASD-specific classrooms.

A typical day for Jackie consists of language and articulation "pull-out" treatment, when she works with students on a one-on-one basis or in small groups, and "push-in" treatment, provided to students in self-contained classrooms. A big part of Jackie's job includes scheduling treatment sessions, data collection, and recordkeeping. When needed, she also assists her supervising SLP with in-class observations and screenings.

Rewards

For Jackie, her greatest reward as an SLPA is developing relationships with students and observing their progress. She believes this comes from providing ongoing services and keeping accurate records.

Challenges

Jackie finds scheduling treatment for students in multiple grade levels, each with individual needs, to be one of the most challenging aspects of her job.

Words of Wisdom

Jackie's words of wisdom for a new SLPA are to "set yourself apart by having an area of specialty (e.g., autism, augmentative and alternative communication (AAC), sign language)." She believes that to be a successful SLPA, you must learn as much as you can during and after your training. Jackie attends professional development workshops on a regular basis to enhance her skills. In California, SLPAs are required to complete 12 hours of continuing professional development (CPD) every 2 years (ASHA, n.d.). Jackie accrues well over this minimum and feels it has been the secret to her success. She also believes being a team player is critical and recommends that new SLPAs be open to completing any and all tasks within their scope of practice.

Reference

American Speech-Language-Hearing Association (ASHA). (n.d.). *ASHA state-by-state*. Retrieved from https://www.asha.org/Advocacy/state/info/CA/California-Support-Personnel-Requirements/

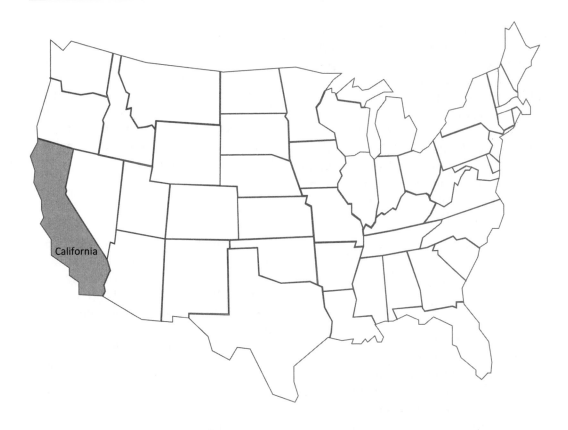

California

A DAY IN THE LIFE OF SUSAN

A Bilingual SLPA

Susan is a licensed SLPA in the state of California. Susan has an associate's degree in speech-language pathology assisting and completed 216 hours of clinical practicum with both children and adults as part of her training.

Susan works in a public school setting in California with children ages 3 to 12 years, many of who have articulation problems, language delays, or both. She also works with individuals with Down syndrome, ASD, and other disabilities. The students at her school have diverse cultural and linguistic back-grounds. Many come from low-income households.

Susan works an 8-hour day. She spends 2 hours per day completing paperwork, preparing materials for therapy sessions, performing recordkeeping, and working with the office manager to contact parents, teachers, and representatives from other disciplines to schedule individualized educational plan (IEP) meetings, and preparing notices and documents for IEP meetings. She also assists her supervisor in preparing materials to share with parents. Often these materials go beyond solely speech and language domains, such as activities for parents to do with their children outside of school and resources for affordable clothing and low-cost medical and dental services. The remainder of her day is spent providing therapy to students in small groups or one-on-one. She also assists her supervising SLP with screenings and assessment of Spanish-speaking students.

Susan is an English-Spanish bilingual SLPA. According to ASHA's (2013) scope-of-practice document, bilingual SLPAs who have been provided with adequate training, planning, and supervision may perform the following tasks (Service Delivery, para. 1):

- Assist the SLP with bilingual translation during screening and assessment activities exclusive of screening and assessment interpretation;
- Serve as interpreter for patients, clients, students, and families who do not speak English;
- Provide services under SLP supervision in another language for individuals who do not speak English and for English-language learners.

Susan performs each of these tasks at her school sites on a regular basis. She is also called to assist with bilingual assessment at the eight other schools within her district and received training as a district translator. She has learned to be flexible in her role as a bilingual SLPA and notes that "one size does fit all." She has noticed that often materials are not available in other languages and in these cases, she works with her supervising SLP to translate information for her clients and their families. She feels that this is critical to connecting with her client's families and granting them equal access to resources. She also conducts the majority of her treatment sessions in Spanish.

Rewards

According to Susan, the most rewarding part of her job is seeing growth in the students she works with and helping them successfully exit the speech program. She looks forward to hearing about their achievements as they transition from middle school to high school.

Challenges

Susan's greatest challenge is not always having the right or current tools to work with her students, such as computer programs, iPads, or materials in general. She has at times spent her own money on materials, supplies, and reinforcements for her students, as her school district does not consistently provide these items.

Words of Wisdom

Susan thinks those training to be an SLPA should have a realistic picture of what it means to be an SLPA. She says it is not always like textbooks and classes make it seem. There are real challenges, such as when you may not have the resources or tools you need to do your job effectively. Susan's advice is not to become an SLPA for the money but because you love working with children, especially those with disabilities and behavioral challenges. She has also found it very valuable to get to know as much as she can about the clients she works with. She reads their reports carefully and tries to get a sense of their family life and circumstances, such as who they live with, whether they are immigrants and which country they are from, their economic background, whether multiple families live in the home, and whether they live in a house, apartment, or motel. She finds this helps her to understand her clients better and to find ways to motivate them to do their best and be successful.

Reference

American Speech-Language-Hearing Association (ASHA). (2013). *Speech-language pathology assistant scope of practice*. Retrieved from http://www.asha.org/policy/SP2013-00337/

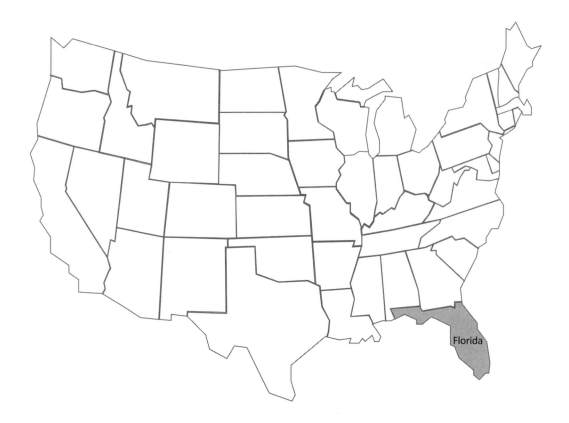

Florida

A DAY IN THE LIFE OF LAURE

An Amazing Field

Laure is a licensed SLPA in Florida. In Florida, to be certified as an SLPA, among other requirements, one must complete the following:

A bachelor's degree from a regionally accredited college or university, including completion of 24 semester hours as specified by the board from a Council for Higher Education–accredited institution

SLPAs also receive on-the-job training by a licensed SLP who maintains responsibility for all services performed by the SLPA (ASHA, n.d.). SLPAs in Flor-

ida must complete 20 CEU per biennium certificate renewal (two of these hours must be in an approved course related to the prevention of medical errors; ASHA, n.d., para. 1).

Laure has a bachelor's degree in management information systems. She also completed more than 200 hours of practicum (24 semester hours) to obtain her license as an SLPA. Laure is currently enrolled in a master's program in communication science and disorders. She has three semesters left in completing her master's degree.

She currently works in a private practice setting with children ranging in age from 3 to 13 years. Half of her caseload consists of individuals with SSD and specifically, those with articulation goals. She also works with individuals who have delays in receptive and/or expressive language skills. A typical day for Laure consists of providing therapy services as directed by her supervising SLP, often using play-based, child-directed approaches. For the most part, Laure sees clients individually, but there are times when she also works with small groups of students.

Rewards

Laure really enjoys the relationship she has been developing with her supervising SLP. She has also been able to develop an excellent rapport with her clients, their parents, and school personnel. She loves seeing her clients' progress and watching them grow and develop both personally and academically.

Challenges

Laure finds that the most challenging aspect of her job is managing client behavior, especially for students with severe developmental delays who may exhibit high levels of frustration, and for younger children who need consistent structure and redirection. She has noticed that sometimes helping a client participate and remain on task may be as simple as discovering the client's likes and dislikes

and determining what learning modality works best for the client. For example, she has found that some children do not respond well to auditory-visual stimulation, and in that case, they may need a more kinesthetic approach where they are allowed to touch and do things themselves. Other children may just need positive, visual reinforcement, which gives them instant reward for small successes.

Words of Wisdom

Laure's advice to new SLPAs is to "hang in there because this is an amazing field." Laure recalls that when she first started, she was "so green," with little experience. However, after working as an SLPA for the past year, she has found it to be truly rewarding and cannot help but tell others who are considering going into this field, especially those who may be struggling to get through their training, that it is well worth it!

Reference

American Speech-Language-Hearing Association (ASHA). (n.d.). *ASHA state-by-state*. Retrieved from https://www.asha.org/Advocacy/state/info/FL/Florida-Support-Personnel-Requirements/

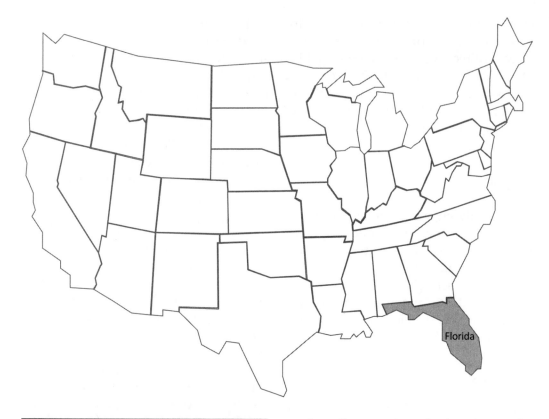

Florida

A DAY IN THE LIFE OF ALYSON

There Are No Wrong Questions

Alyson is a licensed SLPA in the state of Florida. She has a bachelor's degree in communicative disorders and completed 20 hours of clinical practicum as part of her training to become an SLPA. Alyson works part-time for a private practice, providing services to individuals ages 3 to 12 years with primarily SSD and language impairments. She is currently working and applying to graduate schools as she hopes to complete her master's degree and become a fully certified SLP.

Rewards

Alyson says the most rewarding aspect of her job as an SLPA is seeing the progress her clients make, whether they make small or big gains.

Challenges

For Alyson, the most challenging aspects of working as an SLPA are finding the right activities and materials to work effectively with each client. She feels that without the clinical and educational background that comes with a master's degree, she does not always know where to begin.

Words of Wisdom

Alyson recommends that SLPAs, regardless of their experience, should "ask lots of questions." She often faces problems or situations that she is not sure how to address, but she feels fortunate to work in a friendly and safe environment where everyone is willing to help one another. She regularly seeks the guidance of her supervising SLP. She feels there are no wrong questions, but the important thing is to ask.

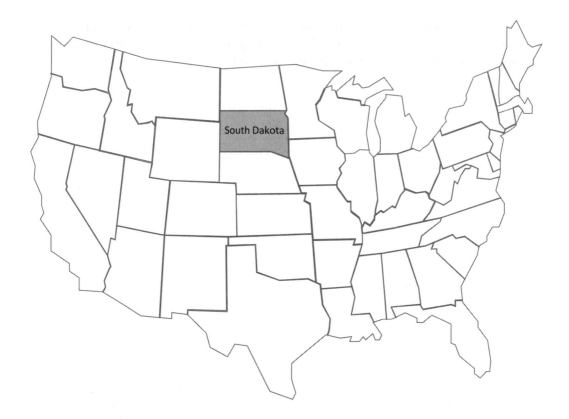

A DAY IN THE LIFE OF JENNIFER

Two Sites and Two Supervisors

Jennifer is a licensed SLPA in the state of South Dakota. To obtain a license in South Dakota, individuals must (ASHA, n.d.):

■ hold an associate's degree in SLPA or a bachelor's degree with major emphasis in speech-language pathology or communication disorders from an accredited academic institution;

■ complete a minimum of 100 clock hours of supervised clinical practicum as an SLPA, while either on the job or during academic preparation; and

■ have committed no act for which disciplinary action is justified.

SLPAs in South Dakota must be supervised by a licensed SLP with at least 3 years of experience (ASHA, n.d.). Jennifer has an associate's degree in speech-language pathology assisting, which included both observation and 100 hours of clinical experience as an SLPA.

Jennifer works in an elementary school setting, with children in kindergarten through third grade. She primarily works with individuals with SSD, and in particular, students with goals targeting articulation. She also provides services to students with fluency and language disorders. Jennifer's time is split between two different school sites, each with a designated supervising SLP. Her supervising SLPs see the clients she treats once per week. She meets with both supervisors once per week to discuss clients, materials, and anything else that might come up during the week.

Most days, Jennifer provides treatment to students back to back, with a short break in her day for lunch and to travel between sites. She plans for her treatment sessions after school or one afternoon a week designated for paperwork and planning. Her treatment is usually provided to small groups of students who share similar goals.

Rewards

For Jennifer, the most rewarding aspect of being an SLPA is getting to see the progress students make from one year to the next. She also feels fortunate to have supervisors who have different styles so she can learn from both.

Challenges

Jennifer finds that the most challenging aspect of her job as an SLPA is working with students who have challenging behaviors. She says you never know what type of day a student is having and need to be prepared.

Words of Wisdom

Jennifer's words of wisdom for new SLPAs are to remember that each student is unique. She believes you can find the right way to help each student if you keep in mind that every little thing is a learning experience for that student. If you do not feel like they accomplished enough during a specific session, Jennifer encourages new SLPAs to remember that more sessions are ahead (and to try again).

Reference

American Speech-Language-Hearing Association (ASHA). (n.d.). *ASHA state-by-state*. Retrieved from https://www.asha.org/Advocacy/state/info/SD/South-Dakota-Support-Personnel-Requirements/

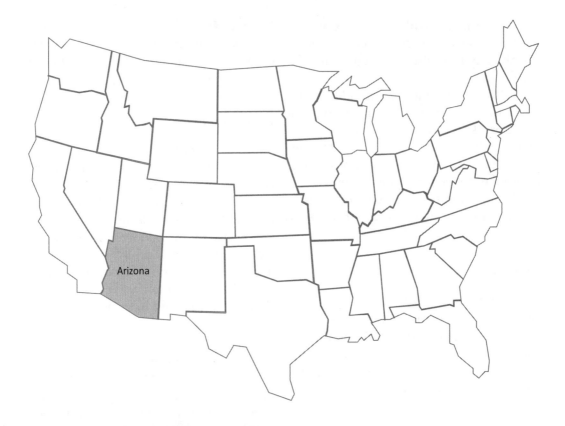

Arizona

A DAY IN THE LIFE OF ELISE

Making It Work, Even in Less Than Ideal Circumstances

Elise has a bachelor's degree in speech and hearing science and is attending school to complete her master's degree in speech-language pathology. Elise holds licensure as an SLPA in Arizona. In Arizona, for all settings, SLPAs must be licensed with the state's Department of Health Services (ASHA, n.d.). To be eligible for licensure, SLPAs must complete an approved training program (or the equivalent) from a nationally or regionally accredited college or university. Requirements include

■ A minimum of 60 semester credit hours and a minimum of

100 hours of clinical interaction under the supervision of a licensed master's level SLP (ASHA, n.d., Statutory and Regulatory Requirements)

Elise received her training as an SLPA while completing her bachelor's degree in speech and hearing science, including 25 observation hours and 100 supervised clinical interaction hours as an SLPA. She currently works in an elementary school.

A typical day for Elise starts at 7:00 AM and ends at 2:30 PM. Elise works with individuals or small groups of students (two to four), providing therapy for articulation, language, and pragmatic disorders. Under the direction of her supervising SLP, she plans the groups and records data on student performance. She also attends parent or IEP meetings with her supervising SLP for the children on her caseload.

Rewards

What Elise finds most rewarding is working with students.

Challenges

Elise's supervisor makes her schedule. She sometimes wishes the children were grouped differently, but there are constraints on when students are available. She often has groups of students with mixed goals; some with articulations goals, some with language, and so forth. She finds this challenging at times and wishes she could work with certain students in one-on-one sessions. She is also at two different schools, one of which does not have a dedicated speech room. This means she must provide services in grade level pods where there are distractions from other small groups and people walking by while she is working with her students.

Words of Wisdom

Elise's words of wisdom for future SLPAs is to establish clear expectations for students. Elise carries a laminated page that says "speech expectations." Her students love reciting the expectations to her at the beginning of the group. Elise also always has at least three activities planned for each session. This way if one is not working well, she can easily move on to another activity. Elise also recommends that SLPAs try to observe many different SLPs. She encourages other SLPAs not to be afraid to contact SLPs in their specialty area and ask to observe their sessions. She cold called several SLPs and found it to be a great learning experience.

Reference

American Speech-Language-Hearing Association (ASHA). (n.d.). *ASHA State-by-State.* Retrieved from https://www.asha.org/Advocacy/state/info/AZ/Arizona-Support-Personnel-Requirements/

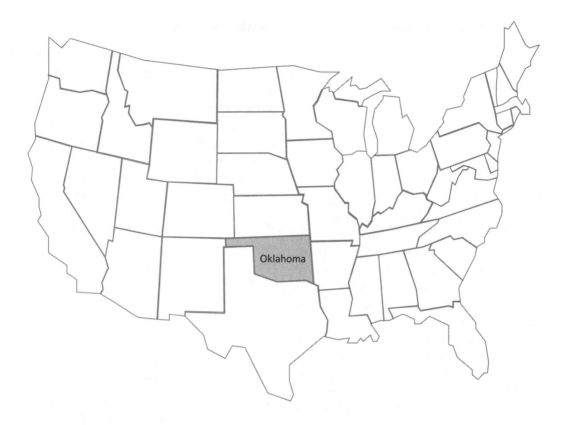

A DAY IN THE LIFE OF BEATRICE

Being Open to Advice Is Key

Beatrice has an associate's degree in speech-language pathology assisting from a community college and a license in Oklahoma as an SLPA. In Oklahoma, effective 2013, SLPA licensure requires that SLPAs have at least an associate's degree (or equivalent), with a major emphasis in speech-language pathology from an accredited academic institution (ASHA, n.d.). SLPAs must also complete 100 clock hours of clinical experience supervised by an SLP who has been fully licensed for a minimum of two years (ASHA, n.d.).

Beatrice works in a secondary school. A typical day for her consists of helping to schedule and attend IEP meetings with her supervisor, scheduling sessions, creating therapy activities, providing one-on-one and group therapy sessions, co-leading social skills groups for students not on IEPs, and attending professional development trainings.

Rewards

Beatrice says the most rewarding part of her job is "helping kids, especially in the secondary grades, find their voice [because] they are past the age where articulation issues are cute." She notes that her students use figurative language and slang to communicate so giving them the confidence they need through communication skills training helps to shape the adults they will become.

Challenges

Beatrice finds scheduling session times very challenging. She also finds that paperwork demands more of my attention than she initially thought it would.

Words of Wisdom

Beatrice recommends that SLPAs take advantage of their clinical hours. She encourages all SLPAs to not just observe during these hours, but to work with their clinical supervisor to try new things and importantly, to be open to any and all advice. Beatrice also recommends that SLPAs take advantage of free trainings, webinars, and other avenues for developing their skills as SLPAs.

Reference

American Speech-Language-Hearing Association (ASHA). (n.d.). *ASHA State-by-State.* Retrieved from https://www.asha.org/Advocacy/state/info/OK/Oklahoma-Support-Personnel-Requirements/

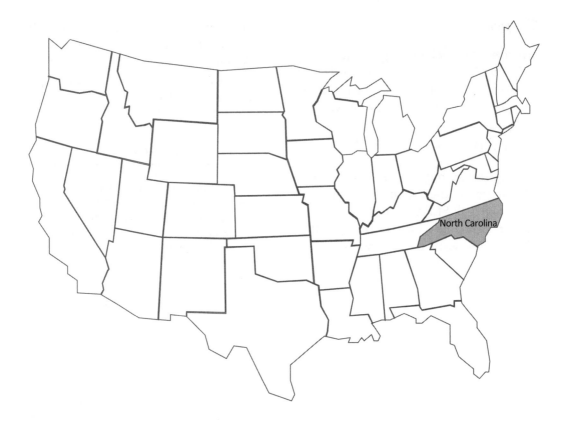

North Carolina

Changing Perceptions: ASHA Certification for SLPAs

Kelly has a bachelor's degree in early childhood education and associate's degree in speech-language pathology assisting from a community college. She is currently working in North Carolina (NC) with registration from NC Board of Examiners for SLPA. In North Carolina, SLPA must register with the North Carolina Board of Examiners for Speech and Language Pathologists and Audiologists (ASHA, n.d.). Qualifications to do so include (ASHA, n.d., Statutory and Regulatory Requirements)

■ An associate's degree in speech-language pathology assisting,

or completion of a bachelor's degree with courses in speech-language assisting developed by the North Carolina Department of Community Colleges; and

■ A passing score on a competency test approved by the NC Board of Examiners.

North Carolina also requires that SLPAs wear a badge noting their title and that the patient receiving services from an SLPA be informed as such in writing (ASHA, n.d.).

For the past 3 years, Kelly has worked primarily in early intervention settings with children birth to 3 years of age. Prior to that, she was employed for 8 years in a private practice setting with a caseload of children 0 to 18 years of age. Prior to that, and in her first 3 years of work as an SLPA, she was employed by a private practice that contracted with elementary and high schools.

Kelly's work as an SLPA consists of seeing children in daycares, homes, and in the clinic. She begins work around 8:30 a.m. and ends somewhere between two and four in the afternoon (later if she is serving as an interpreter for an evaluation). The children she serves at the moment are dual language learners and those with autism, speech and language delays, and Down syndrome. Kelly reports that at this point, she sets and manages her time during the day independently, juggling a wide ranges of duties and activities, including

- Creating client files,
- Maintaining daily notes,
- Creating activities to address goals provided by her supervisor,
- Maintaining communication with her supervisor regarding clients,
- Making calls to families as necessary to schedule sessions,
- Collecting data, and
- Serving as an interpreter for evaluations.

Rewards

Kelly states that the most rewarding part of her work is having the opportunity to work one-on-one with children, and knowing that for some, she may be the only bright spot in their day.

Challenges

Kelly finds it challenging that as an SLPA she is not as well respected or as independent as certified occupational therapy assistants (COTAs) and physical therapy assistants (PTAs). She believes that not having an ASHA certification behind her (and supporting the work of all SLPAs) is a barrier to advancing the standing of assistants in the field of speech-language pathology. She is hopeful this will change when ASHA pursues formal certification for SLPAs.

Words of Wisdom

Kelly's words of wisdom to future SLPAs is to love what you do and make sure that you like children if you plan to work with them as an SLPA.

Reference

American Speech-Language-Hearing Association (ASHA). (n.d.). *ASHA state-by-state*. Retrieved from https://www.asha.org/Advocacy/state/info/NC/North-Carolina-Support-Personnel-Requirements/

APPENDIX 1–E
Sample Job Description—Medical Setting

SPLA JOB DESCRIPTION

Medical Facility Example

General Summary

The speech-language pathology assistant, as a member of an interdisciplinary team, works under the supervision of a certified speech-language pathologist in implementation of services for the rehabilitation of patients with speech, language, cognitive, swallowing, oral muscular, and augmentative alternative communication disorders, and hearing impairments.

Essential Duties and Responsibilities

1. Prepares patients for treatment.
2. Prepares treatment areas and equipment for use.
3. Implements documented treatment plans developed by speech-language pathologists.
4. Accurately collects and records subjective and objective data.
5. Records patient status with regard to established objectives as stated in the treatment plan and reports this information to the supervising speech-language pathologist.
6. Assists the speech-language pathologist in the assessment of patients.
7. Orders supplies and equipment.
8. Engages in various clerical tasks including entry of orders for patient care, filing, billing, and ordering equipment and supplies.
9. Maintains and cleans equipment, adhering to infection control protocol.
10. Maintains the confidentiality of information pertaining to patients and their families.
11. Behaves in accordance with the mission and values of the organization.
12. Participates in quality improvement initiatives as directed by the speech-language pathologist.
13. Respects and appropriately considers age, gender, cultural background, and related factors when providing services.

Supplemental Duties and Responsibilities

1. Participates in educational activities for patients, families, and other health professionals.
2. Participates in organizational committees as time, interest, and necessity permits and dictates.

Required Education, Experience, and Licensure

1. The SLPA must meet state requirements for health.
2. The SLPA must have one of the following:
   - Associate's degree from a speech-language pathology assistant program;
   - Bachelor's degree in speech-language pathology;
   - Completion of a college-based speech-language pathology assistant certificate program; or

■ Required education as designated by the state licensing board or other regulatory agency.

Required Skills and Abilities

1. Knowledge of speech-language pathology treatment and equipment.
2. Ability to follow oral and written directions, including treatment plans.
3. Ability to work under direct and indirect supervision.
4. Ability to show excellent judgment for continuation or discontinuation of a patient's treatment under conditions of pain or discomfort.
5. Analytical skills necessary to identify and report changes in the patient and equipment.
6. Flexibility and adaptability, as the job combines patient care, clinic/equipment maintenance, and clerical responsibilities.
7. Ability to pay close attention to visual and auditory detail.
8. Ability to use a variety of computer programs for documentation and patient treatment.
9. Ability to push wheelchair-bound patients and assist ambulatory patients.
10. Ability to walk and stand up for 90% of the work day.

Working Conditions

1. Work is a combination of sedentary and physical activities completed in a normal patient care and office environment.
2. Travel in a company or personal vehicle may be required.
3. Exposure to body fluids is frequent. Exposure to blood-borne pathogens and other infectious material is possible.
4. Exposure to verbally and/or physically aggressive patients is possible.

Reporting Relationships

The SLPA is directly and indirectly supervised by a certified speech-language pathologist. The supervising SLP maintains legal and moral responsibility for all services provided by the SLPA and ensures that such services are in compliance with the ASHA Code of Ethics, ASHA Guidelines for Speech-Language Pathology Assistants, and state licensure laws.

APPENDIX 1–F
Sample Job Description—Educational Setting

SLPA JOB DESCRIPTION

Educational Facility Example

General Summary

The speech-language pathology assistant, as a member of an educational team, works under the supervision of a certified speech-language pathologist in implementation of services for children/students with speech, language, cognitive, voice, swallowing, oral muscular, and augmentative/alternative communication disorders, and hearing impairments.

Essential Duties and Responsibilities

1. Prepares work area and materials for use.
2. Accompanies the student from the classroom to the service area or prepares classroom for service delivery.
3. Implements documented treatment/intervention plans developed by the speech-language pathologist.
4. Accurately collects and records subjective and objective data.
5. Records student's status with regard to established objectives as stated in the treatment plan and reports this information to the supervising speech-language pathologist.
6. Assists the speech-language pathologist in the assessment of students.
7. Orders supplies and equipment.
8. Engages in various clerical tasks, including filing and copying.
9. Maintains and cleans equipment, adhering to infection control protocol.
10. Maintains the confidentiality of information pertaining to students and their families.
11. Behaves in accordance with the educational facility guidelines.
12. Respects and appropriately considers age, gender, cultural/linguistic background, and related factors when providing services.

Supplemental Duties and Responsibilities

1. Participates in educational facility activities and committees as requested by the speech-language pathologist.
2. Participates in classroom activities as requested by the speech-language pathologist.
3. Participates in conferences as requested by the speech-language pathologist.

Required Education, Experience, and Licensure

1. The SLPA must meet state and facility requirements for health.
2. The SLPA must have one of the following:
   - Associate's degree from a speech-language pathology assistant program;
   - Bachelor's degree in speech-language pathology;
   - Completion of a college-based speech-language pathology assistant certificate program; or

- Required education as designated by the state licensing board or other regulatory agency.

Required Skills and Abilities

1. Knowledge of speech-language pathology equipment, materials, and procedures.
2. Ability to follow oral and written directions, including intervention plans.
3. Ability to work with students individually and in groups.
4. Ability to interact appropriately with others involved in the student's program, including the teacher, parent, and other personnel.
5. Analytical skills necessary to identify and report changes in the student or equipment.
6. Flexibility and adaptability, as the job combines direct intervention, classroom work, equipment/materials maintenance, and clerical responsibilities.
7. Ability to pay close attention to visual and auditory detail.
8. Ability to use a variety of computer programs for intervention and documentation.

9. Ability to walk and stand up for 90% of the work day.

Working Conditions

1. Work is a combination of sedentary and physical activities completed in a normal educational environment.
2. Travel between educational facilities in a personal vehicle may be required.
3. Exposure to body fluids and other infectious material is possible.
4. Exposure to verbally and/or physically aggressive students is possible.

Reporting Relationships

The SLPA is directly and indirectly supervised by a certified speech-language pathologist. The supervising SLP maintains legal and moral responsibility for all services provided by the SLPA, and ensures that such services are in compliance with the ASHA Code of Ethics, ASHA Guidelines for Speech-Language Pathology Assistants, state regulatory and licensure laws, and educational facility guidelines.

APPENDIX 1–G

Example of Competency-Based Assessment

SLPA Scope of Responsibilities Competency Assessment*

PROFESSIONAL CONDUCT

	Does Not Meet	*Needs Improvement*	*Meets Requirements*	*Exceeds Requirements*	*Far Exceeds Requirements*	*COMMENTS*
Refrains from performing tasks or activities that are the sole responsibility of the SLP; performs only those tasks prescribed by the supervising SLP.						
Adheres to all applicable state licensure laws and rules regulating the practice of speech-language pathology, such as those requiring licensure or registration of support personnel.						
Conducts oneself ethically, within the scope of practice and responsibilities for an SLPA.						
Actively participates with the SLP in the supervisory process.						
Actively pursues continuing education and professional development activities.						

64

SERVICE DELIVERY

	Does Not Meet	Needs Improvement	Meets Requirements	Exceeds Requirements	Far Exceeds Requirements	COMMENTS
Identifies self as an SLPA to families, students, patients, clients, staff, and others.						
Maintains client confidentiality; exhibits compliance with HIPAA and (FERPA) regulations, reimbursement requirements, and SLPAs' responsibilities.						
Assists with speech, language, and hearing screenings without clinical interpretation.						
Assists during assessment of students, patients, and clients, exclusive of test administration and/or interpretation.						
Assists with bilingual translation during screening and assessment activities exclusive of interpretation.						
Follows documented treatment plans or protocols developed by the supervising SLP.						

continues

	Does Not Meet	Needs Improvement	Meets Requirements	Exceeds Requirements	Far Exceeds Requirements	COMMENTS
Provides guidance and treatment via telepractice to students, patients, and clients, as directed by the supervising SLP.						
Documents student, patient, and client performance (e.g., tallying data for the SLP to use; preparing charts, records, and graphs) and reports this information to the supervising SLP.						
Programs and provides instruction in the use of AACs devices.						
Demonstrates or shares information with patients, families, and staff regarding feeding strategies developed and directed by the supervising SLP.						
As applicable, serves as interpreter for students/patients/clients/and families who do not speak English.						
As applicable, provides services under SLP supervision in another language for individuals who do not speak English and English-language learners.						

ADMINISTRATIVE SUPPORT

	Does Not Meet	Needs Improvement	Meets Requirements	Exceeds Requirements	Far Exceeds Requirements	COMMENTS
Assists with clerical duties, such as preparing materials and scheduling activities.						
Performs checks and maintenance of equipment.						
Assists with departmental operations (scheduling, recordkeeping, safety/maintenance of supplies and equipment).						

PREVENTION AND ADVOCACY

	Does Not Meet	Needs Improvement	Meets Requirements	Exceeds Requirements	Far Exceeds Requirements	COMMENTS
Presents primary prevention information to individuals and groups known to be at risk for communication disorders and other appropriate groups; promotes early identification and early intervention activities.						

continues

Appendix 1–G. *continued*

	Does Not Meet	Needs Improvement	Meets Requirements	Exceeds Requirements	Far Exceeds Requirements	COMMENTS
Advocates for individuals and families through community awareness, health literacy, education, and training programs to promote and facilitate access to full participation in communication, including the elimination of societal, cultural, and linguistic barriers.						
Provides information to emergency response agencies for individuals who have communication and/or swallowing disorders.						
Advocates at the local, state, and national levels for improved public policies affecting access to services and research funding.						
Supports the supervising SLP in research projects, in-service training, public relations programs, and marketing programs.						
Participates actively in professional organizations.						

Note: Competencies based on American Speech-Language-Hearing Association. (2013). *Speech-language pathology assistant scope of practice.* Retrieved from http://www.asha.org/policy/SP2013-00337/

Recommendations for additional training/education: _____

APPENDIX 1–H
Technical Proficiency Checklist

Verification of Technical Proficiency of a Speech-Language Pathology Assistant

Speech-Language Pathology Assistant Name: _____

Supervisor(s) Name: _____

Program/Facility Name: _____

Skills	Achievement of Skill	
	Yes	No
Clerical/Administrative Skills		
Assists with clerical skills and departmental operations (e.g., preparing materials, scheduling activities, keeping records)		
Participates in in-service training		
Performs checks, maintenance, and calibration of equipment		
Supports supervising SLP in research projects and public relations programs		
Collects data for quality improvement		
Prepares and maintains patient/client charts, records, graphs for displaying data		
Interpersonal Skills		
Uses appropriate forms of address with patient/client, family, caregivers, and professionals (e.g., Dr., Mr., Mrs., Ms.)		
Greets patient/client, family, and caregiver and identifies self as a speech-language pathology assistant		
Restates information/concerns to supervising SLP as expressed by patient/client, family, and caregivers, as appropriate		
Directs patient/client, family, and caregivers to supervisor for clinical information		
Is courteous and respectful in various communication situations		
Uses language appropriate to a patient/client, family, or caregiver's education level, communication style, developmental age, communication disorder, and emotional state		
Demonstrates awareness of patient/client needs and cultural values		
Conduct in Work Setting		
Recognizes own limitations within the ASHA SLPA Scope of Practice		
Upholds ethical behavior and maintains confidentiality as described in the ASHA SLPA Scope of Practice		

continues

Skills	Achievement of Skill	
	Yes	No
Maintains client records in accordance with confidentiality regulations/laws as prescribed by supervising SLPs		
Discusses confidential patient/client information only at the direction of supervising SLP		
Identifies self as an assistant in all written and oral communication with the client/patient, family, caregivers, and staff		
Demonstrates ability to explain to supervising SLP the scope of information that should be discussed with the patient/client, family, caregivers, and professionals		
Arrives punctually and prepared for work-related activities		
Completes documentation and other tasks in a timely manner		
Maintains personal appearance and language expected for the specific work setting		
Evaluates own performance		
Uses screening instruments and implements treatment protocols only after appropriate training and only as prescribed by supervising SLP		
Seeks clarification from supervising SLP as needed to follow the prescribed treatment or screening protocols		
Actively participates in interaction with supervisor demonstrating use of supervisor's feedback		
Maintains accurate records representing assigned work time with patients/clients		
Implements appropriate infection control procedures and universal precautions consistent with the employer's standards and guidelines		
Implements injury prevention strategies consistent with employer's standards and guidelines		
Uses appropriate procedures for physical management of clients according to employer's standards and guidelines and state regulations		
Technical Skills as Prescribed by Supervising SLP		
Accurately administers screening instruments, calculates and reports the results of screening procedures to supervising SLP		
Provides instructions that are clear, concise, and appropriate to the client's developmental age, level of understanding, language use, and communication style		
Follows treatment protocol as developed and prescribed by supervising SLP		
Provides appropriate feedback to patients/clients as to accuracy of their responses		
Identifies and describes relevant patient/client responses to supervising SLP		
Identifies and describes relevant patient/client, family, and caregiver behaviors to supervising SLP		
Uses appropriate stimuli, cues/prompts with the patient/client to elicit target behaviors as defined in the treatment protocol		

Skills	Achievement of Skill	
	Yes	No
Maintains on-task or redirects off-task behavior of patients/clients in individual or group treatment, consistent with the patient/client's developmental age, communication style, and disorder		
Provides culturally appropriate behavioral reinforcement consistent with the patient/client's developmental age and communication disorder		
Accurately reviews and summarizes patient/client performance		
Uses treatment materials that are appropriate to the developmental age and communication disorder of the patient/client and the culture of the patient/client/family		
Starts and ends the treatment session on time		
Obtains cosignature of supervising SLP on documentation		
Accurately records target behaviors as prescribed by supervising SLP		
Accurately calculates chronological age of the patient/client		
Correctly calculates and determines percentages, frequencies, averages, and standard scores		
Uses professional terminology correctly in communication with supervising SLP		
Maintains eligible records, log notes, and written communication		
Appropriately paces treatment session to ensure maximum patient/client response		
Implements designated treatment objectives/goals in specific appropriate sequence		

Source: American Speech-Language-Hearing Association. (2013). *Practical tools and forms for supervising speech-language pathology assistants (SLPAs).* Copyright 2013 American Speech-Language-Hearing Association. All rights reserved. Reprinted with permission.

APPENDIX 1–I
Direct Observation of Skills Brief Checklist—Medical Setting

Speech-Language Pathology Assistant: _____

Supervising SLP: _____

Patient/Client Observed: _____

Date/Time of Observation: _____

Rate the following on a scale of 1 (disagree) to 5 (agree).

Interpersonal Skills

1. Maintains appropriate patient/client relationship.   ○1 ○2 ○3 ○4 ○5
2. Demonstrates appropriate level of self-confidence.   ○1 ○2 ○3 ○4 ○5
3. Considers patient's needs.   ○1 ○2 ○3 ○4 ○5
4. Considers patient's cultural values.   ○1 ○2 ○3 ○4 ○5
5. Uses language appropriate for patient's age and education. ○1 ○2 ○3 ○4 ○5
6. Is courteous and respectful at all times.   ○1 ○2 ○3 ○4 ○5

Personal Qualities

1. Arrives punctually for treatment sessions.   ○1 ○2 ○3 ○4 ○5
2. Arrives prepared for treatment sessions.   ○1 ○2 ○3 ○4 ○5
3. Appearance is appropriate for treatment sessions.   ○1 ○2 ○3 ○4 ○5
4. Recognizes professional boundaries during treatment sessions. ○1 ○2 ○3 ○4 ○5
5. Stays within professional boundaries during treatment sessions. ○1 ○2 ○3 ○4 ○5

Technical and Treatment Skills

1. Completes assigned tasks within designated treatment sessions. ○1 ○2 ○3 ○4 ○5
2. Uses appropriate materials based on treatment plan.   ○1 ○2 ○3 ○4 ○5
3. Uses materials that are age and culturally appropriate.   ○1 ○2 ○3 ○4 ○5
4. Uses materials that are motivating.   ○1 ○2 ○3 ○4 ○5
5. Prepares the treatment/intervention settings to meet the   ○1 ○2 ○3 ○4 ○5
   needs of the patient/client.
6. Accurately determines correct vs. incorrect responses.   ○1 ○2 ○3 ○4 ○5
7. Provides appropriate feedback as to the response accuracy. ○1 ○2 ○3 ○4 ○5
8. Verbally reports the session.   ○1 ○2 ○3 ○4 ○5
9. Provides appropriate documentation of the session.   ○1 ○2 ○3 ○4 ○5

Comments:

Source: American Speech-Language-Hearing Association. (2013). *Practical tools and forms for supervising speech-language pathology assistants (SLPAs).* Copyright 2013 American Speech-Language-Hearing Association. All rights reserved. Reprinted with permission.

Direct Observation Skills Brief Checklist—Educational Setting

Speech-Language Pathology Assistant: _____

Supervising SLP: _____

Student Observed: _____

Date/Time of Observation: _____

Rate the following on a scale of 1 (disagree) to 5 (agree).

Interpersonal Skills

1. Maintains appropriate relationship with student   ○1 ○2 ○3 ○4 ○5
2. Demonstrates appropriate level of self-confidence.   ○1 ○2 ○3 ○4 ○5
3. Considers the student's cultural/linguistic needs.   ○1 ○2 ○3 ○4 ○5
4. Uses language appropriate for student's age and education.   ○1 ○2 ○3 ○4 ○5
5. Is courteous and respectful at all times.   ○1 ○2 ○3 ○4 ○5

Personal Qualities

1. Arrives punctually for the intervention session.   ○1 ○2 ○3 ○4 ○5
2. Arrives prepared for the intervention session.   ○1 ○2 ○3 ○4 ○5
3. Appearance is appropriate for the intervention session.   ○1 ○2 ○3 ○4 ○5
4. Recognizes professional boundaries during the intervention session.   ○1 ○2 ○3 ○4 ○5
5. Stays within professional boundaries during the intervention session.   ○1 ○2 ○3 ○4 ○5

Technical and Intervention Skills

1. Completes assigned tasks within the designated session.   ○1 ○2 ○3 ○4 ○5
2. Uses appropriate materials based on treatment plan.   ○1 ○2 ○3 ○4 ○5
3. Uses materials that are age and culturally appropriate.   ○1 ○2 ○3 ○4 ○5
4. Uses materials that are motivating.   ○1 ○2 ○3 ○4 ○5
5. Prepares the intervention setting to meet the needs of the student.   ○1 ○2 ○3 ○4 ○5
6. Accurately determines correct vs. incorrect responses.   ○1 ○2 ○3 ○4 ○5
7. Provides appropriate feedback as to the response accuracy.   ○1 ○2 ○3 ○4 ○5
8. Verbally reports the session.   ○1 ○2 ○3 ○4 ○5
9. Provides appropriate documentation of the session.   ○1 ○2 ○3 ○4 ○5

Comments:

APPENDIX 1–K
Skills Proficiency Checklist

SLPA: _____   Supervising SLP: _____

Skills or Proficiency	Self-Rating			Supervising SLP Rating			
	Date	Proficiency Level		Date	Proficiency Level	How Learned	Demonstrated

Competence Levels
1. Little or no experience
2. Some experience, requires practice/assist.
3. Proficient with occasional supervision
4. Proficient with independent performance

How Learned
Observation
On-the-job training
Class
Video
Policy/procedure

Demonstrated
Direct observation
Test (written/verbal)
Certificate/license
Discussion
Other

CHAPTER 2

Defining Roles:
Supervision and Mentoring

People seldom improve when they have no other model but themselves to copy.
—Oliver Goldsmith (Irish poet and playwright)

SUPERVISION

Role of Your Supervisor

Speech-language pathology assistants (SLPAs) operate under the supervision of a qualified speech-language pathologist (SLP). As an SLPA, an important question to ask is, "What is the role of my supervisor?" Understanding the role of your supervisor allows you to practice as an SLPA given prescribed regulations. The American Speech-Language-Hearing Association (ASHA) has recommended

guidelines for supervising SLPAs and the roles and responsibilities of those who supervise them (ASHA, 2013). The overarching theme in these recommendations casts the primary role of the supervisor as the decision maker in directing the nature of services provided and as the individual responsible for providing oversight to protect the patient's or client's safety and ensure the highest quality of care. The SLPA's goal is also to maintain the highest quality care for the individuals she or he serves. In this context, as the image at the start of the chapter suggests, the supervisor and SLPA are partners in bringing excellent care to individuals with communicative disorders. Ultimately, though, "diagnosis and treatment for the students, patients, and clients served remains the legal and ethical responsibility of the supervisor" (ASHA, 2013, Guidelines for SLP Supervision of SLPAs, para. 1). The responsibility for patient care cannot be delegated to an SLPA. The SLPA's services should be viewed as an extension of the SLP, not an alternative to services provided by the SLP. The purpose of SLPA services should not be to significantly increase the caseload size of the SLP (ASHA, 2013). This means that SLPAs should be used to deliver services only to those individuals on the supervising SLP's caseload. Importantly, as discussed in Chapter 1, ASHA details that "under no circumstances should an assistant have his or her own caseload" (ASHA, 2013, Guidelines for SLP Supervision of SLPAs, para. 2).

Just as you are expected to be very familiar with your roles and responsibilities, you should also be familiar with those of your supervisor. ASHA expects that SLPA supervisors will do the following (ASHA, 2013, Qualifications of an SLPA, para. 2):[1]

- Conduct ongoing competency evaluations of the SLPA.
- Provide and encourage ongoing education and training opportunities for the SLPA consistent with competency, skills, and needs of the students, patients, or clients served.
- Develop, review, and modify treatment plans for students, patients, and clients that SLPAs implement under the supervision of the SLP.

- Make all case management decisions.
- Adhere to the supervisory responsibilities for SLPs.
- Retain the legal and ethical responsibility for all students, patients, and clients served.
- Adhere to the principles and rules of the ASHA Code of Ethics.
- Adhere to applicable licensure laws and rules regulating the practice of speech-language pathology.

Amount and Type of Supervision

Another question asked is, "How much will I be supervised?" or "How much supervision is required?" ASHA also provides detailed recommendations in this area (Box 2–1; ASHA, 2013). ASHA categorizes the type of supervision, as either *direct supervision*, which is onsite, in-view observation and guidance, or *indirect supervision*, which is conducted without direct observation and guidance, such as during record review, review and evaluation of audio- or videotaped sessions, and so forth (ASHA, 2013). As outlined in Box 2–1, within the first 90 days of working, ASHA recommends that SLPAs receive a total of at least 30% direct and indirect supervision weekly (with no less than 20% supervision for direct patient or client contact activities). After the first 90 days, ASHA recommends a minimum of 1 hour per week of direct supervision and as much indirect supervision as is needed to maintain quality of service.

ASHA states that the supervisor must make herself or himself available to the SLPA for immediate contact while SLPAs are performing their duties. SLPAs may

> ### Box 2–1. Minimum Frequency and Amount of Supervision
> #### (ASHA, 2013, Minimum Requirements for Frequency
> #### and Amount of Supervision, para. 1)[1]
>
> ■ *First 90 workdays:* A total of at least 30% supervision, including at least 20% direct and 10% indirect supervision, is required weekly. Direct supervision of student, patient, and client care should be no less than 20% of the actual student, patient, and client contact time, weekly for each SLPA.
> ■ Direct supervision should be scheduled so that all students, patients, and clients seen by the assistant are directly supervised in a timely manner. Supervision days and time of day (e.g., morning or afternoon) may be alternated to ensure that all students, patients, and clients receive some direct contact with the SLP at least once every 2 weeks.
> ■ *After first 90 workdays:* The amount of supervision can be adjusted if the supervising SLP determines the SLPA meets appropriate competencies and skill levels with a variety of communication and related disorders.
> ■ A minimum of 1 hour of direct supervision weekly and as much indirect supervision as needed to facilitate the delivery of quality services must be maintained.
> ■ One hundred percent direct supervision of SLPAs for medically fragile students, patients, or clients is required.

not perform tasks when "a supervising SLP cannot be reached by personal contact, phone, pager, or other immediate or electronic means" (ASHA, 2013, Minimal Requirements for the Frequency and Amount of Supervision, para. 11). This means that if your supervising SLP is not available, your service provision to clients must be discontinued until adequate supervision can be obtained, including things like extended absences due to maternity leave, illness, or if your supervisor leaves that site to accept employment elsewhere (ASHA, 2013).

ASHA guidelines detail the *minimum* level of supervision recommended. Each supervisor will be responsible for determining the actual amount and nature of supervision an SLPA receives, taking into consideration things such as an SLPA's experience, the clients served, the setting, and the tasks assigned. It is anticipated that more supervision will be needed when you begin a position or when you perform tasks that are new to you. ASHA recommends that supervisors establish a schedule that allows them to review the data collected on every client seen by the SLPA on a weekly basis (ASHA, 2013). Furthermore, to ensure adequate supervision, ASHA recommends that the supervisor has direct contact with every client seen by the SLPA at least every 2 weeks and that SLPs not supervise more than two full-time equivalent SLPAs in any setting or combination thereof (ASHA, 2013). Remember, too, that individual state regulating agencies may differ in the minimal levels of supervision required. As discussed in Chapter 1, you should familiarize yourself with all applicable regulations in your individual state relative to minimum levels of supervision. Chapter 1 contains details on how to obtain this information.

Supervisor Training and Credentials

ASHA guidelines also contain recommendations for supervisor qualifications (Box 2–2). As shown in Box 2–2, ASHA recommends that supervisors have an ASHA Certificate of Clinical Competence (CCC) and applicable state licensure, as well as at least 2 years' experience as an SLP, following certification. Preservice training and at least 10 hours of continuing education on the topic of supervision are also recommended. It is also important that supervisors have a desire to supervise SLPAs and that they have the time and resources needed to do so. It is important to ask how much supervision you will receive when interviewing and considering employment as an SLPA.

Documenting Supervision

ASHA recommends that supervisors document the actual amount and nature of supervision an SLPA receives and that the supervisor participate in performance appraisals of the SLPA (ASHA, 2013). In the case of direct contact activities, documentation should include a description of the nature of services provided by the SLPA, at least every 60 calendar days for each client served.

How supervision is documented varies across settings and supervisors. Appendices 2–A to 2–C have examples of forms used for recording supervision. Chapter 1 contains additional details on common evaluation practices, such as competency-based assessment and samples of ASHA-recommended proficiency checklists and observation forms.

Box 2–2. Qualifications of a Supervising SLP
(ASHA, 2013, Qualifications for Supervising SLP, para. 1)[1]

- Hold a CCC in Speech-Language Pathology from ASHA and/or state licensure (where applicable)
- Have an active interest in and desire to use support personnel
- Have practiced speech-language pathology for at least 2 years following ASHA certification
- Have completed or be currently enrolled in at least one course or workshop in supervision for at least 1.0 continuing education units (CEUs; 10 clock hours)

Supervisory Relationship

When discussing rules and regulations applicable to supervision, often missed is the importance of the relationship between you and your supervisor. Remember that both you and your supervisor are responsible for establishing a good working relationship. It is a two-way street. The level of service you provide depends heavily on the nature of the supervisory relationship you develop together. Ideally, the relationship is one of reciprocity or, as McCready (2007) described, a relationship in which both the SLPA and the supervisor give and take mutually and complement one another professionally. Active listening and good conflict resolution skills will be at the heart of this relationship (McCready, 2007). The sections that follow address expectations, supervisory conferences, and feedback, each of which is important to fostering a good working relationship with your supervisor.

Expectations

Expectations set the stage for all workplace behaviors. Your supervisor will have expectations for you in the performance of your duties as an SLPA. You will also have expectations of your supervising SLP in the execution of her or his duties as your supervisor. These expectations will likely have multiple levels and change given specific circumstances. It is impossible to list everything that will be expected of you or what you can expect of your supervisor. As such, it is critical that you have an ongoing dialogue about these expectations. Many work place conflicts occur between a supervisor and a supervisee because there is a misun-

derstanding about what is expected of each person. A good rule of thumb is to never assume you know what is expected. Rather, directly clarifying expectations is the best course of action.

Supervisory Conferences

Supervisory conferences are a critical part of supervision. A fair amount of research has been conducted on the nature of supervisory conferences in the field of speech-language pathology, most of it directed at supervisors in terms of their role in these conferences (e.g., supervisor training, communication, style; McCrea & Brasseur, 2003). From a supervisee's perspective, though, it is important that you also look closely at your role in shaping supervisory conferences. First, realize that a supervisory conference is not a static, once per year event, like a performance review. Rather, they are an ongoing dialogue between you and your supervisor. These interactions can take many forms, depending on your setting, such as formal weekly or daily meetings or more informal discussions with your supervisor. These conferences are an opportunity to receive feedback, share and clarify expectations, address clinical issues and concerns, develop goals, seek avenues of skill development, and further shape the nature of the relationship between you and your supervisor. Some ways you can contribute to this process are as follows:

1. *Work with your supervisor to establish a routine schedule for conferences.* It is most effective to establish a routine schedule for conferences versus, for example, meeting as available or as needed (Dowling, 2001).

2. *Help to develop the agenda for your conferences by providing questions and suggested items to discuss in advance of the next conference.* Make a list of any pressing questions you may have for your supervisor. If possible, providing this to your supervisor in advance of the conference time will be helpful. As time is often limited, select your questions carefully to maximize the productivity of your conference time.

3. *Take notes about items discussed and things that require follow-up.* Keep a journal of conferences, recording questions, answers, to-do lists, and any other important aspects of this process; however, you should not record any personal information about your clients in this journal. If you want to make clinical notes, use initial or client pseudonyms.

4. *Contribute actively to the discussion during the conference.* Use this opportunity to ask questions and clarify information presented. This is also an opportunity for you to share your perspectives on related issues.

5. *Employ good interpersonal communication and good listening skills.*

6. *After the conference, take time to reflect on the content as well as your contributions and ways to enhance conferences in future.* Use your notes to reflect back on the discussion and document any additional observations, questions, comments, or concerns to be addressed at the next conference.

Feedback

As may be evident at this point, feedback is a key component of the supervisory process (McCrea & Brasseur, 2003; Nelson, 2009). Box 2–3 highlights characteristics of effective feedback. Supervisees across all levels of training generally recognize the value of *effective* feedback (Moss, 2007). In two recent studies by Moss (2007), feedback was specifically highlighted by SLPAs and SLPAs in training as important to both clinical success and satisfaction with training and supervision (Ostergren, 2012; Ostergren & Aguilar, 2012).

As an SLPA, you will receive feedback from your supervisor in a variety of ways. As discussed above, these may include formal feedback through com-

---

Box 2–3. Characteristics of Effective Feedback

Effective feedback is

- Given for a good reason,
- Specific and descriptive,
- Relevant,
- About behavior that can be changed,
- Given at appropriate time (usually right after observation but in an appropriate setting),
- Open to discussion, and
- A balance of positive and negative

petency assessments and performance evaluation tools. You will also receive feedback via informal methods, including verbal comments and discussion during supervisory conferences and/or informal written notes from your supervisor (McCrea & Brasseur, 2003). Feedback may occur after task completion, or during, such as commenting and guiding your behavior if a supervisor participates in a therapy session with you. As an SLPA, you should seek both formal and informal feedback from your supervisor. Both will be important for helping develop your skills and providing the highest quality of care for the clients you serve.

It is critical that you receive this feedback in a way that is productive in shaping your skills, but also in a manner that shapes the nature of future feedback. Providing and receiving feedback, especially negative feedback, is not always easy, particularly if the feedback involves aspects of the supervisory relationship or personal issues (Nelson, 2009). Some suggestions for ways you can enhance this process are the following:

- *Don't take it personally!* SLPAs who develop exceptional skills are those who realize that no matter what the task, there is always room for improvement and *effective* feedback helps you improve. If your supervisor suggests areas to improve, view this as an opportunity to change and grow in your skills.
- *Keep an open mind and to try to see your supervisor's perspective in the feedback provided.*
- *Use reflection when you receive feedback.* Listen or read (in the case of written feedback) and

attempt to understand *before* you react or respond.
- *Know yourself and let your supervisor know your preference for the method of feedback.* Do you prefer feedback to be verbal, written, or a combination of both? It is okay to let your supervisor know your preference, but be careful to take into consideration the demands on your supervisor in this respect. For example, receiving extensive written feedback on every task performed is not realistic, but working with your supervisor to identify tasks where specific written feedback may be helpful to you is.
- *Seek modifications to feedback, as needed.* If you are receiving feedback that is overly critical or overly positive, discuss this with your supervisor. Similarly, if the feedback is not specific or descriptive, ask for clarification. If the feedback is not given in time for you to implement changes, problem solve with your supervisor to change the timing of feedback in the future. Remember to employ good interpersonal communication skills and tact when requesting modifications to feedback.

Supervisory conferences are an excellent time to discuss the nature of the feedback you receive. As an SLPA, you will receive feedback, but you can also offer feedback to your supervisor about the supervisory process. In preparation for discussions about the feedback, it is helpful to reflect back on the nature of effective feedback. Are you receiving positive and negative feedback? Is it given about behaviors that you can change and at an appropriate time so that you can incorporate change into future performance? Is it specific, descriptive, and relevant? These are all areas that can be discussed with your supervisor to optimize feedback.

MENTORING

Mentoring is defined as "a developmental partnership through which one person shares knowledge, skills, information, and perspective to foster the personal and professional growth of someone else" (ASHA, n.d.-a, p. 3). SLPAs often view their supervisor as a mentor, but it is important to remember that *supervisor* and *mentor* are not synonymous roles (ASHA, 2008). The primary role of a supervisor, as discussed above, is to ensure client safety and the highest quality of care. This is done by providing oversight and accountability to the process including for example, "providing grades or conducting performance evaluations or documenting professional behavior and clinical performance" (ASHA, 2008, Mentoring in Supervision, para. 1). Mentors, on the other hand, are individuals who are not necessarily charged with this oversight but take an active role in fostering the development of your professional growth, personal growth, or both. Having a professional mentor is important and has been shown to be related to increases in work satisfaction and career-related motivation and involvement, as well as to a more positive self-image of the mentee and more positive attitudes toward workplace interpersonal relationships (Eby, Allen, Evans, Ng, & DuBois, 2008).

It may be that your supervisor views herself or himself as a mentor to you. If so, this is excellent. You can foster this relationship by taking into consideration the roles of a mentee (Box 2–4), as well as the roles of a mentor (Box 2–5). If your supervisor does not view her or his role as your mentor, this is okay too. In that case, this is an opportunity to develop a mentoring relationship with another individual. Ideally, as an SLPA, it is highly valuable to develop relationships with multiple mentors who each have a vested interest in shaping your professional and personal growth. Remember, too, that a mentor is not necessarily *all purpose*. Mentors can serve different roles, either personal, professional, or both depending on their goals and yours.

Finding a mentor can seem like an intimidating and mysterious task. The truth is that some mentoring relationships develop naturally and others require work on your part to identify and cultivate a suitable mentoring relationship. It is also true that a certain amount of chemistry, in terms of connecting personally with that person, is an important part of this process (ASHA, n.d.-a). There may also be failed attempts where a mentor-mentee relationship looks promising but does not expand to its fullest potential for a variety of reasons. Do not let this discourage you from seeking mentors.

The mentee is the driver of a mentoring relationship. As such, the first step in this process is for you to identify your personal and professional goals. That is, "What do you hope to accomplish from a mentoring relationship?" or "What skills or knowledge do you hope to gain?" Next, you can explore formal and informal channels for identifying individuals who may have an interest in helping you to accomplish your goals.

Box 2–4. Roles of a Mentee

- **Driver of Relationship**
  Identify the skills, knowledge, and goals that you want to achieve and communicate them to your mentor. Bring up new topics that are important to you at any point and give feedback to your mentor.
- **Development Planner**
  Maintain a mentoring plan and work with your mentor to setup goals, developmental activities, and time frames.
- **Resource Partner**
  Work with your mentor to seek resources for learning; identify people and information that might be helpful.
- **Teacher**
  Look for opportunities to give back to your mentor; share any information that you think might be valuable.
- **Continuous Learner**
  Take full advantage of this opportunity to learn.

Box 2–5. Roles of a Mentor

- **Coach and Adviser**
  Give advice and guidance, share ideas, and provide feedback. Share information on "unwritten rules for success" within the environment and organization.
- **Source of Encouragement and Support**
  Act as a sounding board for ideas and concerns about school and career choices, providing insight into possible opportunities. Provide support on personal issues if appropriate.
- **Resource Person**
  Identify resources to help the mentee enhance personal development and career growth. Expand the mentee's network of contacts.
- **Champion**
  Serve as an advocate for the mentee whenever the opportunity presents itself. Seek opportunities to increase visibility of the mentee.
- **Devil's Advocate**
  When appropriate, play devil's advocate to help the mentee think through important decisions and strategies.

Professional organizations, such as ASHA, are often a good place to explore more formal channels of mentoring. At the writing of this text, ASHA had mentoring programs for student members and also for professional SLP and audiology members but not yet for ASHA associates. It may be that these programs are now available, so check ASHA's website for additional information. Even if formal programs are not specifically structured for ASHA associates, ASHA's resources can still be helpful in this area. Another avenue in identifying formal mentoring programs is through state speech, language, and hearing associations. You can explore their websites or contact your regional representative to see if formal mentoring programs are available to you. Similarly, if you are employed in a large company or school district, check with your human resources department to see if there are any formal mentoring programs offered to employees.

You can also seek mentors through more informal channels. Start by making a list of individuals in your professional and personal environments or those you have met at various points in your career or education who may be potential mentors. Compare this list to your personal and professional goals and see if there are any potential matches. If someone listed has not already reached out to you as a mentor, make first contact to initiate the relationship. Try first to develop an open line of communication and personal contact with the person before jumping into questions about mentoring (Hannon, n.d.). Getting to know each other's personal styles allows you and your potential mentor to see if your personalities are a good fit. The next step is to share your interests and related professional or personal goals with that person. Starting out with a, "Will you be my mentor?" question can be too formal and may seem like a big commitment. You can begin instead by asking for advice on a single issue or problem and then build from there (Hannon, n.d.). If the person seems receptive to answering your questions and offering insight, keep the relationship going. Acknowledge the person's assistance and look for ways you can offer support or information to your mentor in turn. Try to establish regular contact with the person, keeping in mind the roles of mentor and mentee as you continue to foster the relationship.

Regardless of how you identify a mentor (formally or informally), be active in growing the relationship. Box 2–6 contains a few additional suggestions for maintaining a successful mentoring relationship.

Lastly, once you have a mentor and have established a positive working relationship, it is important to set goals that you and your mentor can work to accomplish (ASHA, n.d.-b). You should write them down in a journal or calendar to keep track of your progress in achieving your goals. ASHA (n.d.-b) recommends the following tips for successful goal writing:

1. Be specific about your goals.
2. Set a goal for something you really want to accomplish.
3. Break up your goals into manageable subgoals.
4. Give yourself credit when you accomplish a goal.
5. Categorize your goals by the areas of your life that you would like to improve (e.g., financial, career, educational, social).
6. Review your goals daily.
7. Involve family, friends, and colleagues for support, motivation, and resources.

Box 2–6. Guidelines for Mentoring Success

■ Be sure you are clear about how often you will communicate; whether it will be by phone, e-mail, or both; how quickly you will respond; and confidentiality.

■ Make contact frequently, especially during the first few weeks, to build a trusting relationship.

■ Respect your mentor's experience and views even if you don't agree.

■ Follow up when you make a commitment to get information or take action.

■ Don't ever leave your mentor hanging. If you don't respond, the mentor will feel that he or she wasn't helpful. You never want to leave someone who has volunteered to help with this kind of impression.

■ Be appreciative of whatever you get from your mentor; learn his or her strengths and seek advice in those areas.

■ Work hard to make the relationship a two-way street. This means you should always be on the lookout for information and resources that might be of interest to your mentor (e.g., articles you read or information you come across).

■ Be flexible and enjoy the experience!

REFERENCES

American Speech-Language-Hearing Association. (n.d.-a). *The power of passionate mentoring: The ASHA gathering place mentoring manual*. Rockville, MD: Author. Retrieved from http://asha.org/uploadedFiles/students/gatheringplace/ MentoringManual.pdf

American Speech-Language-Hearing Association. (n.d.-b). *Writing mentoring goals and objectives*. Retrieved from http://www.asha.org/students/gatheringplace/step/goals/

American Speech-Language-Hearing Association. (2008). *Clinical supervision in speech-language pathology* [Technical report].Retrieved from http://www.asha.org/policy

American Speech-Language-Hearing Association. (2013). *Speech-language pathology assistant scope of practice*. Retrieved from http://www.asha.org/policy

Dowling, S. (2001). *Supervision: Strategies for successful outcomes and productivity*. Boston, MA: Allyn & Bacon.

Eby, L. T., Allen, T. D., Evans, S. C., Ng, T., & DuBois, D. L. (2008). Does mentoring matter? A multidisciplinary meta-analysis comparing mentored and non-mentored individuals. *Journal of Vocational Behavior*, 72(2), 254–267.

Hannon, K. (n.d.). How to find a mentor. *Forbes*. Retrieved from http://www.forbes.com/sites/kerryhannon/2011/10/31/how-to-find-a-mentor

McCrea, E., & Brasseur, J. (2003). *The supervisory process in speech-language pathology and audiology*. Boston, MA: Pearson Education.

McCready, V. (2007, May 8). Supervision of speech-language pathology assistants: A reciprocal relationship. *ASHA Leader*. Retrieved from http://www.asha.org/Publications/leader/2007/070508/f070508b/

Moss, L. B. (2007). Supervisory feedback: A review of the literature. *Perspectives on Administration and Supervision*, 17(1), 10–12.

Nelson, L. (2009). Feedback in supervision. *Perspectives on Administration and Supervision*, 19(1), 19–24.

Ostergren, J. (2012). Bachelor 's level speech-language pathology assistants (SLPAs) in California: A bachelor 's level clinical practicum course. *Contemporary Issues in Communication Sciences and Disorders, 39*, 1–11.

Ostergren, J., & Aguilar, S. (2012). A survey of speech-language pathology assistants in California: Current trends in demographics, employment, supervision, and training. *Contemporary Issues in Communication Sciences and Disorders, 39*, 121–136.

CHAPTER ENDNOTES

1. American Speech-Language-Hearing Association. (2013). *Speech-language pathology assistant scope of practice*. Available from http://www.asha.org/policy © Copyright 2013 American Speech-Language-Hearing Association. All rights reserved. Reprinted with permission.

APPENDIX 2–A
Supervisor Log of Direct and Indirect Observations

Week ending: _____

SLPA: _____

Supervising SLP: _____

Patient	Mon.	Tues.	Wed.	Thurs.	Fri.	Sat./Sun.
Other Activities						
Billing						
Equipment Maintenance						
Documentation						
Conferences/Inservices						
Other clerical						

Indicate DO for direct observation + time
Indicate IDO for indirect observation + time

Comments:

APPENDIX 2–B
SLPA Weekly Activity Log

Week ending: _____

SLPA: _____

Supervising SLP: _____

Patient	Mon.	Tues.	Wed.	Thur.	Fri.	Sat./Sun.
Total treatment time						
Total direct supervision						

	Mon.	Tues.	Wed.	Thur.	Fri.	Sat./Sun.
Documentation time						
Meeting with supervisor						
Other meetings/conferences						
Observation of sessions						
Equipment maintenance						
Clerical tasks						

S indicates supervised session.

Source: American Speech-Language-Hearing Association. (2013). *Practical Tools and Forms for Supervising Speech-Language Pathology Assistants (SLPAs)*. Copyright 2013 American Speech-Language-Hearing Association. All rights reserved. Reprinted with permission.

APPENDIX 2–C
SLPA Weekly Activity Record

SLPA: _____

Supervising SLP: _____

Week ending: _____

Total hours week: _____

Activity	Time Spent
1. Direct patient treatment/intervention	_____
2. Observation of other sessions	_____
3. Meeting with supervising SLP	_____
4. Other meetings/conferences (list)	_____
_____	
_____	
_____	
_____	
5. Equipment/materials maintenance	_____
6. Documentation	_____
7. Clerical activities	_____
A. Total time directly observed by the SLP	_____
B. Total treatment time provided this week	_____
Percent of time directly observed by the SLP (A/B)	_____

CHAPTER 3

Ethical Conduct

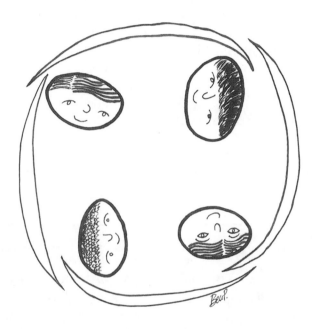

Action indeed is the sole medium of expression for ethics.

—Jane Addams
(first American woman to receive the Nobel Peace Prize)

ETHICS, MORALS, AND LAW

Webster's dictionary defines *ethics* as "the discipline dealing with what is good and bad and with moral duty and obligation" (Merriam-Webster, 2003). Hence, at its very core, ethics is the study of morality, or what is good and bad and right and wrong. *Morals* form the ground rules for society's laws. In contrast, *laws* are enforceable, written rules based on the concepts of justice and equality (Horner, 2003). In the simplest terms, laws dictate what we must do, whereas morals (and thereby ethics) address what we should do (Horner, 2003). A related term, *integrity,* refers to an adherence to high moral standards. As such, a person with professional integrity is someone who adheres to ethical principles in the execution of his or her professional duties.

Often, when students (and professionals) hear that what follows is a discussion of ethics, they brace themselves for a long, difficult discussion of these complex and intertwined terms. However, as Chabon and Morris (2004) highlight, "Ethics is really about helping one to make good decisions" (para. 2). In this light, the study of ethics and an understanding of ethical conduct can be a compass to navigate your professional obligations as a speech-language pathology assistant (SLPA).

ASHA CODE OF ETHICS

The concept of professional ethics refers to the "principles of conduct governing an individual or a group" (Merriam-Webster, 2003). The American Speech-Language Hearing Association (ASHA) has a professional Code of Ethics (ASHA, 2016a). According to ASHA, the purpose of this code is to "ensure the welfare of the consumer and protect the reputation and integrity of professions" (ASHA, 2016a, Preamble, para. 1). The code consists of four ethical principles and related rules of ethics that form the basic moral foundation of the code. Appendix 3-A contains ASHA's complete Code of Ethics. The four ethical principles of this code are listed in Box 3–1.

ASHA's Code of Ethics states that members, nonmember certificate holders, and individuals who are applying for membership or certification shall

---

Box 3–1. ASHA's Four Ethical Principles (ASHA, 2016a)[1]

Principle I (Responsibility to Persons Served Professionally and to Research Participants, both Human and Animal)
Individuals shall honor their responsibility to hold paramount the welfare of persons they serve professionally or who are participants in research and scholarly activities, and they shall treat animals involved in research in a humane manner.

Principle II (Responsibility for One's Professional Competence)
Individuals shall honor their responsibility to achieve and maintain the highest level of professional competence and performance.

Principle III (Responsibility to the Public)
Individuals shall honor their responsibility to the public when advocating for the unmet communication and swallowing needs of the public and shall provide accurate information involving any aspect of the professions.

Principle IV (Responsibility for Professional Relationships)
Individuals shall uphold the dignity and autonomy of the professions, maintain collaborative and harmonious interprofessional and intraprofessional relationships, and accept the professions' self-imposed standards.

observe these principles as "affirmative obligations under all conditions of professional activity," (ASHA, 2016a, Preamble, para. 5). ASHA maintains a Board of Ethics (BOE), charged with the responsibility of reviewing, publishing, and amending its Code of Ethics and developing educational programs and materials applicable to ethical conduct (ASHA, 2016b).

As discussed in Chapter 1, SLPAs can apply to become ASHA associates. This is an optional designation for qualified support personnel in audiology and speech-language pathology. Individuals with this designation must agree to follow all ASHA policies regarding support personnel, working only under the supervision of a qualified CCC-SLP or CCC-A. ASHA associates can access ASHA resources and many ASHA benefits but are not fully designated ASHA "members" or "certificate holders." Hence, although the spirit and moral foundation of ASHA's Code of Ethics are applicable to SLPAs, the exact language of many of the rules of ethics is not consistent with the scope of an SLPA (ASHA, 2013). As such, a question that arises is, "How does ASHA's Code of Ethics apply to SLPAs?" ASHA addressed this issue in its recent revision of the SLPA Scope of Practice (ASHA, 2013, Ethical Considerations, para. 2) stating,

> Although some SLPAs may choose to affiliate with ASHA as associates, the Code of Ethics does not directly apply to affiliates. However, any individual who is working in a support role (technician, aide, assistant) under the supervision of an SLP or speech scientist must be knowledgeable about the provisions of the code. It is imperative that the supervising professional and the assistant behave in a manner

that is consistent with the principles and rules outlined in the ASHA Code of Ethics.

This document also reiterates that the ethical responsibility for patient care cannot be delegated to the SLPA, and as such, the supervisor is responsible for the actions of the assistant during service provision. Furthermore, the document specifically states that "if the assistant engages in activities that violate the Code of Ethics, the supervising professional may be found in violation of the code if adequate oversight has not been provided" (ASHA, 2013, Ethical Consideration, para. 2).

For the purpose of this book, ASHA's Code of Ethics is discussed next in relation to SLPAs. Even though not specifically written for SLPAs, analysis of the code as it applies to the conduct of SLPAs is highly valuable. Box 3–2 lists key ethical principles and rules that have language consistent with the service provision of an assistant. This is not an exhaustive list of all applicable ASHA ethical principles or rules. Any principles that refer to determining the nature of services provided are not included. This is intentional, given that SLPAs do not determine if, when, or how services are provided, nor can they engage in any service provision without the explicit direction and supervision of an SLP (ASHA, 2013). Those listed in Box 3–2 were deemed core concepts important to any level of service provision, such as confidentiality, competence, nondiscrimination, patient safety, support of the profession and other professionals, and accuracy in public statements. The section that follows provides a framework for how to use this information when making ethical decisions in your work as an SLPA.

Box 3–2. Examples of ASHA's Ethical Principles Potentially Applicable to SLPAs (ASHA, 2016a)[1]

Principle of Ethics I

A. Individuals shall provide all services and scientific activities competently.

C. Individuals shall not discriminate in the delivery of professional services or the conduct of research and scholarly activities on the basis of race, ethnicity, sex, gender identity/gender expression, sexual orientation, age, religion, national origin, disability, culture, language, or dialect.

J. Individuals shall accurately represent the intended purpose of a service, product, or research endeavor and shall abide by established guidelines for clinical practice and responsible conduct of research.

O. Individuals shall protect the confidentiality and security of records of professional services provided, research and scholarly activities conducted, and products dispensed. Access to these records shall be allowed only when doing so is necessary to protect the welfare of the person or of the community, is legally authorized, or is otherwise required by law.

P. Individuals shall protect the confidentiality of any professional or personal information about persons served professionally or participants involved in research and scholarly activities and may disclose confidential information only when doing so is necessary to protect the welfare of the person or of the community, is legally authorized, or is otherwise required by law.

Q. Individuals shall maintain timely records and accurately record and bill for services provided and products dispensed and shall not misrepresent services provided, products dispensed, or research and scholarly activities conducted.

R. Individuals whose professional practice is adversely affected by substance abuse, addiction, or other health-related conditions are impaired practitioners and shall seek professional assistance and, where appropriate, withdraw from the affected areas of practice.

S. Individuals who have knowledge that a colleague is unable to provide professional services with reasonable skill and safety shall report this information to the appropriate authority, internally if a mechanism exists and, otherwise, externally.

Principle of Ethics II

C. Individuals who engage in research shall comply with all institutional, state, and federal regulations that address any aspects of research, including those that involve human participants and animals.

D. Individuals shall enhance and refine their professional competence and expertise through engagement in lifelong learning applicable to their professional activities and skills.

G. Individuals shall ensure that all technology and instrumentation used to provide services or to conduct research and scholarly activities are in proper working order and are properly calibrated.

Principles of Ethics III

A. Individuals shall not misrepresent their credentials, competence, education, training, experience, and scholarly contributions.

B. Individuals shall avoid engaging in conflicts of interest whereby personal, financial, or other considerations have the potential to influence or compromise professional judgment and objectivity.

C. Individuals shall not misrepresent research and scholarly activities, diagnostic information, services provided, results of services provided, products dispensed, or the effect of products dispensed.

D. Individuals shall not defraud through intent, ignorance, or negligence or engage in any scheme to defraud in connection with obtaining payment, reimbursement, or grants and contracts for services provided, research conducted, or products dispensed.

E. Individuals' statements to the public shall provide accurate and complete information about the nature and management of communication disorders, about the professions, about professional services, about products for sale, and about research and scholarly activities.

F. Individuals' statements to the public shall adhere to prevailing professional norms and shall not contain misrepresentations when advertising, announcing, and promoting their professional services and products and when reporting research results.

G. Individuals shall not knowingly make false financial or nonfinancial statements and shall complete all materials honestly and without omission.

Principle of Ethics IV

A. Individuals shall work collaboratively, when appropriate, with members of one's own profession and/or members of other professions to deliver the highest quality of care.

C   Individuals' statements to colleagues about professional services, research results, and products shall adhere to prevailing professional standards and shall contain no misrepresentations.

D. Individuals shall not engage in any form of conduct that adversely reflects on the professions or on the individual's fitness to serve persons professionally.

E. Individuals shall not engage in dishonesty, negligence, fraud, deceit, or misrepresentation.

G. Individuals shall not engage in any form of harassment, power abuse, or sexual harassment.

J. Individuals shall assign credit only to those who have contributed to a publication, presentation, process, or product. Credit shall be assigned in proportion to the contribution and only with the contributor's consent.

K. Individuals shall reference the source when using other persons' ideas, research, presentations, results, or products in written, oral, or any other media presentation or summary. To do otherwise constitutes plagiarism.

L. Individuals shall not discriminate in their relationships with colleagues, assistants, students, support personnel, and members of other professions and disciplines on the basis of race, ethnicity, sex, gender identity/gender expression, sexual orientation, age, religion, national origin, disability, culture, language, dialect, or socioeconomic status.

M. Individuals with evidence that the Code of Ethics may have been violated have the responsibility to work collaboratively to resolve the situation where possible or to inform the Board of Ethics through its established procedures.

O. Individuals shall not file or encourage others to file complaints that disregard or ignore facts that would disprove the allegation; the Code of Ethics shall not be used for personal reprisal, as a means of addressing personal animosity, or as a vehicle for retaliation.

P. Individuals making and responding to complaints shall comply fully with the policies of the Board of Ethics in its consideration, adjudication, and resolution of complaints of alleged violations of the Code of Ethics.

Q. Individuals involved in ethics complaints shall not knowingly make false statements of fact or withhold relevant facts necessary to fairly adjudicate the complaints.

R. Individuals shall comply with local, state, and federal laws and regulations applicable to professional practice, research ethics, and the responsible conduct of research.

S. Individuals who have been convicted; been found guilty; or entered a plea of guilty or nolo contendere to (1) any misdemeanor involving dishonesty, physical harm—or the threat of physical harm—to the person or property of another, or (2) any felony, shall self-report by notifying ASHA Standards and Ethics in writing within 30 days of the conviction, plea, or finding of guilt. Individuals shall also provide a certified copy of the conviction, plea, nolo contendere record, or docket entry to ASHA Standards and Ethics within 30 days of self-reporting.

T. Individuals who have been publicly sanctioned or denied a license or a professional credential by any professional association, professional licensing authority or board, or other professional regulatory body shall self-report by notifying ASHA Standards and Ethics in writing within 30 days of the final action of disposition. Individuals shall also provide a certified copy of the final action, sanction, or disposition to ASHA Standards and Ethics within 30 days of self-reporting.

ETHICAL DECISION MAKING

Armed with a discussion of ethics in general and a review of ASHA's Code of Ethics, we now revisit the concept of ethics as a compass that helps you navigate decisions about what you should do in the execution of your daily duties as an SLPA. Rarely do threats to ethical conduct in our professional (or personal) lives present themselves in conveniently identified and easily resolved scenarios. Careful and thoughtful reflection is often required, both in identifying the param-

eters of a conflict and in suggesting a potential course of action.

Several authors in the field of speech-language pathology have suggested ways of approaching this task using frameworks for ethical decision making (Body & McAllister, 2009; Chabon & Morris, 2004; Irwin, Pannbacker, Powell, & Vekovius, 2007). One framework that appears particularly applicable is Chabon and Morris's (2004) discussion of consensus building in ethical decision making. These concepts have been applied to represent the unique elements of service provision as an SLPA (Figure 3–1). The sample scenario

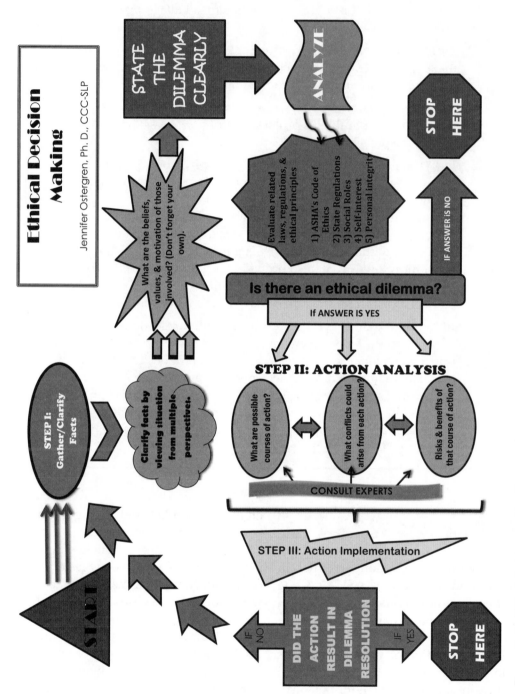

Figure 3–1. Ethical decision–making framework.

described in Box 3–3 is a hypothetical one for the purpose of describing the use of Chabon and Morris's framework. A worksheet that can be used in addressing ethical principles using this framework is available on the companion website of this textbook. A completed version of this worksheet for this particular case can be found in Appendix 3–B so you can follow along as you read the description below.

The initial phase of ethical decision making is the information gathering and

Box 3–3. Sample Scenario

Amber is an SLPA employed in a large, urban elementary school setting. She has worked in this setting for more than a year. She is currently supervised by an experienced SLP who has an ASHA Certificate of Clinical Competence (CCC). Amber herself is an ASHA associate. Amber's supervisor has one of the highest caseloads in their district. Next week, her supervisor has several individualized educational plan (IEP) meetings scheduled. She has expressed to Amber that she is behind schedule in writing documentation for these meetings and in performing follow-up assessments. Amber's supervisor just asked her to perform a diagnostic assessment on a client in preparation for an upcoming IEP meeting. Amber has observed her supervisor administering assessments and has frequently taken part in assisting her supervisor during assessments, such as preparing materials and helping to record data during the assessment; however, consistent with her scope of duties, Amber has not administered these tests independently, nor has she interpreted or summarized the results. Amber and her supervisor have a good working relationship. Amber wants to help her supervisor, but Amber is concerned that this request violates her licensing regulations and ASHA's Code of Ethics. She is unsure how to address this situation.

clarification phase (see Figure 3–1). You can start by making sure that you understand the circumstances of a situation accurately and gather any additional facts needed to understand the situation fully. In our sample scenario, it is important to clarify if, in fact, the supervisor meant for Amber to perform the assessment on her own (i.e., collecting, summarizing, and interpreting the data). Alternatively, perhaps there had been some form of miscommunication and Amber's supervisor only meant to request that Amber help administer or prepare for testing (as Amber has done previously).

As Figure 3–1 indicates, in this phase, it is important to view the circumstances from all perspectives, considering carefully your own motives and role, as well as those of others involved. In the sample scenario, it is important to think about why the supervisor made the request and if there are extenuating circumstances surrounding it. It appears from the details that time and several impending IEP meetings and reports may be factors. The fact that Amber had assisted with tests previously may be relevant to the situation. Amber's role as the assistant and her relationship with her supervisor are also facts to consider further. Amber and her supervisor appear to have a good working relationship, and as such, Amber likely has a desire to help her supervisor, but Amber may also be concerned that telling her supervisor that she cannot do something may affect her job or this relationship. The sample scenario indicates that this is indeed a concern for Amber and that she wants to help her supervisor if she can. Of course, none of these factors necessarily makes the situation ethical, but they are nonetheless important to consider and may play a role in helping to identify a possible course of action.

Also in this phase, it is important to review any relevant rules, laws, and ethical principles (see Figure 3–1). As a general rule, some important documents for SLPAs to consider are ASHA's Scope of Practice for SLPAs (see Appendix 1–A in Chapter 1; ASHA, 2013), ASHA's Code of Ethics (see Appendix 3–A; ASHA, 2016a), applicable state regulations and laws governing SLPAs and their supervisors, and any employer documents regarding policies and procedures. In the sample scenario, the supervisor is an ASHA CCC-SLP. As such, ASHA's Code of Ethics is important to consider and directly relates to the supervisor's actions in this matter. Several principles that apply to this situation include:[1]

- **Principle of Ethics I, Rule F:** Individuals who hold the Certificate of Clinical Competence shall not delegate tasks that require the unique skills, knowledge, judgment, or credentials that are within the scope of their profession to aides, assistants, technicians, support personnel, or any nonprofessionals over whom they have supervisory responsibility.
- **Principle of Ethics II, Rule E:** Individuals in administrative or supervisory roles shall not require or permit their professional staff to provide services or conduct research activities that exceed the staff member's certification status, competence, education, training, or experience.
- **Principle of Ethics IV, Rule I:** Individuals shall not knowingly allow anyone under their

supervision to engaged in any practice that violates the Code of Ethics.

In Amber's case, she is an ASHA associate and therefore has agreed to abide by ASHA rules and regulations regarding SLPA use. ASHA's Scope of Practice for SLPAs specifically states that SLPAs should not "perform standardized or nonstandardized diagnostic tests, formal or informal evaluations, or swallowing screenings/checklists" (ASHA, 2013, Responsibilities Outside the Scope for SLPAs, para. 2). From Amber's perspective as an SLPA, the following two ethical principles seem most related to this situation.

- **Principle of Ethics I, Rule A:** Individuals shall provide all services and scientific activities competently.
- **Principle of Ethics II, Rule E:** Individuals in administrative or supervisory roles shall not require or permit their professional staff to provide services or conduct research activities that exceed the staff member's certification status, competence, education, training, or experience.

Furthermore, Amber is registered as an SLPA in her state, and her state regulations prohibit SLPAs from performing diagnostic assessments.

At the end of the gather/clarify information phase, the next step is to ask yourself, "Is this an ethical dilemma?" (see Figure 3–1). If the answer is no, then you are not facing an ethical dilemma. If the answer is yes, then the next step is to begin the action analysis phase by identifying a plausible course of action. Ask yourself, "What actions can I take?" For each course of action, think about the following:

1. What does that course of action entail? Is it feasible?
2. Who will be affected by that course of action (either negatively or positively)?
3. What are the risks and benefits of that course of action?
4. Will that action result in an ethical resolution to the dilemma at hand?

Obviously, the final consideration in this phase (whether action will result in an ethical resolution) is the most important; however, sometimes it is helpful to start with listing all courses of action.

Ideally, the action analysis phase reveals a course of action which can resolve the ethical dilemma (see Figure 3–1). If not, then an additional branching step may be required, which involves consulting with experts, supervisors, or colleagues. This in fact can occur at any step in the process when additional assistance or insight is needed, but it is important to remember that self-analysis is key. You are likely the person closest to this situation, as it affects you personally or professionally. As such, you are the first expert to analyze the situation, bringing in additional insight from outside perspectives as needed.

A word of caution as well in seeking additional opinions: SLPAs must maintain confidentiality, particularly when discussing any situation that involves clients or their families. Federal regulations prohibit you from discussing personal information about the clients you serve (Annett, 2001). ASHA's Code of Ethics (2016a) also specifically addresses the matter of client confidentiality and confidentiality in relationships with colleagues. Appendix 3–C contains a copy of ASHA's statement on confidentiality. This topic is also given additional consideration at the end of this chapter.

In the sample scenario, as highlighted in Table 3–1, there are several potential courses of action.

The final stage in this process is the action implementation phase (see Figure 3–1). In this stage, you implement the course of action decided on in the action analysis phase. At the end of the action implementation phase, hopefully the situation is resolved and the ethical dilemma eliminated. If not, this process starts over again, as you restart the gather and clarify facts, action analysis, and action implementation phases until a satisfactory conclusion is reached. In the sample scenario, the action selected for implementation is bolded in Table 3–1. Amber plans to speak directly with her supervisor about her concerns regarding performing assessments, highlighting that this activity is outside the scope of responsibilities of an SLPA according to ASHA and state regulations.

In light of this, Amber will rearrange her schedule so that she can assist her supervisor during administration of the assessment and offer to stay late to prepare test materials. Furthermore, Amber has identified a few clerical tasks she can perform to help decrease the demands on her supervisor's schedule so that the supervisor has time to complete the assessment.

As this case illustrates, ethical decision making requires careful consideration from multiple perspectives. Making decisions based on ethics takes practice. Using a structured framework like the one discussed in this chapter is a first step in developing your skills in this area. Appendix 3–D contains additional ethical scenarios samples applicable to SLPAs. Use the worksheet and framework provided to practice your skills in this area. Taking it a step further by discussing your conclusions with others in the profession is also an excellent way to hone your skills in this area.

Table 3–1. Potential Courses of Action for Sample Scenario

Possible Course of Action	Benefits	Risks	Ethical Resolution? (Yes/No)
Amber could assess the client (as requested) but not tell anyone and allow her supervisor to sign the report as if the speech-language pathologist (SLP) conducted this assessment.	• Amber avoids conflict with her supervisor by not having to tell her that assessment is outside Amber's scope of responsibilities.	• Violation of ethical principles for both Amber and her supervisor. • Negative impact on quality of care for the client. • Potential for sanctions from state licensing board, for both Amber and her supervisor. • Potential for sanctions from the American Speech-Language-Hearing Association's (ASHA's) Board of Ethics for Amber's supervisor	No

Table 3–1. *continued*

Possible Course of Action	Benefits	Risks	Ethical Resolution? (Yes/No)
Amber can tell her supervisor that assessment is not within Amber's scope of responsibilities and as such Amber is not able to assess the client as requested. She can, however, offer to assist in the assessment and in any other duties within Amber's scope of responsibilities so that the supervisor has additional time to assess the client.	• No violation of ethical principles. • Quality of client care is maintained, as Amber has reduced the supervisor's workload in other ways; the client can be assessed by the SLP, who is qualified to do so.	• Amber's supervisor may disagree or may be upset that Amber has refused to do something requested. If good interpersonal skills are used in addressing this situation, this risk may be mitigated.	Yes
Amber could assess the client (as requested) but report her supervisor's conduct to the state licensing board, ASHA's Board of Ethics, and their employer.	• Amber avoids direct conflict with her supervisor by not having to tell the supervisor that assessment is outside Amber's scope of responsibilities.	• Violation in ethical principles for both Amber and her supervisor.* • Negative impact on quality of care for the client. • Potential for sanctions from state licensing board for both Amber and her supervisor. *NOTE: Although Amber reported her supervisor to ASHA's Board of Ethics, Amber would still be engaging in unethical conduct by performing the assessment, which was not in the best interest of the client.	No
Amber could avoid mentioning this conflict to her supervisor and call in sick the day the assessment is scheduled so she does not have to do it.	• Amber avoids direct conflict with her supervisor by not having to tell her that assessment is outside Amber's scope of responsibilities. • No sanctions from state licensing board for either Amber or her supervisor as the assessment is not performed by Amber.	• Potential negative impact on quality of care as the assessment may not be performed as needed, which isn't in the best interest of the client. Alternatively, the supervisor may simply reschedule the assessment for another day when Amber is available and in that case the issue has not been resolved and will resurface when Amber returns.	No

Finally, a discussion of ethical conduct would not be complete without highlighting the role of good interpersonal skills and conflict resolution in resolving ethical dilemmas professionally. Chapter 4 addresses this topic in greater detail, including several guiding principles for resolving conflict effectively.

CONFIDENTIALITY

Before we close the chapter on ethics, let's take a closer look at the topic of confidentiality. As highlighted above, when discussing ethical matters, you should maintain confidentiality of client information, confidentiality in your relationships with colleagues, and confidentiality regarding every other aspect of your role as an SLPA. This issue of confidentiality, however, goes beyond discussing an ethical dilemma (Annett, 2001; ASHA, 2018; O'Neil-Pirozzi, 2001). Appendix 3–C presents ASHA's confidentiality statement, which includes confidentiality of client information and confidentiality in relationships with peers and colleagues..

Confidentiality of Client Information

Confidentiality of client information encompasses both verbal and written information. In addition, beyond ASHA's Code of Ethics, the privacy and security of documentation are governed by federal regulations outlined in the Health Insurance Portability and Accountability Act (HIPAA) and Family Educational Rights and Privacy Act (FERPA; U.S. Department of Education, n.d.; U.S. Department of Health and Human Services, n.d.). HIPAA regulations outline rules pertaining to health care providers and health-related information. FERPA regulations outline rules applicable to school personnel and educational records. Both require specific and explicit consent for providers to use and disclose protected information. They also stipulate that individuals have a right to review and correct their official records, be notified of disclosure history, and receive notice of policies regarding disclosure of protected information. As such it is critical that SLPAs maintain confidentiality of all client information including all aspects of a client's care. This means that you must not share the details about any aspect of your services with anyone other than your supervising SLP, those specifically granted access to this information by your client (in writing), or as expressly required by law. This confidentiality includes verbal information, written materials, and audio and video recordings. Written documents and audio and visual recordings must be kept in a secure location and may not be stored, electronically or in hard copy form, in locations where those without specific permission are able to view this information. It is crucial that you take confidentiality seriously. Some reminders to ensure your client's confidentiality include the following:

1. Do not share information about your client with anyone not specifically granted access to this information. This includes sharing information about your client with your family or friends, as they are not specifically authorized service providers.
2. Do not speak in public locations about your client.
3. Do not remove any documents (written, audio, or visual) from clinical or educational locations.

4. Get specific permission to forward or copy any information about your client.

5. If you are given passwords or access codes to confidential information, do not share this information with others and do not store this information in a public location.

6. Do not dispose of client information without first adequately destroying or removing all confidential information. Your employer should have specific procedures for doing so.

Confidentiality in Relationships with Peers and Colleagues

Confidentiality in relationships with colleagues, peers, and other professionals takes on several meanings (ASHA, 2016a; ASHA, 2018). First, you should be careful not to misrepresent yourself or others in your verbal or written communications. In addition, when conflicts arise, you should limit discussion of these matters to those involved. This means you should not discuss conflict with colleagues and peers in public locations. If you must seek additional guidance, do so with discretion and confidentiality. Chapter 4 provides additional details about confidentiality in written communications.

REFERENCES

American Speech-Language-Hearing Association. (2013). *Speech-language pathology assistant scope of practice.* Retrieved from http://www.asha.org/policy

American Speech-Language-Hearing Association. (2016a). *Code of ethics* [Ethics]. Available at from https://www.asha.org/Code-of-Ethics/

American Speech-Language-Hearing Association. (2016b). *Practices and procedures of the board of ethics.* Retrieved from http://www.asha.org/policy

American Speech-Language-Hearing Association. (2018). *Issues in Ethics: Confidentiality.* Retrieved from http://www.asha.org/policy

Annett, M. M. (2001, February 20). Law concerns privacy, transfer of patient data: New regulations will affect SLPs, audiologists across settings. *ASHA Leader.* Retrieved from http://www.asha.org/Publications/leader/2001/010220/privacy.htm

Body, R., & McAllister, L. (2009). *Ethics in speech and language therapy.* Somerset, NJ: John Wiley.

Chabon, S. S., & Morris, J. F. (2004, February 17). A consensus model for making ethical decisions in a less-than-ideal world. *ASHA Leader.* Retrieved from http://www.asha.org/Publications/leader/2004/040217/040217e.htm

Horner, J. (2003). Mortality, ethics, and law: Introductory concepts. *Seminars in Speech and Language, 24,* 263–274.

Irwin, D., Pannbacker, M., Powell, W., & Vekovius, G. (2007). *Ethics for speech-language pathologists and audiologists: An illustrative casebook.* Clifton Park, NY: Thomson Delmar Learning.

Merriam-Webster. (2003). *Merriam-Webster's collegiate dictionary* (11th ed.). Springfield, MA: Author.

O'Neil-Pirozzi, T. M. (2001). Please respect patient confidentiality. *Contemporary Issues in Communication Sciences and Disorders, 28,* 48–51.

U.S. Department of Education. (n.d.). *Family Educational Rights and Privacy Act (FERPA): General information.* Retrieved from http://www2.ed.gov/policy/gen/guid/fpco/ferpa/index.html

U.S. Department of Health and Human Services. (n.d.). *Summary of HIPPA security rules.* Retrieved from http://www.hhs.gov/ocr/privacy/hipaa/understanding/summary/index.html

CHAPTER ENDNOTE

1. American Speech-Language-Hearing Association. (2016). *Code of ethics* [Ethics]. Available from http://www.asha.org/policy Copyright 2016 American Speech-Language-Hearing Association. All rights reserved. Reprinted with permission.

APPENDIX 3–A
ASHA Code of Ethics

PREAMBLE

The American Speech-Language-Hearing Association (ASHA; hereafter, also known as "The Association") has been committed to a framework of common principles and standards of practice since ASHA's inception in 1925. This commitment was formalized in 1952 as the Association's first Code of Ethics. This code has been modified and adapted as society and the professions have changed. The Code of Ethics reflects what we value as professionals and establishes expectations for our scientific and clinical practice based on principles of duty, accountability, fairness, and responsibility. The ASHA Code of Ethics is intended to ensure the welfare of the consumer and to protect the reputation and integrity of the professions.

The ASHA Code of Ethics is a framework and focused guide for professionals in support of day-to-day decision making related to professional conduct. The code is partly obligatory and disciplinary and partly aspirational and descriptive in that it defines the professional's role. The code educates professionals in the discipline, as well as students, other professionals, and the public, regarding ethical principles and standards that direct professional conduct.

The preservation of the highest standards of integrity and ethical principles is vital to the responsible discharge of obligations by audiologists, speech-language pathologists, and speech, language, and hearing scientists who serve as clinicians, educators, mentors, researchers, supervisors, and administrators. This Code of Ethics sets forth the fundamental principles and rules considered essential to this purpose and is applicable to the following individuals:

- a member of the American Speech-Language-Hearing Association holding the Certificate of Clinical Competence (CCC)
- a member of the Association not holding the Certificate of Clinical Competence (CCC)
- a nonmember of the Association not holding the Certificate of Clinical Competence (CCC)
- an applicant for certification, or for membership and certification

By holding ASHA certification or membership, or through application for such, all individuals are automatically subject to the jurisdiction of the Board of Ethics for ethics complaint adjudication. Individuals who provide clinical services and who also desire membership in the Association must hold the CCC.

The fundamentals of ethical conduct are described by Principles of Ethics and by Rules of Ethics. The four Principles of Ethics form the underlying philosophical basis for the Code of Ethics and are reflected in the following areas: (I) responsibility to persons served professionally and to research participants, both human and animal; (II) responsibility for one's professional competence; (III) responsibility to the public; and (IV) responsibility for professional relationships. Individuals shall honor and abide by these Principles as affirmative obligations under all conditions of applicable professional activity. Rules of Ethics are specific statements of minimally acceptable as well as unacceptable professional conduct.

The code is designed to provide guidance to members, applicants, and certified individuals as they make professional decisions. Because the code is not intended to address specific situations and is not inclusive of all possible ethical dilemmas, professionals are expected to follow the written provisions and to uphold the spirit and purpose of the code. Adherence to the Code of Ethics and its enforcement results in respect for the professions and positive outcomes for individuals who benefit from the work of audiologists, speech-language pathologists, and speech, language, and hearing scientists.

TERMINOLOGY

ASHA Standards and Ethics: The mailing address for self-reporting in writing is American Speech-Language-Hearing Association, Standards and Ethics, 2200 Research Blvd., #313, Rockville, MD 20850.

Advertising: Any form of communication with the public about services, therapies, products, or publications.

Conflict of interest: An opposition between the private interests and the official or professional responsibilities of a person in a position of trust, power, and/or authority.

Crime: Any felony; or any misdemeanor involving dishonesty, physical harm to the person or property of another, or a threat of physical harm to the person or property of another. For more details, see the "Disclosure Information" section of applications for ASHA certification found on www.asha.org/certification/AudCertification/ and www.asha.org/certification/SLPCertification/

Diminished decision-making ability: Any condition that renders a person unable to form the specific intent necessary to determine a reasonable course of action.

Fraud: Any act, expression, omission, or concealment—the intent of which is either actual or constructive—calculated to deceive others to their disadvantage.

Impaired practitioner: An individual whose professional practice is adversely affected by addiction, substance abuse, or health-related and/or mental health-related conditions.

Individuals: Members and/or certificate holders, including applicants for certification.

Informed consent: May be verbal, unless written consent is required; constitutes consent by persons served, research participants engaged, or parents and/or guardians of persons served to a proposed course of action after the communication of adequate information regarding expected outcomes and potential risks.

Jurisdiction: The "personal jurisdiction" and authority of the ASHA Board of Ethics over an individual holding ASHA certification and/or membership, regardless of the individual's geographic location.

Know, known, or knowingly: Having or reflecting knowledge.

May vs. shall: May denotes an allowance for discretion; shall denotes no discretion.

Misrepresentation: Any statement by words or other conduct that, under the circumstances, amounts to an assertion that is false or erroneous (i.e., not in accordance with the facts); any statement made with conscious ignorance or a reckless disregard for the truth.

Negligence: Breaching of a duty owed to another, which occurs because of a failure to conform to a requirement, and this failure has caused harm to another individual, which led to damages to this person(s); failure to exercise the care toward others that a reasonable or prudent person would take in the circumstances, or taking actions that such a reasonable person would not.

PRINCIPLE OF ETHICS I

Individuals shall honor their responsibility to hold paramount the welfare of persons they serve professionally or who are participants in research and schol-

arly activities, and they shall treat animals involved in research in a humane manner.

Rules of Ethics

A. Individuals shall provide all services and scientific activities competently.

B. Individuals shall use every resource, including referral and/or interprofessional collaboration when appropriate, to ensure that quality service is provided.

C. Individuals shall not discriminate in the delivery of professional services or the conduct of research and scholarly activities on the basis of race or ethnicity, gender, gender identity/gender expression, sexual orientation, age, religion, national origin, disability, culture, language, or dialect.

D. Individuals shall not misrepresent the credentials of aides, assistants, technicians, support personnel, students, research interns, Clinical Fellows, or any others under their supervision, and they shall inform those they serve professionally of the name, role, and professional credentials of persons providing services.

E. Individuals who hold the Certificate of Clinical Competence may delegate tasks related to provision of clinical services to aides, assistants, technicians, support personnel, or any other persons only if those persons are adequately prepared and are appropriately supervised. The responsibility for the welfare of those being served remains with the certified individual.

F. Individuals who hold the Certificate of Clinical Competence shall not delegate tasks that require the unique skills, knowledge, judgment, or credentials that are within the scope of their profession to aids, assistants, technicians, support personnel, or any nonprofessionals over whom they have supervisory responsibility.

G. Individuals who hold the Certificate of Clinical Competence may delegate tasks related to provision of clinical services that require the unique skills, knowledge, and judgment that are within the scope of practice of their profession only if those students are adequately prepared and are appropriately supervised. The responsibility for the welfare of those being served remains with the certified individual.

H. Individuals shall obtain informed consent from the persons they serve about the nature and possible risks and effects of services provided, technology employed, and products dispensed. This obligation also includes informing persons served about possible effects of not engaging in treatment or not following clinical recommendations. If diminished decision-making ability of persons served is suspected, individuals should seek appropriate authorization for services, such as authorization from a spouse, other family member, or legally authorized/appointed representative.

I. Individuals shall enroll and include persons as participants in research or teaching demonstrations only if participation is voluntary, without coercion, and with informed consent.

J. Individuals shall accurately represent the intended purpose of a service, product, or research endeavor and shall abide by established guidelines for clinical practice and the responsible conduct of research.

K. Individuals who hold the Certificate of Clinical Competence shall evaluate the effectiveness of services provided, technology employed, and products dispensed, and they shall provide services or dispense products only when benefit can reasonably be expected.

L. Individuals may make a reasonable statement of prognosis, but they shall not guarantee—directly or by implication—the results of any treatment or procedure.

M. Individuals who hold the Certificate of Clinical Competence shall use independent and evidence-based clinical judgment, keeping paramount the best interests of those being served.

N. Individuals who hold the Certificate of Clinical Competence shall not provide clinical services solely by correspondence, but may provide services via telepractice consistent with professional standards and state and federal regulations.

O. Individuals shall protect the confidentiality and security of records of professional services provided, research and scholarly activities conducted, and products dispensed. Access to these records shall be allowed only when doing so is necessary to protect the welfare of the person or of the community, is legally authorized, or is otherwise required by law.

P. Individuals shall protect the confidentiality of any professional or personal information about persons served professionally or participants involved in research and scholarly activities and may disclose confidential information only when doing so is necessary to protect the welfare of the person or of the community, is legally authorized, or is otherwise required by law.

Q. Individuals shall maintain timely records and accurately record and bill for services provided and products dispensed and shall not misrepresent services provided, products dispensed, or research and scholarly activities conducted.

R. Individuals whose professional practice is adversely affected by substance abuse, addiction, or other health-related conditions are impaired practitioners and shall seek professional assistance and, where appropriate, withdraw from the affected areas of practice.

S. Individuals who have knowledge that a colleague is unable to provide professional services with reasonable skill and safety shall report this information to the appropriate authority, internally if a mechanism exists and, otherwise, externally.

T. Individuals shall provide reasonable notice and information about alternatives for obtaining care in the event that they can no longer provide professional services.

PRINCIPLE OF ETHICS II

Individuals shall honor their responsibility to achieve and maintain the highest level of professional competence and performance.

Rules of Ethics

A. Individuals who hold the Certificate of Clinical Competence shall engage in only those aspects of the professions that are within the scope of their professional practice and competence, considering their certification status, education, training, and experience.

B. Members who do not hold the Certificate of Clinical Competence may not engage in the provision of clinical services; however, individuals who are in the certification application process may engage in the provision of clinical services consistent with current local and state laws and regulations and with ASHA certification requirements.

C. Individuals who engage in research shall comply with all institutional, state, and federal regulations that address any aspects of research, including those that involve human participants and animals.

D. Individuals shall enhance and refine their professional competence and expertise through engagement in lifelong learning applicable to their professional activities and skills.

E. Individuals in administrative or supervisory roles shall not require or permit their professional staff to provide services or conduct research activities that exceed the staff member's certification status, competence, education, training, and experience.

F. Individuals in administrative or supervisory roles shall not require or permit their professional staff to provide services or conduct clinical activities that compromise the staff member's independent and objective professional judgment.

G. Individuals shall make use of technology and instrumentation consistent with accepted professional guidelines in their areas of practice. When such technology is not available, an appropriate referral may be made.

H. Individuals shall ensure that all technology and instrumentation used to provide services or to conduct research and scholarly activities are in proper working order and are properly calibrated.

PRINCIPLE OF ETHICS III

Individuals shall honor their responsibility to the public when advocating for the unmet communication and swallowing needs of the public and shall provide accurate information involving any aspect of the professions.

Rules of Ethics

A. Individuals shall not misrepresent their credentials, competence, education, training, experience, and scholarly contributions.

B. Individuals shall avoid engaging in conflicts of interest whereby personal, financial, or other considerations have the potential to influence or compromise professional judgment and objectivity.

C. Individuals shall not misrepresent research and scholarly activities, diagnostic information, services provided, results of services provided, products dispensed, or the effects of products dispensed.

D. Individuals shall not defraud through intent, ignorance, or negligence or engage in any scheme to defraud in connection with obtaining payment, reimbursement, or grants and contracts for services provided, research conducted, or products dispensed.

E. Individuals' statements to the public shall provide accurate and complete information about the nature and management of communication dis-

orders, about the professions, about professional services, about products for sale, and about research and scholarly activities.

F. Individuals' statements to the public shall adhere to prevailing professional norms and shall not contain misrepresentations when advertising, announcing, and promoting their professional services and products and when reporting research results.

G. Individuals shall not knowingly make false financial or nonfinancial statements and shall complete all materials honestly and without omission.

PRINCIPLE OF ETHICS IV

Individuals shall uphold the dignity and autonomy of the professions, maintain collaborative and harmonious interprofessional and intraprofessional relationships, and accept the professions' self-imposed standards.

Rules of Ethics

A. Individuals shall work collaboratively, when appropriate, with members of one's own profession and/or members of other professions to deliver the highest quality of care.

B. Individuals shall exercise independent professional judgment in recommending and providing professional services when an administrative mandate, referral source, or prescription prevents keeping the welfare of persons served paramount.

C. Individuals' statements to colleagues about professional services, research results, and products shall adhere to prevailing professional standards and shall contain no misrepresentations.

D. Individuals shall not engage in any form of conduct that adversely reflects on the professions or on the individual's fitness to serve persons professionally.

E. Individuals shall not engage in dishonesty, negligence, fraud, deceit, or misrepresentation.

F. Applicants for certification or membership, and individuals making disclosures, shall not knowingly make false statements and shall complete all application and disclosure materials honestly and without omission.

G. Individuals shall not engage in any form of harassment, power abuse, or sexual harassment.

H. Individuals shall not engage in sexual activities with individuals (other than a spouse or other individual with whom a prior consensual relationship exists) over whom they exercise professional authority or power, including persons receiving services, assistants, students, or research participants.

I. Individuals shall not knowingly allow anyone under their supervision to engage in any practice that violates the Code of Ethics.

J. Individuals shall assign credit only to those who have contributed to a publication, presentation, process, or product. Credit shall be assigned in proportion to the contribution and only with the contributor's consent.

K. Individuals shall reference the source when using other persons' ideas, research, presentations, results, or products in written, oral, or any other media presentation or summary. To do otherwise constitutes plagiarism.

L. Individuals shall not discriminate in their relationships with colleagues, assistants, students, support personnel, and members of other professions and disciplines on the basis of race, ethnicity, sex, gender identity/gender expression, sexual orientation, age, religion, national origin, disability, culture, language, dialect, or socioeconomic status.

M. Individuals with evidence that the Code of Ethics may have been violated have the responsibility to work collaboratively to resolve the situation where possible or to inform the Board of Ethics through its established procedures.

N. Individuals shall report members of other professions who they know have violated standards of care to the appropriate professional licensing authority or board, other professional regulatory body, or professional association when such violation compromises the welfare of persons served and/or research participants.

O. Individuals shall not file or encourage others to file complaints that disregard or ignore facts that would disprove the allegation; the Code of Ethics shall not be used for personal reprisal, as a means of addressing personal animosity, or as a vehicle for retaliation.

P. Individuals making and responding to complaints shall comply fully with the policies of the Board of Ethics in its consideration, adjudication, and resolution of complaints of alleged violations of the Code of Ethics.

Q. Individuals involved in ethics complaints shall not knowingly make false statements of fact or withhold relevant facts necessary to fairly adjudicate the complaints.

R. Individuals shall comply with local, state, and federal laws and regulations applicable to professional practice, research ethics, and the responsible conduct of research.

S. Individuals who have been convicted; been found guilty; or entered a plea of guilty or nolo contendere to (1) any misdemeanor involving dishonesty, physical harm—or the threat of physical harm—to the person or property of another, or (2) any felony, shall self-report by notifying ASHA Standards and Ethics (see Terminology for mailing address) in writing within 30 days of the conviction, plea, or finding of guilt. Individuals shall also provide a certified copy of the conviction, plea, nolo contendere record, or docket entry to ASHA Standards and Ethics within 30 days of self-reporting.

T. Individuals who have been publicly sanctioned or denied a license or a professional credential by any professional association, professional licensing authority or board, or other professional regulatory body shall self-report by notifying ASHA Standards and Ethics (see Terminology for mailing address) in writing within 30 days of the final action or disposition. Individuals shall also provide a certified copy of the final action, sanction, or disposition to ASHA Standards and Ethics within 30 days of self-reporting.

APPENDIX 3–B
Sample SLPA Ethical Decision–Making Worksheet

STEP 1: GATHER/CLARIFY FACTS*

- Who is involved in this situation?
  Amber and her supervisor.

- Who is affected by this situation?
  Amber, her supervisor, and the client and his or her family (if Amber performs the assessment).

- What are the motives and roles of others involved in this situation?
  Amber's supervisor appears to be motivated by currently pressing issues in terms of a large number of reports and assessments that need to be done soon. Additional clarification may be needed as to why this particular client was highlighted as a person Amber should be involved in assessing. Perhaps Amber and this client have a positive relationship or there is some input Amber's supervisor feels will be valuable from Amber in terms of assessment or the client's progress report. Related to this, Amber can also clarify her supervisor's intent with this request. Was the request that Amber assist in this assessment or that Amber perform this assessment independently? The role of Amber's supervisor is that of Amber's superior, which is a position of power in terms of Amber's employment and performance evaluation, as well as potential future supervision.

- What is *your own* motive (role) in the situation?
  Amber's role is that of an assistant who works under the direction of her supervisor. Amber may be concerned how her supervisor will react if she tells her she cannot do something, both personally because they appear to have a good relationship, but also from an employment and supervision standpoint. Amber may be concerned she will lose her job or be rated poorly on evaluations if she tells her supervisor that assessment is outside of her scope of practice.

- Describe applicable state regulations and laws (if any).
  Regulations for Amber's state licensure specifically state she may not independently assess a client. They do state she can assist with assessment. Similarly, state regulations governing Amber's supervisor also specifically state that she may not delegate tasks such as assessment to support personnel.

■ Describe applicable employer policies and/or procedures (if any).
No specific employer-related policies or procedures on this matter were identified.

■ List applicable ASHA ethical principles and rules of ethics (if any):

Ethical Principle	Ethical Rule
Applicable to Amber	
Principle of Ethics I	*Rule A: Individuals shall provide all services and scientific activities competently.*
Principle of Ethics II	*Rule E: Individuals in administrative or supervisory roles shall not require or permit their professional staff to provide services or conduct research activities that exceed the staff member's certification status, competence, education, training, and experience.*
Applicable to Amber's Supervisor	
Principle of Ethics I	*Rule F: Individuals who hold the Certificate of Clinical Competence shall not delegate tasks that require the unique skills, knowledge, judgment, or credentials that are within the scope of their profession to aides, assistants, technicians, support personnel, or any nonprofessionals over whom they have supervisory responsibility.*
Principle of Ethics II	*Rule E: Individuals in administrative or supervisory roles shall not require or permit their professional staff to provide services or conduct research activities that exceed the staff member's certification status, competence, level of education, training, and experience.*
Principle of Ethics IV	*Rule I: Individuals shall not knowingly allow anyone under their supervision to engage in any practice that violates the Code of Ethics.*

*Note: At the end of Step 1 (gather/clarify facts), you should be able to describe the nature of the problem accurately and in depth, factoring in each of the facts in Step 1. If not, continue to gather additional information. If by clarifying the facts, the ethical dilemma no longer exists, stop here. If not, proceed to Step 2 (action analysis).

STEP 2: ACTION ANALYSIS

Possible Course of Action	Benefits	Risks
Amber could assess the client (as requested) but not tell anyone and allow her supervisor to sign the report as if the SLP was the one who conducted this assessment.	■ Amber avoids conflict with her supervisor by not having to tell the supervisor that assessment is outside Amber's scope of responsibilities.	■ Violation of ethical principles, for both Amber and her supervisor. ■ Negative impact on quality of care for the client. ■ Potential for sanctions from state licensing boards, for both Amber and her supervisor. ■ Potential for sanctions from the American Speech-Language-Hearing Association (ASHA's) Board of Ethics for Amber's supervisor.
Amber can tell her supervisor that assessment is not within her scope of responsibilities, and as such, she is not able to assess the client (as requested). She can offer to assist in the assessment and in any other duties within Amber's scope of responsibilities so that her supervisor has additional time to assess the client.	■ No violation in ethical principles. ■ Quality of client care is maintained, as Amber has reduced the supervisor's workload in other ways so that the client can be assessed by the SLP, who is qualified to do so.	■ Amber's supervisor may disagree or may be upset that Amber has refused to do something requested. If good interpersonal skills are utilized in addressing this situation, this risk may be mitigated.

Possible Course of Action	Benefits	Risks
Amber could assess the client (as requested) but report her supervisor's conduct to the state licensing board, ASHA's Board of Ethics, and their employer.	■ Amber avoids direct conflict with her supervisor by not telling her that assessment is outside Amber's scope of responsibilities.	■ Violation of ethical principles for both Amber and her supervisor.+ ■ Negative impact on quality of care for the client. ■ Potential for sanctions from state licensing board, for both Amber and her supervisor. +*Note*: Although Amber reported her supervisor to ASHA's Board of Ethics, Amber would still be engaging in unethical conduct as she performed the assessment, which was not in the best interest of the client.
Amber could not mention this conflict to her supervisor but call in sick the day the assessment is scheduled, so she does not have to assess the client.	■ Amber avoids direct conflict with her supervisor by not having to tell her supervisor that assessment is outside Amber's scope of responsibilities. ■ No sanctions from the state licensing board for either Amber or her supervisor as the assessment is not performed by Amber.	■ Potential negative impact on quality of care as the assessment may not be performed as needed, which isn't in the best interest of the client. Alternatively, the supervisor may simply reschedule the assessment for another day when Amber is available. and in that case, the issue has not been resolved and will resurface when Amber returns.

Consult Experts[++]

- Who are sources of assistance in problem solving this matter (e.g., supervisor, employer, coworker, etc.)?
  Amber has another SLP she has worked closely with in the same district. She may be an additional resource on the matter, given of course that Amber discusses this issue in confidence.

- What are the opinions of experts on your course(s) of action?
  After evaluating the possible course of actions, Amber decided there was only one that resulted in an ethical resolution. She decided not to involve her former supervisor in the matter at this time. For this particular issue, Amber felt she could resolve it without consulting others.

[++]*Note:* In consulting with others about the situation, you must do so with discretion and complete confidentiality. This is particularly true when the conflict involves a client. Federal law prohibits you from discussing any personal information about your client with anyone other than the SLP responsible for that client's care and those specifically authorized (typically in writing). When consulting, use only generic descriptions, without any names or personal information specifically identifying the individuals involved. Have this discussion in a private location where others cannot overhear your conversation.

STEP 3: ACTION IMPLEMENTATION[+++]

- What action did you implement?
  Amber expressed to her supervisor that assessment was not within her scope of responsibilities, and as such, she was not able to assess the client, as requested. She offered to assist in the assessment by preparing the materials. Amber also indicated that she would be willing to stay late to assist with other scheduling and clerical duties needed in preparation for the upcoming IEPs.

- What was the outcome of your action?
  Amber's supervisor assessed the client and, with the additional help that Amber provided, was able to meet all her obligations in terms of upcoming IEPs. Amber's professional approach and good interpersonal skills preserved their relationship and helped Amber feel confident in addressing conflict in the future ethically.

[+++]*Note:* The outcome of your action should resolve the ethical dilemma. If not, restart this process at Step 1 (gather/clarify facts) and proceed to Step 2 (action analysis) and Step 3 (action implementation) until an ethical resolution is achieved.

APPENDIX 3–C
ASHA Issues in Ethics: Confidentiality Statement (ASHA 2018)

members and certificate holders can benefit from additional analysis and instruction concerning a specific issue of ethical conduct. Issues in Ethics statements are intended to heighten sensitivity and increase awareness. They are illustrative of the *Code of Ethics* (2016) (hereinafter, the "Code") and are intended to promote thoughtful consideration of ethical issues. They may assist members and certificate holders in engaging in self-guided ethical decision making. These statements do not absolutely prohibit or require specified activity. The facts and circumstances surrounding a matter of concern will determine whether the activity is ethical.

ABOUT THIS DOCUMENT

Published 2018. This Issues in Ethics statement is a revision of *Confidentiality* (originally published in 2001, and revised in 2004 and 2013). It has been updated to make any references to the Code of Ethics consistent with the *Code of Ethics* (2016). The Board of Ethics reviews Issues in Ethics statements periodically to ensure that they meet the needs of the professions and are consistent with ASHA policies.

ISSUES IN ETHICS STATEMENTS: DEFINITION

From time to time, the Board of Ethics (hereinafter, the "Board") determines that

INTRODUCTION

Professional persons in health care delivery fields (including those working in the public schools) have legal and ethical responsibilities to safeguard the confidentiality of information regarding the clients in their care. Scholars and those involved in human research have legal and ethical obligations to protect the privacy of persons who agree to participate in clinical studies and other research projects. Children and adults who are legally incompetent have the same right to privacy enjoyed by adults who are competent, although their rights will be mediated by a designated family member or a legal guardian.

There are federal statutes binding on all ASHA members who treat clients or patients, whether they work in health care facilities (where the Health Insurance Portability and Accountability Act [HIPAA] privacy and security rules apply), schools (which operate under the Family Educational Rights and Privacy Act [FERPA] as well as HIPAA), or private practice. There are also stringent federal statutes governing the treatment of human subjects in medical and other forms of scientific research. Individual states also have statutes governing the confidentiality of patient and client information, the protection of data gathered in research, and the privacy of students. It is the responsibility of all members of the audiology and speech-language pathology professions to know these laws and to honor them. Because state laws may vary, professionals moving from one state to another should take special care to familiarize themselves with the legal requirements of the new place of practice or residence. Educational institutions preparing professionals in the Communication Sciences and Disorders (CSD) discipline should give significant attention to informing all those entering the discipline about these legal requirements and should model good practice in their handling of confidential information concerning the students enrolled in their programs. Owners of businesses and managers of facilities should regularly review these legal requirements with the professionals and the staff whom they employ.

Institutions and facilities within which professionals see clients or pursue research may have their own policies concerning safeguarding privacy and maintaining confidential records. It is incumbent on the professionals in such settings to familiarize themselves with such workplace policies and regulations and to perform their work in conformity with these requirements. Owners and managers should make sure that such policies are readily available to their employees. Workplace training is desirable, and periodic reviews are recommended.

The Code identifies the confidentiality of information pertaining to clients, patients, students, and research subjects as a matter of ethical obligation, not just as a matter of legal or workplace requirements. Respect for privacy is implicitly addressed in *Principle of Ethics I* because to hold paramount the welfare of persons served is to honor and respect their privacy and the confidential nature of the information with which they entrust members of the professions. This broad, general obligation is further specified in both *Rule O* and *Rule P.*

Principle I, Rule O: Individuals shall protect the confidentiality and security of records of professional services provided, research and scholarly activities conducted, and products dispensed. Access to these records shall be allowed only when doing so is necessary to protect the welfare of the person or of the community, is legally authorized, or is otherwise required by law.

Principle I, Rule P: Individuals shall protect the confidentiality of any professional or personal information about persons served professionally or participants involved in research and scholarly activities and may disclose confidential information only when doing so is necessary to protect the welfare of the person or of the community, is legally authorized, or is otherwise required by law.

If there is variation among the different sources of rules on privacy, the professional should follow the most restrictive rule; for example, if the law seems to allow an action that the Code seems to prohibit, follow the Code. If there is conflict between sources, do what the law requires; for example, if workplace policies conflict on some point with legal requirements for confidential handling of records, the law takes precedence.

CONFIDENTIALITY ISSUES IN RESEARCH

Discussion

Attention to the protection of privacy begins with the planning of a research project, is crucial to the way research on human subjects is conducted, and extends through the review of research results (on both human and animal subjects) for publication and the sharing of data sets. Everyone involved—researchers, human subjects, support personnel, editors, reviewers, and data managers—should be aware of the ethical and legal requirements regarding privacy and should not compromise confidentiality for any reason.

Institutional review boards must be consulted about any research involving human subjects, and informed consent forms must be obtained and honored. Human subjects have a right to expect that their personal information will not be divulged when the results of a study are published or when data sets from a research project are shared with other investigators. Protecting the privacy of research subjects is an obligation for all those who are involved in the research.

Guidance

Data and the personal identities of individual participants in research studies must be kept confidential. There should be careful supervision of staff to make sure that they, too, are adhering to best practices in protecting the confidentiality of all participant data. Some reasonable precautions that should be taken to protect and respect participants' confidentiality include

- disseminating research findings without disclosing personal identifying information;
- storing research records securely and limiting access (i.e., records may be accessed only by authorized personnel);
- removing, disguising, or coding personal identifying information; and
- obtaining written informed consent from the participant (or, in the case of a child, the parent or guardian) to disseminate findings that include photographic/video images or audio voice recordings that might reveal personal identifying information.

Because legal requirements in this area are very strict and because institutions monitor research on human subjects carefully, professionals should seek further guidance directly from the appropriate personnel in their home institutions.

During the peer review of submitted manuscripts, all findings, information, and graphics in the manuscripts must be treated as highly confidential, and reviewers and editors alike have an obligation to protect findings from any form of premature disclosure. In a blind-review process, researchers' identities must be protected. In a double-blind review process, the anonymity of authors and reviewers alike must be scrupulously preserved. Editors and reviewers should make no prepublication use of information that they learn from submitted manuscripts.

CONFIDENTIALITY OF CLIENT INFORMATION

Discussion

Clients must be assured that all aspects of their communication with an audiologist or speech-language pathologist regarding themselves or their family members will be held in the strictest confidence. Clients who cannot trust professionals to treat information as confidential may withhold information that is important to assessment and treatment. When professionals disregard the privacy of their clients, the clients are injured in obvious and/or subtle ways. Evaluations, treatment plans and therapy, discussions with the client or the client's relatives, consultations with the family or with other professionals, treatment records, and payment negotiations should all be treated as confidential. All persons who come into possession of client information are equally bound by this requirement. Therapists, supervisors, assistants, and support staff in schools, facilities, and firms overseeing billing services are all prohibited from revealing client information to unauthorized third parties. ASHA members have a responsibility not only for monitoring their own conversations, securing records, and sharing client information, but also for ensuring that supervisees and support staff are adhering to ethical requirements regarding privacy. ASHA members who oversee facilities delivering services should have in place policies and sanctions regarding violations of confidentiality by their employees or by students working under supervision.

Guidance With Respect to Verbal Communication

In the case of a competent adult, no one other than the client herself or himself has the right to authorize the release of information. In the case of a child, only the parent of record or guardian ad litem has this right. It should be noted that there will be cases (e.g., in custody disputes or under custody agreements) in which a biological or adoptive parent has neither the right to know client information nor the right to authorize disclosures. In the case of an incompetent adult, only the designated family member(s) or legal guardian has the right to authorize disclosure. Good practice suggests the following:

- In all treatment situations, a written form specifying disclosure of information should be provided to, and signed by, the client or client representative at the beginning of treatment.
- Every client record should contain a clear, specific, up-to-date, and easily located statement indicating who has the right of access to client information and who may authorize the release of such information to other parties.

For any release of information other than that specified in the preliminary privacy agreement or as required by law (e.g., a subpoena), audiologists and speech-language pathologists must obtain a release-of-information agreement from clients or their designated representatives. This includes obtaining permission to share information with another professional. It is prudent to obtain this permission in writing rather than rely on verbal assent.

In rare cases, courts or administrative bodies with subpoena power may legitimately require the disclosure of confidential information. When a court serves an organization or individual with a subpoena requiring records or other information as evidence in a legal proceeding, typically the professional complies with the request; however, it is often prudent for professionals to seek legal advice in such situations.

Professionals are prohibited from discussing clients in public places—such as elevators, cafeterias, staff lounges, restrooms, or clinical/business sites— with others, specifically including the practitioner's family members and friends. Practitioners sometimes think that if they do not use the client's name such discussions are acceptable, but this is not true. Any description of, or comment about, a client who is being served constitutes disclosure of confidential information.

The same restrictions that apply to face-to-face conversation also apply to digital and electronic forms of communication with professionals, colleagues, and friends.

Guidance With Respect to Written Records

Written records have a durability and reproducibility distinct from spoken information; therefore, additional concerns about the protection and handling of paper files or computerized records. These concerns and challenges have become more complex and intense as a result of the digitizing of information. Breaches of confidentiality can occur as a result of the way records are created, stored, or transmitted.

Ordinarily, professionals should not create, update, or store records on their personal electronic devices (e.g., computers, cell phones, and flash drives) or on personal online accounts. If a workplace is aware of and allows such off-site handling of records, then privacy safeguards, such as password protection and anonymized client identifications, should be meticulously observed. Records on portable devices should not be opened and read in public places such as coffee shops or on public transportation.

All therapists who practice independently and all businesses should have clear written policies concerning client records. Workplace policies concerning records management should typically address

- record accuracy and content;
- record storage, both electronic and paper;
- ownership of records;
- record access—both with respect to personnel who may read and manipulate the record and with respect to rights of access by clients;
- record review and retention and related statutes of limitation;
- transfer of information, including transfer by electronic means;
- procedures for handling requests for information by someone other than the client or the client's representative;

- use of client records for research; and
- destruction of material removed from records.

These policies should be observed without variance. Failure to comply with the requirements designed to protect client records not only puts client welfare at risk but also makes the practitioner vulnerable to ethics complaints and legal action.

It is particularly important for professionals serving clients in institutions and facilities to be aware of who owns the record. Usually, in a medical setting, the medical facility owns the record. In a private practice, the individual who is legally responsible for the practice owns the record. In a school setting, the school district owns the record. A report prepared by an audiologist or a speech-language pathologist in the course of employment in a particular setting is not owned by that audiologist or speech-language pathologist, and he or she may not remove or copy such confidential records while employed, upon termination of employment, or if the practice closes.

It is important for the professional to be aware of what information is necessary and appropriate for inclusion in the client's legal record and to exercise professional judgment in making notations in the client's record.

Appropriate steps must be taken to ensure the confidentiality and protection of electronic and computerized client records and information. All information should be password protected, and only authorized persons should have access to the records and information. Computerized records should be backed up routinely, and there should be plans for protecting computer systems in case of emergencies.

STUDENT PRIVACY ISSUES

Discussion

Many academic programs prepare audiologists and speech-language pathologists for entry into the CSD discipline. At all levels of professional education, students and student clinicians have privacy rights that educators must respect. Many of these rights are specifically protected by federal law (e.g., FERPA), and there may also be relevant state statutes. But, once again, safeguarding the privacy of information entrusted to a teacher, program administrator, or institution is an ethical and not just a legal obligation. Professional regard for students and student clinicians involves respecting each student as the arbiter of what personal information may be divulged and to whom it may be divulged.

Guidance With Respect to Students in Classes

Most academic institutions have very specific policies regarding access to, storage of, and release of confidential student academic and disciplinary records. Academic institutions are less likely to have written policies concerning appropriate conversations and communications among educators with respect to the students at that institution. Students do, however, have a right to assume that the knowledge that the faculty have of their academic achievements and personal situations will not be widely or carelessly shared. Verbal and electronically mediated discussion of a student's performance should be carefully restricted to those directly responsible for the student's education.

Student performance and personal disclosures should not be discussed in public places, such as elevators, hallways, cafeterias, coffee shops, restrooms, or campus transportation vehicles. Graded student work and records of student achievement must be carefully safeguarded; access to grades in electronic files stored on mobile devices should be password protected if the device is carried outside the faculty member's campus office. Sensitive personal information that a faculty member may possess should not be shared at all in the absence of a clear and compelling need to know on the part of the person making inquiries.

Guidance With Respect to Student Clinicians

Maintaining the confidentiality of information is a complex challenge in the case of student clinicians. Those who supervise student clinicians must ensure the privacy of client and student clinical records and should model high regard for client privacy and best practices in recording, securing, and storing client records. Supervisors and mentors must treat the performance, records, and evaluations of student clinicians as confidential.

Supervisors of student clinicians must be familiar with the rules for viewing and sharing client information in a teaching setting. For example, a student supervisor's discussion of a patient record for the purposes of education in a university clinic is not a violation of confidentiality, but a student's discussion of the same patient with other students or friends would constitute a violation of confidentiality.

When student clinicians work with clients, persons unrelated to the client may request information about the client's communication problem. Requests might come from an off-site clinic supervisor, clinical fellowship mentor, or a professional who supervises student teachers. Patient or client information cannot be disclosed without a signed release.

CONFIDENTIALITY IN RELATION TO PEERS AND COLLEAGUES

Discussion

Issues of confidentiality also arise for ASHA members and certificate holders in their relationships with colleagues as a result of information that they obtain as they serve in roles such as site visitor, consultant, supervisor, administrator, or reviewer of documents such as manuscripts, grant proposals, and fellowship applications. All of these roles allow access to peer information of a personal and confidential nature. These activities are covered broadly under *Principle of Ethics IV*, which states, "Individuals shall uphold the dignity and autonomy of the professions, maintain collaborative and harmonious interprofessional and intraprofessional relationships, and accept the professions' self-imposed standards."

Guidance

Information about colleagues and professional peers that is gathered or revealed in the course of evaluations, assessments, or reviews should be treated with the same care and respect that are appropriate to information about clients and research subjects.

When a colleague shares sensitive information or when one participates in committees or other groups that discuss sensitive or controversial matters, participants should clarify in a candid conversation what level of confidentiality is expected and scrupulously maintain the desired level. Records of such conversations should be appropriately secured with agreement as to their storage and disposal.

Matters that may result in disciplinary action by some body, board, or institution deserve special comment. Individuals reporting or responding to alleged violations of codes of ethics or professional codes of conduct are also dealing with confidential matters and acting in a confidential relationship with the adjudicating body. It would be prudent to consider all aspects of a matter confidential until a final decision is rendered. Once a final determination has been reached, it is important for the adjudicating body to clarify what information can now be shared and what information must remain confidential.

Adjudicating bodies themselves typically follow rules of confidentiality (some dictated by law and regulation, some dic-

tated by the organization's internal governance policies and procedures) while the case is under consideration.

With respect to disclosure of decisions by adjudicating bodies, individuals need to inform themselves of pertinent laws and organizational policies. It would not be prudent simply to assume that the outcome can in all cases be made public. Even when the outcome can be made public, it is often the case that earlier filings, testimony, and deliberations must be maintained in confidence.

ASHA members who either place a complaint before the Board or find themselves responding to such a complaint have specific responsibilities to preserve the confidentiality of all materials relevant to the adjudication of complaints. *Principle of Ethics IV, Rule P,* is specific about this ethical obligation and states, "Individuals making and responding to complaints shall comply fully with the policies of the Board of Ethics in its consideration, adjudication, and resolution of complaints of alleged violations of the Code of Ethics."

Source: American Speech-Language-Hearing Association. (2018). *Issues of Ethics: Confidentiality.* Available from http://www.asha.org/policy. Copyright 2018 American Speech-Language-Hearing Association. All rights reserved. Reprinted with permission.

*Note: The ASHA ethical principles referenced in particular are those of the ASHA Code of Ethics for 2013. ASHA revised this code in 2016. This revised version of ASHA's Code of Ethics (ASHA, 2016) is available in Appendix 3–A of this chapter.

APPENDIX 3–D
SLPA Ethical Dilemma Scenarios

Scenario 1: You are a newly hired SLPA in a public school setting. This is your first SLPA position and your first job in a public school. Your supervisor trained you for approximately 1 week, consisting of showing you paperwork and having you observe her providing services to students. She then became seriously ill and has taken an extended medical leave. The district supervisor has asked you to work until they can find a replacement supervisor for you, including providing treatment services to the students on the supervisor's caseload.

Scenario 2: You are an SLPA in a public school setting and attending graduate school for your master's degree in SLP. You have been employed as an SLPA for approximately 6 months under the supervision of an SLP. There is an opening for an SLP position at another school site, and the district supervisor tells you they would like to hire you for this position. She says that they will request a "waiver" for you to work in this position as an SLP, but in the meantime, she indicates that they need you to begin working in this position immediately, so until the paperwork is official, you will need to perform evaluation and treatment at the new school setting.

Scenario 3: You are an SLPA working in a medical setting that bills Medicare for services provided to patients. Your supervisor has trained you to work with individuals in this setting and you feel relatively competent in doing so, under her supervision. One day she mentions to you that SLPA services are not "billable" under Medicare, but she states that this setting allows you to provide services, as long as the paperwork indicates that the SLP provided the services. As such, your supervisor tells you not to document your services in official records but to let her know the status of the treatment sessions and she will enter that information into the system for you.

Scenario 4: You are an SLPA working in a private practice. Your supervisor has trained you to work with individuals in this setting and you feel competent doing so under her supervision. You are assigned a new client to work on treatment goals addressing memory and attention. When you read the client's chart, you see that she is HIV positive. You are pregnant and concerned that you will contract HIV/AIDS, so you tell your supervisor that you do not feel comfortable working with this client.

Scenario 5: You are an SLPA working in a public school setting. You have been working in this setting for 3 months. Thus far, you have received excellent training. You have a close relationship with one particular student and her family. The student's mother does not get along with your supervising SLP. As a result, the student's mom approaches you one afternoon and asks to speak with you about her child's goals, progress, and future recommendations for the student. She tells you that you "know her child best," and as such, she wants to know your opinion, not your supervisor's opinion, on the topic.

CHAPTER 4

Professional Conduct

Learn from yesterday, live for today, hope for tomorrow.
The important thing is not to stop questioning.

—Albert Einstein (renowned physicist)

Being employed as a speech-language pathology assistant (SLPA) means that you enter into a professional community in which you are expected to conform to community-accepted standards for professional conduct. Although your training provides you with the technical skills and competencies needed to perform your SLPA duties, there are still "soft skills" required to interface successfully within the professional community and to establish your credibility as an SLPA (American Speech-Language-Hearing Association [ASHA], n.d., paragraph 2). ASHA (n.d.) recommends five tips to establish your credibility as an SLPA, including the following:

1. Maintain a positive and pleasant attitude.
2. Project a professional image.
3. Convey a willingness to learn new things.
4. Demonstrate initiative.
5. Exhibit a sense of organization.

Broken down further, many of these skills have behaviors that fall under the categories of appearance, communication (verbal and written), self-assessment, and conflict resolution. Although you remain an individual with unique characteristics and contributions, as in any setting, there will be expectations of you for each of behavioral categories. Actively seeking to improve your skills in these areas will enhance your effectiveness, project professionalism, and increase your credibility as an SLPA. The sections that follow provide additional detail areas about each behavioral category.

APPEARANCE

Your appearance is one example of your ability to establish credibility (ASHA, n.d.; Piasecki, 2003). This does not mean that all SLPAs in all environments dress and look alike, but it does mean you should have a professional appearance. This includes wearing clean, neat, and suitable clothing (ASHA, n.d.; Piasecki, 2003). Wearing clothing that is clean and neat are minimal requirements in any setting, but SLPAs often ask, "What is 'suitable' clothing?" For example, some questions you might ask are whether you must wear a suit and tie, whether jeans are acceptable, whether you can wear jewelry, is perfume appropriate? What is suitable clothing varies across clinical settings, but generally, if you adhere to the following principles, you will be able to project a professional image and meet the appearance standards of your particular setting:

1. *Check the written professional attire policies in your setting.* Many settings have specific rules and regulations that require you to dress a certain way. Make sure you familiarize yourself with these rules and follow them in selecting suitable attire. In some cases you may need to wear setting-specific attire (Piasecki, 2003). For example, in medical settings you may be asked to wear a uniform, such as a lab coat or scrubs.

2. *Fit your clothing to your duties.* Think about what you will be expected to do and what physical positions that might entail. SLPAs may be in a variety of different positions throughout their day, from being seated behind a desk or table, to sitting and playing on the floor with young children, to working in playgroups or other community environments (e.g., grocery stores, parks, libraries), to walking on hospital floors, and many other possible positions. Match your clothing to the physical tasks you will be asked to perform. Consider safety and comfort in your decision. Generally, closed-toe and low-heeled shoes allow for the greatest safety in a variety of settings. Clothing that allows you to move freely in a variety of positions also optimizes safety.

3. *Blend into your environment and do not be a distraction.* Use those in your environment who are respected professionals as a general guideline. Look to your superiors for examples of what is expected. Importantly, do not wear clothing or accessories that will be distracting or draw attention to you. Remember that as an SLPA, you interact with a variety of individuals. Your attire should not be a distraction to your clients or others in your work environment. The emphasis should be on what you do and not what you are wearing.

4. *Be conservative.* This aligns with not being a distraction (above), but also pertains to revealing and tight-fitting clothing. Cultural norms for what is acceptable vary (Piasecki, 2003). In all settings, you should err on the side of being more conservative, which usually translates to wearing clothing that reveals less skin and not wearing clothing that is excessively tight or form fitting.

In addition to attire, you should consider personal hygiene practices. Good personal hygiene is a minimum requirement (Piasecki, 2003), but consider carefully which personal hygiene products you might use. Because SLPAs work with a variety of individuals, you should limit the use of heavily scented personal products, such as perfumes, scented sprays, and body lotions. Some clients may be sensitive to these products or may have adverse medical reactions to them (Piasecki, 2003). Similarly, some clients may be sensitive to the scent of smoke (Piasecki, 2003). If you smoke, you should take steps to ensure no odor is present when you perform your duties as an SLPA.

You should also consider body jewelry (e.g., nose, brow, or lip rings) and exposed tattoos carefully. In some settings they are acceptable, while in others they may be a source of distraction and detract from the performance of your duties. Generally, it is best to minimize or conceal tattoos and body jewelry (Piasecki, 2003).

Lastly, some employers may require you to wear a name tag or ID badge denoting your position and any other relevant employment information (e.g., your department; Piasecki, 2003). ASHA recommends that SLPAs identify themselves verbally, in writing or with titles on name badges (ASHA, 2013). Some state licensure standards for SLPAs have specific regulations about nametags and identifying yourself as an SLPA. Check with your supervisor about how to obtain an identification badge that meets those standards and make sure that you wear it visibly when you are performing your duties.

As with all aspects of your conduct, if you are unsure about what are the acceptable guidelines for appearance in your setting, contact your supervisor for suggestions and guidance.

COMMUNICATION

Verbal Communication

As professionals who specialize in speech and language, SLPAs are expected to communicate with a high level of proficiency. Verbal communication will be the cornerstone of your daily interactions with clients and coworkers in most settings (McNamara, 2007). Defining "professional" communication is not an easy task because the form and content of communication vary given the topic, communication partner(s), and setting (van Servellen, 1997). Generally however, there are a few principles that guide communication in professional settings. First and foremost, remember that communication in employment settings is typically more formal, both in form and content, than in daily interactions, for example, with family and friends outside of work settings. A few tips to remember to enhance the effectiveness of your verbal communication and maintain the required level of formality are as follows:

1. Address individuals according to your environment. When working with adult clients, it is generally acceptable

to address them as Mr., Mrs., Miss, Dr., and so on depending on their life role or title (Piasecki, 2003). With any age individual, client, or coworker, avoid pejorative terms such as sweetie, honey, and so forth (Piasecki, 2003). If you are unclear how someone prefers to be addressed, it is appropriate and courteous to ask him or her.

2. Speak clearly and at a rate appropriate for your communication partner(s). Match vocal loudness to the tone of the conversation (e.g., softer for personal, sensitive, or private matters; van Servellen, 1997).

3. Avoid using slang and profanity in work settings.

4. Be a good listener. Use active listening strategies, such as not interrupting people when they are speaking (van Servellen, 1997). Comment (as appropriate) on what speakers are saying to let them know that you understand and are paying attention to what they have to say.

5. Be mindful of your nonverbal communication and body language. Use welcoming body language, which includes smiling (as appropriate), maintaining good eye contact, not fidgeting when you are speaking or being spoken to, holding your arms and legs in an uncrossed position, and maintaining an appropriate distance in terms of personal space (Piasecki, 2003; van Servellen, 1997).

6. Be culturally sensitivity to differences in communication styles (van Servellen, 1997). Chapter 5 provides additional information about appropriate and effective communication.

In the context of service provision, effective verbal communication is critical (van Servellen, 1997). . When working with clients and their families, be especially careful to reduce *jargon* usage in your verbal communication. Jargon refers to the technical terms used by a group of professionals. Avoiding jargon increases comprehension in communication with the individuals you serve and will ensure that you do not intimidate or offend the individuals you interact with by using words they do not have in common with you.

As an SLPA, service provision requires that you can comprehend specific aspects of spoken language and, in some cases, produce an accurate model of these structures. In terms of accents and nonstandard dialects used by speech-language pathology professionals, ASHA (1998) states that "there is no research to support the belief that audiologists and speech-language pathologists who speak a nonstandard dialect or who speak with an accent are unable to make appropriate diagnostic decisions or achieve appropriate treatment outcomes" (para. 8). Rather, ASHA says that if a professional speaks a nonstandard dialect or speaks with an accent, it will *not* affect treatment if the individual has the required level of knowledge about normal and disordered communication and the expected level of clinical case management skills. If modeling is necessary, the professional can model the target phoneme, grammatical feature, or other aspect of speech and language that targets the client's particular problem. If any of these factors affect your clinical services, speak with your supervisor about remediating these skills so that you can provide effective treatment.

Written Communication

Written communication is also an integral part of your daily interactions in the field of speech-language pathology (Goldfarb & Serpanos, 2009). Similar to the high expectations for verbal communication, as a professional specializing in speech and language SLPAs are expected to be proficient in their written communication skills. These skills develop with time and training but you should be vigilant in developing and enhancing them. Note that writing, as discussed in Chapter 9, is one of the primary modes of communication used by SLPAs. Chapter 9 contains helpful tips for ensuring accuracy of your written clinical notes. SLPAs may be required to write other documents as well. An important practice in ensuring excellent written communication is to proof your work, proof your work, and proof your work again. An advantage of written communication in that it is tangible and can be carefully reviewed and rewritten to achieve a high level of performance. This of course, means that you must plan in advance and allow time for careful proofing. Below are suggestions to help you have effective and professional written communication.

1. *Proof your written language carefully to ensure it is free of errors in grammar and spelling.* Using spell check and grammar check is a minimum step in proofing your written work, but realize that there is no substitute for careful review of any written documents you generate, for any purpose. If you are working in an electronic format, printing a hard copy version to proof may help you catch errors. Reading your written work aloud may also increase the accuracy of your proofing skills.

2. *Use formality in your written communication.* Generally, brief but complete sentences are required in most forms of written communication. Avoid using slang, colloquialisms (e.g., he is *gonna* need, the clinician tried to *get across* the idea), and clichés (e.g., using *tried-and-true* methods, not the client's *cup of tea*; Hegde, 1998). In formal documents, spell out contractions (e.g., *haven't* should be written as *have not, can't* as *cannot*; Hegde, 1998).

3. *Ensure your written content is comprehensible to readers unfamiliar with your field.* Do not assume that readers of your written documents know what you know or share a similar background on a given topic. When you proof your written work, view it from the perspective of a new person reading new information. Does what you wrote make sense and have sufficient detail for a new person reading new information to understand it? If the answer is no, rewrite your document to ensure the content is understandable to an readers.

4. *Use standard forms of medical abbreviations and phonetic notation.* If you do not know the standard abbreviation for a word, spell out the entire word. Appendix 4–A contains a list of common medical abbreviations. Many online sources are also available to search for standard medical abbreviations. Appendix 4–B contains a list of common International Phonetic Alphabet (IPA) symbols. More information about IPA symbols and their use is available in Chapter 13. Many word processors contain font libraries with IPA symbols and you can also access digital IPA symbols through online keyboards, such as http://ipa.typeit.org/

5. *Learn from your mistakes.* You will receive feedback from your supervisor about the content and form of your written communication. You should

save all comments and suggestions and incorporate these recommendations into all future documents. An excellent way to improve your writing is to make a list of the errors you have made and refer to that list when you proof new documents. Similarly, you can use lists of commonly misused (Appendix 4–C) and misspelled words (Appendix 4–D), textbooks, and online sources for common grammatical errors to help refine your writing skills over time.

One area that requires additional attention is electronic forms of written communication, including e-mails and social networking tools, such as Facebook, Twitter, and so on. As Chapter 3 discussed, all professional communication about the clients you serve is to be held in complete confidence. Appendix 3–C in Chapter 3 states ASHA's position on confidentiality. It is critical that you only communicate electronically to or about a client as specifically instructed by your supervisor. Many settings have specific rules and regulations about what type of written information can be sent electronically and how this information is to be transmitted. You should not use personal e-mail accounts for this purpose, nor should you ever post anything about your clients on social networking sites. Remember too, that social networking tools, such as Facebook and Twitter, often serve as a source of information about you to those you interact with professionally, including your clients and their families, your coworkers, and current and prospective employers. Box 4–1 contains helpful tips regarding social media etiquette.

Box 4–1. Social Media Etiquette

- *Pick a professional screen name.*
- *Create a professional profile and maintain a separate personal profile.* Keep your professional contacts separate from your personal contacts, and "do not send winks, pokes, virtual martinis, or invitations to your business contacts" (Ritch & McGary, n.d., para. 3).
- *Be careful with what you post online in any form.* Only post information that will portray you in a positive light to all who view it, including your supervisors, employers, and your clients and their families. Be sure to use privacy settings to limit who can view your personal information, but remember this is not an absolute fail-safe for keeping unflattering information private. The best course of action is to use restraint in posting anything online.
- *Be respectful in all online communication.* In other words, "acknowledge people when they ask a question, apologize if you offend someone, and never ever spam, flame, or trash someone else online" (Ritch & McGary, n.d., para. 3).

Disability–Sensitive Communication

Last, communication in all forms, whether verbal or written, must be sensitive to the needs and rights of people with disabilities. You should use *person-first language* when communicating with or referring to individuals with disabilities (Centers for Disease Control and Prevention, n.d.). This means referring to the person first and their disability second, such as the "person with aphasia" or "individuals with seizure disorders," not "the aphasic person" or "the epileptic." Similarly, you should not indicate that the person with a disability has suffered or is a victim in some way from their disability (Centers for Disease Control and Prevention, n.d.). This means not using phrases such as "the client suffers from a hearing loss," "the patient suffered a stroke," or "the client is afflicted with multiple sclerosis." Instead, you could say, "the client experienced a stroke," or "the patient has a diagnosis of multiple sclerosis." In addition, if you are referring to someone *without* a disability, do not refer to that person(s) as "normal" (Centers for Disease Control and Prevention, n.d.); it implies that the individual with a disability is not normal. Instead, state that the individual(s) is without a specific disability, such as "individuals without aphasia," "individuals without visual impairments," and so on.

Using the correct terminology to refer to a disability is also important. According to the World Health Organization (WHO, 2012), *disability* "is an umbrella term, covering impairments, activity limitations, and participation restrictions" (para. 2). Impairment is a problem in body function or structure, whereas an activity limitation is the difficulty an individual encounters in executing a task or action because of a specific impairment(s). Participation restriction refers to a problem experienced in life situations due to an impairment and activity limitation. Using these classifications, the WHO accounts for the role that personal and environmental factors (not just a person's impairment) play in participation restriction. Importantly, the WHO emphasizes that disability is a universal human experience, in that all human beings can experience a decrement in health and thereby some degree of disability.

In addition, as an SLPA, you need to be able to effectively communicate with individuals with a variety of disabilities. In doing so, it is critical that you view all individuals as unique in their needs, desires, and preferred methods of communication. For example, core principles in communicating with individuals with disabilities include the following (North Dakota Center for Persons with Disabilities, n.d., p. 7):

1. Communicate directly with the person with a disability (versus ignoring the person and communicating instead with their caregiver or interpreter).
2. Offer to shake hands, even if the individual has limited hand movement.
3. Identify yourself when greeting someone who is visually impaired.
4. Wait until the assistance you offer is accepted before acting on behalf of an individual with a disability.
5. Treat adults with disabilities as adults.
6. Protect the personal space of individuals with a disability, including not leaning on their wheelchair or touching a service animal without permission.
7. Listen carefully and wait for an individual with a communication disability to finish speaking before you speak.

8. Position yourself at eye level when speaking with someone in a wheelchair

9. Get the attention of people with a hearing disability by tapping on their shoulder or waving your hand

Remember to relax when communicating with someone with a disability. Each time you meet someone with a disability, as with any person you meet, view it as an opportunity to get to know that person and to find out firsthand his or her preferred methods of communication.

SELF-ASSESSMENT AND SELF-IMPROVEMENT

Self-assessment, or self-evaluation as it is sometimes called, is the process of evaluating your own skills and abilities and then, importantly, seeking avenues for improvement (Moon-Meyer, 2004). This is critical to becoming a highly skilled SLPA and is also part of professional conduct. SLPAs who seek self-improvement through self-assessment act in the best interest of their clients by ensuring the highest quality of care. As discussed in Chapter 3, this is the cornerstone of ASHA's Ethical Principle 1 (Responsibility to Clients Served and Research Participants). SLPAs who engage in self-assessment and self-improvement will continue to grow in their skills over time and thereby reach high levels of proficiency. The evaluations of others, especially your supervisor, will be important in shaping this proficiency, but SLPAs who rely solely on others in their environment to improve their performance will ultimately be limited in their professional growth. Self-assessment and self-improvement can

include any aspect of your performance as an SLPA, including your clinical skills and those skills outside the clinical realm, such as your interpersonal, written and verbal communication, and conflict resolution skills.

The first step in self-improvement is self-assessment. This requires that you carefully observe and reflect on your behaviors. If you are open to the fact that no one is perfect, observation and reflection about your own behaviors will usually reveal potential areas for improvement. Using audio or video recordings can be helpful in evaluating your own behaviors during clinical sessions (Moon-Meyer, 2004). Reflection and taking notes on a task immediately after completion can also be used. Remember, though, that if you are writing notes about what you do as an SLPA, as discussed in Chapter 3, you must do so in a way that protects the confidentiality of your clients. This generally means not recording any identifying information about clients in these written notes and using pseudonyms if you directly reference a client in your written notes. Largely, your notes in the area of self-assessment should be about you, but in some cases, a confidential reference to a clinical interaction may be used to set the context for your narrative. Similarly, if you are recording a clinical session (audio or video), be sure to follow the policies in your setting for doing so, such as requesting permission, using required formats, and protecting the recordings as confidential information.

Individuals new to the process of self-assessment often struggle with what exactly to observe about their own performance or where to begin in the self-assessment process. ASHA forms are available for use as a starting point in the self-evaluation of intervention sessions (see Appendix 4–E and 4–F). Remember, though, that you can self-assess in any area of performance, not just service delivery.

In addition to rating yourself using pre-determined categories and self-rating scales, another good way to focus your self-assessment is to observe and write down aspects of a task you performed that were (a) successful and (b) not successful (Crago, 1987). Once you do this, the next step is to identify what about your own behaviors and actions may have contributed to an area of success, an area of difficulty, or both. This is particularly applicable to clinical sessions but can be applied to any aspect of your professional duties as an SLPA. The topics discussed in Chapter 10 are an excellent starting point for areas to assess in the clinical realm.

A reflection journal can be used to record information about your successful and unsuccessful performance, as well as your own contributions to these outcomes. It can then be extended to reflect on how to improve or change your own behaviors for a more successful outcome, as well as a place to record goals and progress in accomplishing self-improvement. Box 4–2 contains an example of an entry in a reflection journal. The companion website of this text contains a blank form for this.

In many ways, an entry in a reflection journal is similar to a note an SLPA may write about a client's performance. They both describe subjective and objective details about a given task or interaction but an important distinction is that reflection journals focus on your own performance. There is often crossover, however, between discussion of the client's performance and discussion of your own performance. For example, the notes that SLPAs write about a client often include a section devoted to future plans from the SLPA's perspective. As such, observing and recording your own behaviors may help you generate ideas of things to modify in future sessions with a client. This concept is discussed in greater detail in Chapter 9.

Once you have reflected on areas to improve, do not stop there. Set a goal for improvement and continue to monitor your performance, making adjustments until you achieve the desired outcome. Dating your reflection journal entries allows you to track overall patterns and change over time. You might also consider developing your own data collection methods for tracking specific behaviors over time. Chapter 9 discusses data collection methods for tracking client behaviors. Employing similar methods for your own performance is an excellent way to document progress and to improve over time. In addition, if there are more overarching goals that emerge from your self-reflection, such as additional education, training in a specific area, or both, write down these goals and work with your supervising speech-language pathologist (SLP) and/or mentor in developing a plan for improvement in these areas. Lastly, some additional ideas in the areas of self-assessment and self-improvement include the following:

- Review setting-specific methods used to evaluate yourself (Dowling, 2001). Generally, there will be a set of standards by which you are evaluated for employment purposes, in many cases including a list of clinically related skills you are expected to perform. Chapter 1 contains several examples of SLPA performance measures.

Box 4–2. Sample Reflection Journal Entry

Date: *2/14/2018*
Task(s): *10:00 a.m. Small Group Session (JL, AS, TM)*

Successes:
JL and AS participated fully and had high levels of accuracy for target sounds. The session ended on time. The students appeared to enjoy the session and were eager to begin. I felt relaxed and was able to stay focused on each student's targets during the session.

Difficulties:
TM was distracted during the session. He left the table several times to look out the window. I wasn't sure how to shape this behavior other than reminding him that he needed to participate. I had difficulty keeping track of errors and the number and type of cues I gave for sound production. When I listened to the audio recording of the session, I provided many more models than I had noted on my data sheet. I also said "okay" twice when JL's target sound was not correct. The time spent explaining the session's activities took too long (10 minutes). The students argued about which activity to do first and who would go first in each activity.

Areas (Ways) to Improve:
1. *Increase structure of the session at the onset. Make sure to briefly instruct the students in the rules of the activity. Don't allow them to choose the order of the activities. Rotate who goes first per session or have them draw from a deck of cards and whoever gets the highest card goes first.*
2. *Improve data collection methods. Get additional examples of data collection sheets used for group sessions. Check with supervisor about her methods for effectively and quickly noting both errors and cues in group settings. Possibly, rearrange the data collection sheet in advance with a column to place an X under each type of cue. Place a sticky note reminder on my data collection sheet for next time reminding me not to say "okay." Listen to the audio recording from next week's session to record the number of "okays."*
3. *Close the blinds in the room or move the table so the students aren't distracted by the things happening outside the window.*

Look to these evaluation tools for ideas of specific areas to target in self-assessment and self-improvement.

■ Observe experienced clinicians (Dowling, 2001). For SLPAs, this usually means your supervising SLP. It may also mean observing other professionals, such as teachers, occupational therapists, and psychologists, who engage in activities with clients in your setting that are applicable to what you do. It could also mean observing more experienced SLPAs. This can be done once you have identified an area to improve, as a source of additional techniques in this area or as a source of ideas for areas of self-assessment.

- Immerse yourself in the professional community of SLPs and related professionals. This means attending regional or national conferences and workshops in your clinical service area and participating in applicable training and workshops offered in your setting. This will provide you with state-of-the art information applicable to the field of speech-language pathology and related topics that may stimulate ideas for self-assessment or serve as a resource for self-improvement. In fact, as discussed in Chapter 1, one of ASHA's expectations is that SLPAs will "actively pursue continuing education and professional development activities" (ASHA, 2013, Expectations of an SLPA, para. 1). Some state regulating bodies also require formal or informal documentation regarding continuing education (CE) to maintain certification, licensure, or credentials as an SLPA.

As with any long-term goal, it is best to start small with a few attainable goals and work up from there. Similarly, do not attempt to reflect on every task you perform as an SLPA all at once. Start with tasks that are more structured or more in need of improvement and work up from there. Do not expect to achieve perfection overnight, or ever. The entire point of this process is to view self-improvement as a career-long goal, no matter your proficiency.

CONFLICT RESOLUTION

As an SLPA, no matter the setting, you will be required to work collaboratively with a variety of individuals, including your supervising SLP, as well as other SLPAs and SLPs in your specific setting. You will also collaborate with individuals from other disciplines. Table 4–1 contains a listing of some types of professions that SLPAs may work with across a variety of settings (Cascella, Purdy, & Dempsey, 2007).

Conflict occurs when individuals or groups disagree. Conflict is inevitable in any workplace setting (Victors, 2009). How conflicts are addressed will have a dramatic impact on their outcome (Culbertson, 2008). There are four possible outcomes of conflict, as listed in Figure 4–1. The most desirable outcome, when possible, is a win-win outcome for all involved. The best way to accomplish this outcome is to first set aside personal feelings and view the conflict objectively from the perspective of everyone involved.

Good interpersonal skills are also at the heart of positive conflict resolution (Gerrard, Boniface, & Love, 1980). Interpersonal skills are "those skills that promote good relationships between individuals" (p. 2). Several guiding principles to

Table 4–1. Professional Colleagues Across Settings

	Birth to 3 Years Settings	Educational Settings	Medical Settings
Audiologist	X	X	X
Chaplain			X
Childcare worker	X		
Dietician			X
Neuropsychologist			X
Nurse	X	X	X
Nurse's aide			X
Occupational therapist	X	X	X
Pediatric development specialist	X	X	
Physical therapist	X	X	X
Physician	X	X	X
Recreational therapist			X
Rehabilitation therapist			X
School counselor		X	
Social worker	X	X	X
Special education teacher	X	X	
Teacher (general education)	X	X	X

Source: Cascella, Purdy, and Dempsey, 2007, p. 263.

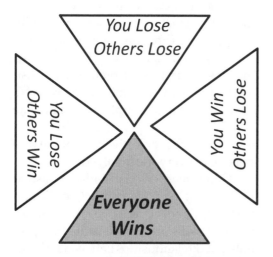

Figure 4–1. Possible outcomes of conflict.

resolving conflict effectively include the following:

1. *Employ active listening and good communication skills.* Communicate openly, clearly, and directly about the conflict to express your feelings, but do so in a way that respects the feelings of others. Using the communication tips discussed previously will help.
2. *When possible, seek resolutions to conflict that result in a positive outcome for all involved.* Let go of the need to be right or an attachment to a specific outcome (McCready, 2007). Place the

conflict in perspective. Do not trivialize or avoid conflict, but also do not make conflict out of trivial matters (Culbertson, 2008).

3. *Be sensitive to the feelings of others and be ready to move on and work collaboratively once a conflict has been resolved.* Do not make the conflict personal. From the outset, separate facts from feelings and opinions and avoid placing blame for conflict (McCready, 2007). At all stages, consider the feelings of everyone involved and do not hold a grudge (Hull, 2003). This means being willing to admit if you are wrong and apologizing and forgiving others who err or have done something wrong.

In addition, Chapter 3 addresses ethical dilemmas and offers suggestions for addressing ethical conflict. These strategies are helpful in problem solving and making decisions during any conflict, not just those that pose an ethical dilemma.

REFERENCES

American Speech-Language-Hearing Association. (n.d.). *Five tips to become a more credible assistant.* Retrieved from http://www.asha.org/associates/Five-Tips-to-Become-a-More-Credible-Assistant/

American Speech-Language-Hearing Association. (1998). *Students and professionals who speak English with accents and nonstandard dialects: Issues and recommendations* [Technical report]. Retrieved from http://www.asha.org/policy

American Speech-Language-Hearing Association. (2013). *Speech-language pathology assistant scope of practice.* Retrieved from http://www.asha.org/policy

Cascella, R., Purdy, M. H., & Dempsey, J. J. (2007). Clinical service delivery and work settings. In R. Paul & P. Cascella (Eds.), *Introduction to clinical methods in communication disorders* (pp. 259–302). Baltimore, MD: Paul H. Brookes.

Centers for Disease Control and Prevention. (n.d.). *Communicating with and about people with disabilities.* Retrieved from http://www.cdc.gov/ncbddd/disabilityandhealth/pdf/DisabilityPoster_Photos.pdf

Crago, M. (1987). Supervision and self-exploration. In M. Crago & M. Pickering (Eds.), *Supervision in human communication disorders: Perspective on a process* (pp. 137–167). San Diego, CA: Singular.

Culbertson, R. (2008). Conflict: Your role in how it ends. *Perspectives on Administration and Supervision, 18*(3), 99–104.

Dowling, S. (2001). *Supervision: Strategies for successful outcomes and productivity.* Needham Heights, MA: Allyn & Bacon.

Gerrard, B. A., Boniface, W. J., & Love, B. H. (1980). *Interpersonal skills for health professionals.* Reston, VA: Reston Publishing.

Goldfarb, R., & Serpanos, Y. C. (2009). *Professional writing in speech-language pathology and audiology.* San Diego, CA: Plural.

Hegde, M. N. (1998). *A coursebook on scientific and professional writing for speech-language pathologists.* San Diego, CA: Singular.

Hull, R. H. (2003). The art of interpersonal persuasion. *ASHA Leader.* Retrieved from http://www.asha.org/Publications/leader/2003/031007/031007f.htm

McCready, V. (2007). Supervision of speech-language pathology assistants: A reciprocal relationship. *ASHA Leader.* Retrieved from http://www.asha.org/Publications/leader/2007/070508/f070508b/

McNamara, K. (2007). Interviewing, counseling, and clinical communication. In R. Paul & P. Cascella (Eds.), *Introduction to clinical methods in communication disorders* (pp. 203–236). Baltimore, MD: Paul H. Brookes.

Moon-Meyer, S. (2004). *Survival guide for the beginning speech-language clinician.* Austin, TX: Pro-Ed.

North Dakota Center for Persons with Disabilities. (n.d.). *Communicating effectively with people who have a disability.* Retrieved from http://www.labor.state.ny.us/workforcenypartners/forms/communication.pdf

Piasecki, M. (2003). *Clinical communication handbook.* Malden, MA: Blackwell.

Ritch, S., & McGary, M. (n.d.). *Social media etiquette for professionals.* Retrieved from http://www.asha.org/associates/Social-Media-Etiquette-for-Professionals/

van Servellen, G. (1997). *Communication skills for health care professionals*. Gaithersburg, MD: Aspen.

Victor, S. (2009, November). *Supervision and conflict resolution*. Paper presented at ASHA 2009 Annual Convention, New Orleans, LA.

file:///C:/Users/000666547/Downloads/1030_Victor_Shelley.pdf

World Health Organization. (n.d.). *Health topics: Disabilities*. Retrieved from http://www.who.int/topics/disabilities/en/

APPENDIX 4–A
Common Medical Abbreviations (ASHA, n.d.)

Aa

ADL: activities of daily living

A&O: alert and oriented

A/P: anterior-posterior

AROM: active range of motion

ASAP: as soon as possible

Bb

b.i.d.: twice a day

BP: blood pressure

BR: bed rest

BS: breath sounds

B/S: bedside

Bx: biopsy

Cc

With: (c with bar above it)

CA: cardiac arrest

ca: carcinoma

CAD: coronary artery disease

CBC: complete blood count

CC: chief complaint

CHI: closed head injury

c/o: complains of

CPR: cardiopulmonary resuscitation

CT: computerized tomography

CV: cardiovascular

CVA: cerebral vascular accident

CXR: chest x-ray

Dd

d/c: discontinue

DC: discharge

DNK: do not know

DNT: did not test

DOB: date of birth

d/t: due to

Dx: diagnosis

Ee

EENT: eye, ear, nose, throat

ENT: ear, nose, throat

ETOH: ethanol (alcohol)

exam: examination

Ff

FH: family history

f/u: follow-up

Gg

GCS: Glasgow Coma Scale

GERD: gastroesophageal reflux disease

GSW: gunshot wound

Hh

H/A: headache

HBP: high blood pressure

HEENT: head, eyes, ear, nose, throat

H_2O: water

h/o: history of

H&P: history and physical

HR: heart rate

HTN: hypertension

Hx: history

Ii

ICCU: intensive coronary care unit

ICU: intensive care unit

imp.: impression

Ll

LBW: low birth rate

LE: lower extremities

LOC: loss of consciousness, level of consciousness

LOS: length of stay

LUE: left upper extremity

Mm

MBSS: modified barium swallow study

MCA: middle cerebral artery

MRI: magnetic resonance imaging

MVA: motor vehicle accident

Nn

NG: nasogastric

NICU: neonatal intensive care unit

NKA: no known allergies

NPO: nothing by mouth

Oo

O_2: oxygen

OM: otitis media

OME: otitis media with effusion

ot.: ear

Pp

PE: physical examination

Ped.: Pediatrics

PEG: percutaneous endoscopic gastrostomy

PET: positron emission tomography

PH: past history

PMH: past medical history

p.o.: by mouth

PRN: as often as necessary, as needed

Qq

Q: every

q.h.: every hour

q.i.d.: four times a day

Rr

rehab.: rehabilitation

RLA: Rancho Los Amigo Scale

R/O: rule out

ROM: range of motion

RUE: right upper extremity

Ss

SCI: spinal cord injury

SH: social history

SOAP: subjective, objective, assessment, and plan

SOB: shortness of breath

s/s: signs and symptoms

Tt

TB: tuberculosis

TBI: traumatic brain injury

TIA: transient ischemic attack

TKR: total knee replacement

Tx: treatment, traction

Uu

UCD: usual childhood diseases

UCHD: usual childhood diseases

Source: American Speech-Language-Hearing Association. (n.d.). *Common medical abbreviations.* Retrieved from http://www.asha.org/uploadedFiles/slp/healthcare/Medicalabbreviations. pdf#search=%22common%22

APPENDIX 4-B
Common International Phonetic Alphabet (IPA) Symbols

CONSONANTS:

IPA SYMBOL	EXAMPLE
/p/	Ha**pp**y
/m/	**M**other
/h/	**H**ello
/n/	**N**ever
/w/	**W**ednesday
/b/	**B**aseball
/k/	**K**ite
/g/	**G**olf
/d/	**D**eliver
/t/	**T**uesday
/ŋ/	Pi**n**k
/f/	**F**all
/j/	**Y**ellow
/r/	Ca**rr**ot
/l/	Ba**ll**oon
/s/	**S**aturday
/tʃ/	**Ch**urch
/ʃ/	**Sh**oe
/z/	**Z**oo
/dʒ/	**J**ewel
/v/	**V**olcano
/θ/	**Th**umb
/ð/	**Th**at
/ʒ/	Vi**s**ion

VOWELS:

IPA SYMBOL	EXAMPLE
/i/	S**ee**
/ɪ/	**I**nsect
/ʊ/	F**oo**t
/u/	B**oo**t
/e/	B**e**d
/ə/ Unstressed	**A**round
/ɜ/	T**u**rn
/ɔ/	L**aw**n
/æ/	**A**pple
/ʌ/ Stressed	h**u**t
/ɑ/	F**a**ther

R-COLORED VOWELS:

IPA SYMBOL	EXAMPLE
/ɝ/	H**er**
/ɚ/	Col**or**

DIPHTHONGS:

IPA SYMBOL	EXAMPLE
/eɪ/	Play
/eə/	Their
/əʊ/	Boat
/ɪə/	Here
/ɔɪ/	Coin
/ʊə/	Tour
/aɪ/	Sky
/aʊ/	House

Examples of Commonly Misused Words and Phrases

Effect ■ *a distinctive impression <the color gives the* effect *of being warm>* ■ *the creation of a desired impression <her tears were purely for* effect>* ■ *the conscious subjective aspect of an emotion considered apart from bodily change* **Affect** ■ *something that inevitably follows an antecedent (as a cause or agent)* ■ *an outward sign* ■ *a set of observable manifestations of a subjectively experienced emotion <patients . . . showed perfectly normal reactions and* affects>*	**Alternate** ■ *occurring or succeeding by turns <a day of* alternate *sunshine and rain>* ■ *arranged one above or alongside the other* ■ *every other: every second <he works on* alternate *days>* **Alternative** ■ *offering or expressing a choice <several* alternative *plans>* ■ *different from the usual or conventional <*alternative *lifestyle>*	**Incidence** ■ *rate of occurrence or influence <a high* incidence *of crime>* **Prevalence** ■ *the degree to which something is prevalent; especially: the percentage of a population that is affected by a particular disease at a given time*
Were ■ *past 2nd person singular, past plural, or past subjunctive of* BE **We're** ■ *we are* **Where** ■ *at, in, or to what place <*where *is the house> <*where *are we going>*	**Farther** ■ *at or to a greater distance or more advanced point <got no* farther *than the first page> <nothing could be* farther *from the truth>* ■ *to a greater degree or extent <see to it that I do not have to act any* farther *in the matter>* **Further** ■ *in addition:* MOREOVER ■ *to a greater degree or extent <*further *annoyed by a second intrusion> <my ponies are tired, and I have* further *to go>*	**Their** ■ *of or relating to them or themselves especially as possessors, agents, or objects of an action <*their *furniture> <*their *verses> <*their *being seen>* **They're** ■ *they are* **There** ■ *in or at that place <stand over* there>* ■ *to or into that place <went* there *after church>* ■ *at that point or stage <stop right* there *before you say something you'll regret>*

continues

Abduct ■ *to draw or spread away (as a limb or the fingers) from a position near or parallel to the median axis of the body or from the axis of a limb* **Adduct** ■ *to draw (as a limb) toward or past the median axis of the body* ■ *to bring together (similar parts)* <adduct *the fingers*>	**Elicit** ■ *to draw forth or bring out* <hypnotism elicited *his hidden fears*> ■ *to call forth or draw out (as information or a response)* <her remarks elicited *cheers*> **Evoke** ■ *to call forth or up:* <evoke *evil spirits*> ■ *to bring to mind or recollection* <this place evokes *memories*> ■ *to re-create imaginatively*	**Its** ■ *of or relating to it or itself, especially as possessor, agent, or object of an action* <going to its *kennel*> <a child proud of its *first drawings*> <its *final enactment into law*> **It's** ■ *it is*
Except ■ *with the exclusion or exception of* <daily except *Sundays*> **Accept** ■ *to receive willingly* <accept *a gift*> ■ *to be able or designed to take or hold (something applied or added)* <a surface that will not accept *ink*> ■ *to give admittance or approval to* <accept *her as one of the group*> ■ *to endure without protest or reaction* <accept *poor living conditions*> ■ *to recognize as true: BELIEVE* <refused to accept *the explanation*> ■ *to make a favorable response to* <accept *an offer*> ■ *to agree to undertake (a responsibility)* <accept *a job*> ■ *to assume an obligation to pay; also: to take in payment* <we don't accept *personal checks*>	**You're** ■ *you are* **Your** ■ *of or relating to you or yourself or yourselves, especially as possessor or possessors* <your *bodies*>, *agent or agents* <your *contributions*>, *or object of an action* <your *discharge*> ■ *of or relating to one or oneself* <when you face the north, east is at your *right*>	**Principal** ■ *most important, consequential, or influential: CHIEF* <the principal *ingredient*> <the region's principal *city*> *NOTE: This can also be a title, such as* <Mr. Thomas is Principal *of Thomas Jefferson Elementary School.*> **Principle** ■ *a comprehensive and fundamental law, doctrine, or assumption* ■ *a rule or code of conduct* ■ *habitual devotion to right principles* <a man of principle>

Personnel

- *a body of persons usually employed (as in a factory or organization)*
- *a division of an organization concerned with personnel*

Personal

- *of, relating to, or affecting a particular person: PRIVATE, INDIVIDUAL* <personal *ambition*> <personal *financial gain*>
- *done in person without the intervention of another; also: proceeding from a single person*
- *carried on between individuals directly* <*a* personal *interview*>
- *relating to the person or body*
- *relating to an individual or an individual's character, conduct, motives, or private affairs often in an offensive manner* <*a* personal *insult*>
- *intended for private use or use by one person* <*a* personal *stereo*>

Then

- *at that time*
- *soon after that: next in order of time* <*walked to the door,* then *turned*>
- *following next after in order of position, narration, or enumeration*
- *being next in a series* <*first came the clowns, and* then *came the elephants*>
- *in addition: BESIDES* <then *there is the interest to be paid*>

Than

- *used as a function word to indicate the second member or the member taken as the point of departure in a comparison expressive of inequality; used with comparative adjectives and comparative adverbs* <*older* than *I am*> <*easier said* than *done*>
- *used as a function word to indicate difference of kind, manner, or identity; used especially with some adjectives and adverbs that express diversity* <*anywhere else* than *at home*>
- *rather than—usually used only after prefer, preferable, and preferably*
- *other than*

Too

- *BESIDES, ALSO* <*sell the house and furniture* too>
- *to an excessive degree: EXCESSIVELY* <too *large a house for us*>
- *to such a degree as to be regrettable* <*this time he has gone* too *far*>: *VERY* <*didn't seem* too *interested*>

Two

- *being one more than one in number*
- *being the second—used postpositively* <*section* two *of the instructions*>

To

- *used as a function word to indicate movement or an action or condition suggestive of movement toward a place, person, or thing reached* <*drove* to *the city*> <*went* to *lunch*>
- *used as a function word to indicate direction* <*a mile* to *the south*>
- *used as a function word to indicate contact or proximity* <*applied polish* to *the table*> <*put her hand* to *her heart*>
- *used as a function word to indicate the place or point that is the far limit* <*100 miles* to *the nearest town*>
- *used as a function word to indicate relative position* <*perpendicular* to *the floor*>
- *used as a function word to indicate purpose, intention, tendency, result, or end* <*came* to *our aid*> <*drink* to *his health*>

continues

		To *(continued)*
		■ *used as a function word to indicate the result of an action or a process <broken all to pieces> <go to seed> <to their surprise, the train left on time>*
		■ *used as a function word to indicate position or relation in time:*
		■ *BEFORE <five minutes to five>: TILL <from eight to five>*
		■ *used as a function word: (1) to indicate a relation to one that serves as a standard <inferior to her earlier works> (2) to indicate similarity, correspondence, dissimilarity, or proportion <compared him to a god>*
		■ *used as a function word to indicate agreement or conformity <add salt to taste> <to my knowledge>*
		■ *used as a function word to indicate a proportion in terms of numbers or quantities <400 to the box> <odds of ten to one>*
		■ *used as a function word to indicate that the following verb is an infinitive <wants to go> and often used by itself at the end of a clause in place of an infinitive suggested by the preceding context <knows more than she seems to>*

Medical Prefix	Medical Prefix	Medical Prefix
Inter- ■ *Among* <inter*dental*> ■ *In the midst of; within* <inter*oceptor*> Intra- ■ *within* <intra*galactic*> ■ *during* <intra*day*> ■ *between layers of* <intra*dermal*>	A-/An- ■ *Not, without, or less* <a*lexia*> <a*phonia*> <an*emia*> <an*oxia*> Dys- ■ *abnormal, difficult, or impaired* <dys*chromia*> <dys*pnea*> <dys*function*>	Hypo- ■ *under* ■ *beneath* ■ *down* <hypo*blast*> <hypo*dermic*> ■ *less than normal or normally* <hyp*esthesia*> <hypo*tension*> Hyper- ■ excessively <hyper*sensitive*> ■ excessive <hyper*emia*> <hyper*tension*>

Definitions provided from Merriam-Webster. (2003). *Merriam-Webster's collegiate dictionary* (11th ed.). Springfield, MA: Author.

APPENDIX 4–D
Commonly Misspelled Words in English

A
acceptable
accidentally
accommodate
acquire
acquit
amateur
apparent
argument

B
believe

C
calendar
category
changeable
column
committed
conscience
conscientious
conscious
consensus

D
definite (ly)
discipline

E
embarrass (ment)
equipment

exceed
existence
experience

F
foreign

G
gauge
guarantee

H
harass
height
hierarchy
humorous

I
ignorance
immediate
independent
indispensable
inoculate
intelligence

J
judgment

L
leisure
liaison

library
license

M
maintenance
maneuver
millennium
minuscule
mischievous
misspell

N
neighbor
noticeable

O
occasionally
occurrence

P
pastime
perseverance
personnel
possession
precede
privilege
pronunciation
publicly

Q
questionnaire

R
receive/receipt
recommend
referred
reference
relevant
restaurant
rhyme
rhythm

S
schedule
separate
supersede

T
threshold
twelfth

U
until

Source: 100 Most Often ~~Mispelled~~ Misspelled Words in English. (2003). In YourDictionary.com. Retrieved from http://grammar.yourdictionary.com/spelling-and-word-lists/misspelled.html

APPENDIX 4–E
Self-Evaluation of Intervention Sessions—Educational Setting

Note: This form may be used in conjunction with the Direct Observation Skills Brief Checklist.

Date/Time of Session:

_____

Rate the following on a scale of 1 (disagree) to 5 (agree).

1. I maintained an appropriate relationship with the student throughout the session. ○1 ○2 ○3 ○4 ○5

2. I was self-confident in this session. ○1 ○2 ○3 ○4 ○5

3. I considered the student's needs in selecting my materials and interacting with this student. ○1 ○2 ○3 ○4 ○5

4. I considered the student's cultural/linguistic needs in selecting my materials and interacting with this student. ○1 ○2 ○3 ○4 ○5

5. I used language appropriate for the student's age and education. ○1 ○2 ○3 ○4 ○5

6. I was courteous and respectful with this student. ○1 ○2 ○3 ○4 ○5

7. I was punctual for the session. ○1 ○2 ○3 ○4 ○5

8. I was prepared for the session. ○1 ○2 ○3 ○4 ○5

9. I was dressed appropriately for this session. ○1 ○2 ○3 ○4 ○5

10. I used time efficiently during this session. ○1 ○2 ○3 ○4 ○5

11. I completed the assigned tasks during this session. ○1 ○2 ○3 ○4 ○5

12. I accurately determined correct versus incorrect responses. ○1 ○2 ○3 ○4 ○5

13. I provided appropriate feedback to the student. ○1 ○2 ○3 ○4 ○5

14. The work area was appropriate for this student. ○1 ○2 ○3 ○4 ○5

15. I was aware of my professional boundaries during this session. ○1 ○2 ○3 ○4 ○5

16. I documented the results of the session appropriately. ○1 ○2 ○3 ○4 ○5

17. I shared the results with my supervision. ○1 ○2 ○3 ○4 ○5

Comments:

SLPA Signature: _____

APPENDIX 4–F
Self-Evaluation of Intervention Sessions—Medical Setting

Note: This form may be used in conjunction with the Direct Observation Skills Brief Checklist.

Date/Time of Session:

_____

Rate the following on a scale of 1 (disagree) to 5 (agree).

1. I maintained an appropriate relationship with the patient throughout the session ○1 ○2 ○3 ○4 ○5

2. I was self-confident in this session. ○1 ○2 ○3 ○4 ○5

3. I considered the patient's needs in selecting my materials and interacting with this patient. ○1 ○2 ○3 ○4 ○5

4. I considered the patient's cultural and linguistic needs in selecting my materials and interacting with this patient. ○1 ○2 ○3 ○4 ○5

5. I used language appropriate for the patient's age and education. ○1 ○2 ○3 ○4 ○5

6. I was courteous and respectful with this patient. ○1 ○2 ○3 ○4 ○5

7. I was punctual for the session. ○1 ○2 ○3 ○4 ○5

8. I was prepared for the session. ○1 ○2 ○3 ○4 ○5

9. I was dressed appropriately for this session. ○1 ○2 ○3 ○4 ○5

10. I used time efficiently during this session. ○1 ○2 ○3 ○4 ○5

11. I completed the assigned tasks during this session. ○1 ○2 ○3 ○4 ○5

12. I accurately determined correct versus incorrect responses. ○1 ○2 ○3 ○4 ○5

13. I provided appropriate feedback to the patient. ○1 ○2 ○3 ○4 ○5

14. The treatment environment was appropriate for this patient. ○1 ○2 ○3 ○4 ○5

15. I was aware of my professional boundaries during this session. ○1 ○2 ○3 ○4 ○5

16. I documented the results of the session appropriately. ○1 ○2 ○3 ○4 ○5

17. I shared the results with my supervision. ○1 ○2 ○3 ○4 ○5

Comments:

SLPA Signature: _____

CHAPTER 5

Cultural and Linguistic Diversity

Carolyn Conway Madding

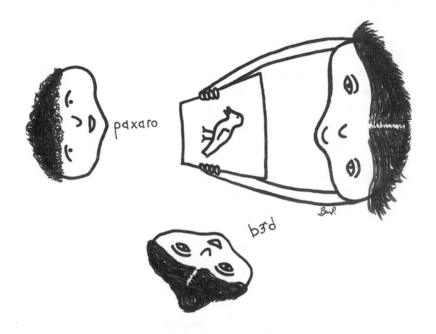

I know there is strength in the differences between us.
I know there is comfort where we overlap.

—Ani DiFranco
(American singer, songwriter, poet,
and women's rights advocate)

DIVERSITY OVERVIEW: IMPORTANT STATISTICS

The United States has been a land of immigrants from its inception, resulting in a demographic collage that demonstrates great diversity. In fact, this country is often referred to as the most diverse nation on earth. According to the 2014 U.S. Population Report, by 2044, more than half of all Americans are projected to belong to a minority group (any group other than non-Hispanic White alone);

and by 2060, nearly one in five of the nation's total population is projected to be foreign born (Colby & Ortman, 2015). With diversity comes the challenge of integrating a multitude of cultures and languages into the fabric of American life. Perhaps the most formidable task is faced in the field of education, in the effort to provide schooling and special services to children using myriad languages and coming from a diversity of cultures.

According to the U.S. Census Bureau (2015), more than 60 million persons (i.e., 60,361,574) in the United States older than 5 years use a language other than English in the home. Seventeen of these home languages encompass 500,000 or more users (Table 5–1). The majority representation, however, lies within the Spanish-using community, numbering approximately 37 million individuals.

The impact of language variations on municipalities, school districts, hospitals, and other community resources will continue to require adaptation in the foreseeable future. Many cities in the United States, as well as small towns, must accommodate to provide best services. Consider these cities with percentages of the population older than 5 years who use a language other than English in the home (Box 5–1).

Regardless of the professional service area covered by speech-language pathologists (SLPs) and speech-language pathology assistants (SLPAs), encountering language and cultural diversity is a certainty. The American Speech-Language-Hearing Association (ASHA) has therefore provided guidelines for assessment, intervention, and family interactions. All speech-language professionals should follow ASHA's mandate for appropriate service provision to culturally and linguistically

Table 5–1. Ranking of Languages Spoken in the United States other than English

Ranking	Language
1	Spanish (over 37 million)
2	Chinese–all dialects
3	Tagalog
4	Vietnamese
5	French
6	Korean
7	German
8	Arabic
9	Other Asian languages
10	African languages
11	Russian
12	Indic languages
13	French Creole
14	Italian
15	Portuguese
16	Hindi
17	Polish (580,153)

Source: U.S. Bureau of the Census, 2015. Available from https://www.census.gov/data/tables/2013/demo/2009-2013-lang-tables.html

Box 5–1. Major U.S. Cities and Percentages of Individuals (Older Than 5 Years) Who Speak a Language Other Than English (U.S. Bureau of the Census, 2012)

El Paso, Texas	73%
Los Angeles, California	61%
San Jose, California	55%
New York, New York	48%
San Francisco, California	45%
Houston, Texas	45%

diverse (CLD) clients and students and avail themselves of continuing education opportunities related to CLD populations. The sections of this chapter to follow, as well as the definitions at the end of this chapter, provide an overview of several important terms and concepts needed to serve CLD populations. After you finish reading this chapter, test your knowledge of this content with the questions in Appendix 5–A (answers provided).

DEFINITIONS, DISCUSSION, AND THE IMPORTANCE IN SERVICE PROVISION

According to Battle (2002), culture refers to "the behaviors, beliefs, and values of a group of people who are brought together by their commonality" (p. 3). Within the confines of the United States, myriad cultures exist, following their own ways of life. Cultural groups may not only be different from each other in their lifestyles and beliefs but may also use languages specific to their groups other than English. Due to the characteristics of life and language, they differ both culturally and linguistically from other groups and from so-called mainstream culture. In contrast, some cultural enclaves may use English but may maintain a *heritage language* for in-group communication and may live within a blend of cultures, consisting of the mainstream and the specific group from which they arise.

However, there are also diverse cultural groups that use English, or a *dialect* of English, as their native or heritage language and differ only in their cultural attributes from so-called mainstream Euro-Americans. They would be designated as culturally diverse but not linguistically diverse.

Dialects

In addition to numerous non-English languages spoken in the United States, dialectal variations of English abound. Dialects are rule-governed variations of a language. They may be spoken by a regional, ethnic, or socioeconomic group. Although dialects of a language are often intelligible to those outside the dialectal group, they may nevertheless vary in form, content, and use. Consider the regional dialects associated with Boston, New Orleans, and New York, as examples. On the other hand, there is Cajun, a dialect of an ethnic, Southern regional group, and African American English, shared by some in widespread African American communities.

Standard American English is the prevalent term for the mainstream dialect of the United States. This is the dialect used in most educational settings and in the media. On the other hand, there are many who use using a nonmainstream dialects. As dialects are rule governed, just as is Standard American English, they do not represent a language deficit, nor should they be described as inferior or substandard. According to ASHA, all dialects represent a functional and effective tool of expression in English.

It is ASHA's position, therefore, that no dialect of American English should be considered as a speech or language disorder (ASHA, 2003). Users of American English dialects do not present with language disorders but rather with language differences and dialectal differences. As such, they are not to be treated by SLPs or SLPAs. If an individual is referred for a screening or assessment and a culturally or linguistically appropriate assessment shows only a dialectal difference from Standard American English, no further intervention is warranted.

Similarly, if a referred client or student is *bilingual* or is an English-language learner, influences of the individual's non-English language should not be construed as a deficit in English but as a *language difference*. As such, the client or student is not within the scope of treatment for the SLP or the SLPA. If the family or client wishes to produce English that is more consistent with Standard American English, a speech-language pathologist specialized in accent modification can assist. In schools, English-language learners should be enrolled in special courses to assist them in the development of English but should not be placed on the caseload of the SLP unless they present with a speech or language disorder in their native language, as well as in the emergence of English.

To differentiate between a language difference and a *language disorder*, the SLP must assess the client or student in all languages spoken. A true language disorder exists across languages as is a language-learning disability. Box 5–2 contains helpful information for use in addressing speech-language disorders in linguistically and culturally diverse populations. If, however, assessment results show problems in only one language, they are indicative of a language difference, not a language-learning disability.

Box 5–2. Speech–Language Disorders in Linguistically and Culturally Diverse Populations

- Most children, even those presenting with language disorders, have the capacity and facility to learn more than one language (ASHA, n.d.-a).
- Learning two languages will not confuse children, although dual-language development may be prolonged. Learning more than one language does not represent a cognitive overload so long as both languages are supported (Genesee, 2003).
- Bilingualism represents a positive effect and supports the acquisition of a second language (Uchikoshi & Maniates, 2010).
- Bilingual children with language-learning disorders experience problems learning and using both languages (Roseberry & Connell, 1991). Thus, bilingual children must be assessed in each of their languages to differentiate between a language difference and a language disorder.
- Parents should be encouraged to maintain and model the home language, as this is their best language model (Mumy, 2012).
- Parents should not be told to stop using the home language or to switch to English in the home. This is both culturally and linguistically inappropriate.

Cultural Competence/Cultural Literacy

In any professional setting, a knowledge and understanding of linguistic and cultural diversity is mandatory for successful intervention. As stated by Lipson and Dibble (2005), "Health care professionals cannot provide good care without assessing both cultural group patterns and individual variation with a cultural group" (p. xi). This can be accomplished through *ethnographic methods,* adept listening, and careful, considerate interviewing techniques. According to Westby, Burda, and Mehta (2003), speech-language professionals "need to see the world through the eyes of the individuals they serve. Ethnographic interviewing provides a means of asking the right questions in the right ways to accomplish this" (p. 1). Ethnographic interviewing, through the clinician's open-ended questions, allows the client, student, or family to offer glimpses of their life and culture (Westby et al., 2003). To provide effective services, professionals must be attuned to all possible aspects of diversity, taking into consideration any issues related to racial or ethnic groups, language, dialect, religion, sexual orientation, age, and country of origin.

Professionals are not required to use the language of those referred for screening, assessment, or treatment, but understanding the basics of the culture is indeed important, even though the interactions may be through the use of an *interpreter.* The ability to understand and relate effectively with individuals from different cultures and language groups is frequently referred to as *cultural competence* (Hoodin, 2011) or *cultural literacy* (Haynes, Moran, & Pindzola, 2012).

Cultural competence within a group other than one's own does not ensue spontaneously with the ability to pro-

duce, listen, comprehend, or read and write a nonnative language. A person must have experience within the community, often but not necessarily in tandem with language proficiency, to develop cultural competence. According to Westby, professionals do not have to speak or understand the language of their clients or students, but need the ability to empathize with them.

When SLPAs decide to learn a second language to work more empathically and appropriately with individuals, their experience is restricted in some ways. Those who are nonnative language users differ from native or heritage language users in that language and culture may be learned linearly by nonnative users, that is, over time. Conversely, native users learn the culture and language cohesively as a developmental process. Thus, they are often unaware of the enmeshing of language and culture. The professional who is learning the language and culture of another group must invest time to be both linguistically and culturally competent (Madding, 2002). Cultural and linguistic competence is often appreciated by individuals and families being served but should not be construed as in-group acceptance.

In summary, language is the principal means through which the socialization process takes place. Culture and language are therefore inextricably intertwined during a child's development (Madding, 2000). To become culturally competent as a person outside the group requires time, attention to cues, and an intense interest in the culture and language. SLPAs, as part of the professional team addressing the needs of each client or student, should avail themselves of opportunities to learn as much as possible about the cultural and language background of every client. Awareness is the first principle, followed by interest, investigation, and learning. SLPAs will be pleasantly surprised when clients react favorably to an interest in their culture, as well as when respect is shown for cultural values. Learning the language of the client, or having the ability to greet clients in their heritage language, represents a significant step in the continuum of cultural competence acquisition.

To learn more about a culture, we must first recognize the characteristics, values, and beliefs of our own culture. Then we can begin to ascertain the ways in which the behaviors and beliefs of others differ from each other and from the one with which we are most familiar. Appendix 5–B contains cultural consciousness activities to help you explore your own cultural mores or rules. Acknowledging your own culture but respecting what is honored and cherished by others is of utmost importance in the practice of speech-language pathology.

We can learn about other cultures and languages through the Internet, from books and journal articles, and from *cultural informants*. The latter are those from the cultural community who can answer questions and provide information that will help the SLPA to approach and interact with clients, students, and families in a culturally appropriate manner. The cultural informant must be knowledgeable about the specific client or student's culture and language community (ASHA, n.d.-b).

LANGUAGES OTHER THAN ENGLISH

According to the U.S. Census Bureau (2015), there are more than 60,361,574 individuals in the country, age 5 years and older, who use a language other than English. Due to the free movement of populations within the United States, professionals in every state may encounter clients or students who use any of these languages. It is therefore an educational priority to know which languages are at the top of this list in terms of number of users and to become acquainted with their basic characteristics and related cultural distinctions when a student or client is referred to the SLP and the SLPA. See Table 5–1 for languages used by the largest number of people in the United States, excluding English (from the largest group, at approximately 37 million, to the last on the list, at 580,000 users).

Languages and Countries— A Guide for the Professional

SLPs and SLPAs can access phonemic inventories for many different languages and dialects at the following ASHA website: http://www.asha.org/practice/multicultural/Phono. Cultural profiles and resources for service providers for a variety of groups are also included, as well as videos of assessment and treatment of bilingual individuals. Phonemic inventories are available for the following languages listed in Table 5–1: Arabic, Mandarin, Cantonese, Haitian Creole (French), Hindi, Korean, Russian, Spanish, Tagalog, and Vietnamese. Phonemic information for African American English and dialects of several other languages also reside at this website (ASHA, n.d.-c).

BILINGUAL SLPS AND SLPAS (DEMOGRAPHICS AND STATISTICS)

In a data snapshot of ASHA *bilingual service providers* in the United States, year-end

2011, ASHA (2012) reported there were a total of 6,282 bilingual ASHA-certified SLPs. The largest contingent of bilingual ASHA-certified SLPs who lived in the United States at that time were in Texas (1,077), New York (1,006), California (857), and Florida (608).. Some bilingual clinicians may not be registered with ASHA. Nevertheless, statistics show the overall dearth of bilingual SLPs, with the subsequent conclusion that many bilingual and non-English-speaking clients or students cannot possibly be served directly, without interpretation, in their home or native language.

ASHA reported the primary work settings of bilingual service providers to be almost equally represented by educational and health care settings (ASHA, 2012).

THE SLPA AS AN INTERPRETER OR TRANSLATOR

As a solution to the relatively small corps of bilingual SLPs to serve CLD populations, ASHA encourages the development of collaborative relationships with *interpreters* and *translators* (ASHA, n.d.-b). Bilingual SLPAs may provide a valuable service to their supervising SLP and to the clients served, either as a direct service provider under supervision or as an interpreter or translator. See definitions at the end of the chapter for differentiation between an interpreter and translator. In fact, ASHA's 2013 SLPA scope-of-practice document acknowledges this role, stating that provided adequate training, planning, and supervision, SLPAs may perform the following tasks (ASHA, 2013, Service Delivery, para. 1):

- Assist the SLP with bilingual translation during screening and assessment activities exclusive of interpretation.
- Serve as interpreter for patients, clients, students, and families who do not use English.
- Provide services under SLP supervision in another language for individuals who do not use English and for English-language learners.

Your Role as an Interpreter or Translator

As an SLPA, to serve as a qualified interpreter or translator you must carefully follow guidelines provided by ASHA (n.d.-d) and others who have written extensively in this area. Box 5–3 provides an overview of these requirements. Subsequent to gaining thorough background knowledge of your role as interpreter or translator, you may begin to work in this capacity, under the guidance of your supervising SLP.

How to Prepare for your Role as an Interpreter or Translator

Box 5–4 outlines helpful tips in preparing to work as an interpreter or translator.

WORKING WITH AN INTERPRETER OR TRANSLATOR

When you are assigned to work with a client or student who is bilingual or whose language is not one you use, your first step is to consult with your supervising SLP.

Box 5–3. Basic Requirements to Serve as Interpreter or Translator (Langdon, 2002)

1. Native or near native proficiency in the student's or client's native language or dialect
2. Ability to provide accurate and complete oral interpretation or written translation
3. Familiarity with and respect for the student's or client's culture and language community
4. Knowledge of professional terminology
5. Maintenance of client, student, or family confidentiality of information
6. High-level oral and written or signing proficiency both in English and the non-English language
7. Maintenance of neutrality between yourself and the client, student, or family
8. Ability to provide interpretation without addition, subtraction, or commentary
9. Knowledge of assessment and therapeutic techniques, with special emphasis on those to be used with bilingual or non-English-speaking clients or students

---

Box 5–4. Helpful Tips in Preparing to Work as an Interpreter or Translator

1. Although you may be bilingual, do not volunteer or allow yourself to be solicited as an interpreter or translator unless you meet all the minimum requirements listed in Box 5–3. SLPs and other team members may urge you to take on the role when they learn of your bilingual skills. Be honest about your abilities and maintain adherence to basic requirements listed in Box 5–3.
2. Do not serve as an interpreter or translator if you are not from the same language community or cultural background as the client or student. Examples of mismatches: You are Mexican American and the client is from Spain or Argentina; you are Egyptian American and your client is from Yemen; you are Mexican American and your client is from a rural, indigenous community in Guatemala. Mismatches such as these may result in inaccurate interpretations, translations, and cultural misunderstandings.

As your supervisor, the SLP is legally and ethically responsible for all clients and students on the caseload and delegates tasks to you, the SLPA (ASHA, 2013). You must have the compliance and permission of the SLP before you can seek the interpreter or translator you need for appropriate intervention (ASHA, 2013). Keeping in mind the ASHA mandates for service provision mentioned earlier in this chapter, express the importance of contacting a qualified interpreter or translator to assist in your interactions with the client or student.

Choosing an Interpreter or Translator

Many school districts, hospitals, and other service sites maintain a bank of interpreters and translators. Inquire if such a list exists and whether the interpreters or translators meet the basic requirements listed in Box 5–4. In cases where no resources are available, it is incumbent upon the supervising SLP to locate and train an interpreter. A cultural informant may assist in locating an appropriate interpreter or translator or one who is willing to be trained. Your employer may provide stipends for interpreters and translators. If no remuneration is available, however, you may need to locate someone who is willing to volunteer his or her services. Family members, and most especially children, should not be solicited for this task for many reasons. Among those may be a vested interest in the case of the client, difficulty in being impartial, and the tendency to cue the client. Children may be embarrassed, cannot be counted on to maintain confidentiality, and do not possess the maturity to follow the basic requirements to be an interpreter

or translator. Whenever possible, choose a trained professional.

Using an Interpreter or Translator

Box 5–5 provides helpful tips for working with an interpreter or translator, including guidelines for before, during, and after treatment sessions.

CHAPTER DEFINITIONS AND OTHER RELEVANT DEFINITIONS

Bilingual: A bilingual individual possesses the ability to use more than one language effectively (Bhatia & Ritchie, 2006). A bilingual person may be fully competent in oral languages (or sign and speech) without the ability to read or write in more than one language. Furthermore, those who comprehends and follow through with instructions in a language other than their native language, even though they do not produce the second language, is considered at least marginally bilingual.

Bilingual Service Provider: Individuals who "speak their primary language and to speak (or sign) at least one other language with native or near-native proficiency in lexicon (vocabulary), semantics (meaning), phonology (pronunciation), morphology/syntax (grammar), and pragmatics (uses) during clinical management. In addition to linguistic proficiency, bilingual service providers must have the specific knowledge and skill sets necessary for the services to be delivered (ASHA, n.d.-e, Bilingual Service Providers, para 1)

Box 5–5. Helpful Tips in Working With an Interpreter or Translator (ASHA, n.d.-d)

Before the Session

1. Meet with the interpreter or translator. Plan sufficient time to review the procedures, goals, professional terminology, and to develop rapport.
2. Remind the interpreter or translator to avoid nonverbal cues such as intonational changes or hand gestures.
3. Ensure that the interpreter or translator will maintain confidentiality.
4. Inquire about specific cultural or linguistic information that may assist you in working with the client, such as greetings in the client's language.

During the Session

1. Define your role as the SLPA and introduce the interpreter or translator to the client.
2. Talk directly to the client and not to the interpreter.
3. Interpreters should also look at the person to whom they are communicating (i.e., the client and then responsively to you).
4. Use short, concise sentences to allow for careful, thorough interpretation or translation.
5. Allow sufficient time for the interpreter to convey your message to the client in the client's language and to relay the client's message back to you in English.

Wrap-Up Session

1. Plan sufficient time at the end of your session to review with the interpreter or translator.
2. If the client or family has brought in written material, ask it to be translated for you. This can be done after the session.
3. Review the session and answer any questions the interpreter or translator may have.
4. Thank interpreter or translator and congratulate him/her on a job well done.

Biliterate: A biliterate person is one who speaks, reads, and writes effectively in more than one language.

Cultural Informant: A cultural informant is a person with whom a professional may consult to learn more about a cultural community, a linguistic community, or both. The cultural informant should be a member of that community. To avoid bias, more than one cultural informant may be used. The goal in using information about the community is to optimize services for the client (ASHA, n.d.-a). The informant may provide information relative to topics such as child-rearing, language and dialect usage, and attitudes toward disabilities (Anderson, 2002).

Dialect: A dialect is defined as "a rule-governed variation of a language used by a definable group of people characterized by their culture, ethnicity, or geographical region" (Haynes, Moran, & Pindzola, 2012, p. 426).

Ethnicity: Ethnicity is variously defined as the affiliation with a population group; having a common cultural heritage or nationality; or distinguished by customs, characteristics, languages, and common history.

Ethnographic Methods or Ethnography: An ethnographic method allows an individual to observe and conscientiously collect information about the life and culture of a specific group. Observations and data collection occur over time and can reveal the mores, beliefs, and interactional styles of a group. Ethnographic or qualitative study is descriptive and thus can be especially useful in understanding linguistically and culturally diverse communities (Brice, 2002). "Ethnography is the social research style that emphasizes encountering unfamiliar worlds and making sense of them" (Agar, 1986, p.12).

Heritage Language: A heritage language, sometimes referred to as the native or home language, is one used by a family, cultural group, or both, , and usually the first language to which a child is exposed.

Interpreter: An interpreter is a bilingual person specially trained to translate *oral* communication or manual communication systems (sign language) from one language to another (ASHA, n.d.-b).

Language Difference: As opposed to a language disorder, a language difference is characterized by variations from Standard American English in phonology, morphology, syntax, semantics, and pragmatics, as the result of the influence of another language or dialect.

Language Disorder: A language disorder is defined as "impaired comprehension and/or use of spoken, written, signed, and/or other symbol systems. The disorder may involve: (1) the form of language (phonology, morphology, syntax), (2) the content of language (semantics), and/or (3) the function of language in communication (pragmatics) in any combination" (ASHA, 1993).

Translator: A translator is a bilingual person specially trained to translate written text from one language to another (ASHA, n.d.-b).

REFERENCES

Agar, M. (1986). *Speaking of ethnography*. Newbury Park, CA: Sage.

American Speech-Language-Hearing Association. (n.d.-a). *The advantages of being bilingual*. Retrieved from http://www.asha.org/about/news/tipsheets/bilingual/

American Speech-Language-Hearing Association. (n.d.-b). *Collaborating with Interpreters* Retrieved from https://www.asha.org/Practice-Portal/Professional-Issues/Collaborating-With-Interpreters/

American Speech-Language-Hearing Association. (n.d.-c). *Phonemic inventories across languages*. Retrieved from http://www.asha.org/practice/multicultural/Phono/

American Speech-Language-Hearing Association. (n.d.-d). *Tips for working with an interpreter.* Retrieved from http://www.asha.org/practice/multicultural/issues/interpret/

American Speech-Language-Hearing Association. (n.d.-e). *Bilingual service delivery.* Retrieved from https://www.asha.org/PRPSpecificTopic.aspx?folderid=8589935225&section=Key_Issues#Bilingual_Service_Providers

American Speech-Language-Hearing Association. (1993). *Definitions of communication disorders and variations.* doi:10.1044/policy.RP1993-00208

American Speech-Language-Hearing Association (ASHA). (2003). *American English dialects* [Technical report]. doi:10.1044/policy.TR2003-00044

American Speech-Language-Hearing Association. (2012). *Demographic profile of ASHA members providing bilingual services August 2012.* Retrieved from http://www.asha.org/uploadedFiles/Demographic-Profile-Bilingual-Spanish-Service-Members.pdf

American Speech-Language-Hearing Association (ASHA). (2013). *Speech-language pathology assistant scope of practice.* doi:10.1044/policy.SP2013-00337

Anderson, R. (2002). Practical assessment strategies with Hispanic students. In A. Brice (Ed.), *The Hispanic child: Speech, language, culture and education* (pp. 143–184). Boston, MA: Allyn & Bacon.

Battle, D. (2002). Communication disorders in a multicultural society. In D. Battle (Ed.), *Communication disorders in multicultural populations* (3rd ed., pp. 33–70). Stoneham, MA: Butterworth-Heinemann.

Bhatia, T., & Ritchie, W. (Eds.). (2006). *The handbook of bilingualism.* Cambridge, UK: Blackwell.

Brice, A. (2002). Clinician as a qualitative researcher. In A. Brice (Ed.), *The Hispanic child: Speech, language, culture, and education* (pp. 85–99). Boston, MA: Allyn & Bacon.

Colby, S. L., & Ortman, J. M. (2015). Projections of the size and composition of the U.S. population: 2014 to 2060. Current Population Reports, *P25–1143.* Washington, DC: U.S. Census Bureau.

Genesee, F. (2003). Rethinking bilingual acquisition. In J. Dewaele, A. Housen, & L. Wei (Eds.), *Bilingualism: Beyond basic principles* (pp. 204–229). Clevedon, UK: Multilingual Matters.

Haynes, W., Moran, M., & Pindzola, R. (2012). *Communication disorders in educational and medical settings: An introduction for speech-language pathologists, educators, and health professionals.* Sudbury, MA: Jones & Bartlett Learning.

Hoodin, R. (2011). *Intervention in child language disorders: A comprehensive handbook.* Sudbury, MA: Jones & Bartlett Learning.

Langdon, H. (2002). Language interpreters and translators: Bridging communication with clients and families. *ASHA Leader, 7,* 14–15. doi:10.1044/leader.FTR4.07062002.14

Lipson, J., & Dibble, S. (2005). *Culture and clinical care.* San Francisco: University of California San Francisco Nursing Press.

Madding, C. (2002). Socialization practices of Latinos. In A. Brice (Ed.), *The Hispanic child: Speech, language, culture, and education* (pp. 66–84). Boston, MA: Allyn & Bacon.

Mumy, A. P. (2012). *Tips for parents raising bilingual children: When the home language differs from the community language.* Retrieved from http://blog.asha.org/2012/08/16/tips-for-parents-raising-bilingual-children-when-the-home-language-differs-from-the-community-language/

Roseberry, C.A., & Connell, P. J. (1991). The use of an invented language rule in the differentiation of normal and language-impaired Spanish-speaking children. *Journal of Speech and Hearing Research, 34,* 596–603. doi:10.1044/jshr.3403.596

Uchikoshi, Y., & Maniates, H. (2010). How does bilingual instruction enhance English achievement? A mixed-methods study of Cantonese-speaking and Spanish-speaking bilingual classrooms. *Bilingual Research Journal, 33*(3), 364–385. doi:10.1080/15235882.2010.525294

U.S. Census Bureau. (2012). *Statistical abstract of the United States.* Washington, DC: U.S. Department of Commerce.

U.S. Census Bureau. (2015). *Detailed languages spoken at home and ability to speak English for the population 5 years and over: 2009–2013.* American Community Survey. Washington, DC: U.S. Department of Commerce. Retrieved from https://www.census.gov/data/tables/2013/demo/2009-2013-lang-tables.html

Westby, C., Burda, A., & Mehta, Z. (2003, April 29). Asking the right questions in the right ways. *ASHA Leader, 8,* 4–17, doi:10.1044/leader.FTR3.08082003.4

APPENDIX 5–A
Chapter Review Self-Test

		T/F
1.	*Interpreter* and *translator* are synonymous terms.	
2.	Interpreters should tell non-English-speaking families to speak to their children in English.	
3.	Being bilingual means that an individual will be an appropriate interpreter or translator.	
4.	Acquiring cultural competence is an ongoing process.	
5.	Only a bilingual speech-language pathology assistant may work with a non-English-speaking client or student.	
6.	The interpreter or translator should be acquainted with the procedures of the upcoming session before it begins.	
7.	It is the speech-language pathology assistant's role to train and prepare the interpreter.	
8.	The interpreter or translator must be neutral, ethical, and maintain confidentiality.	
9.	A bilingual child may have a language disorder in just one of his or her languages.	
10.	A student with a dialectal difference from the mainstream should receive speech-language services in order to develop Standard American English.	

Answers: 1. F; 2. F; 3. F; 4. T; 5. F; 6. T; 7. T; 8. T; 9. F; 10. F.

APPENDIX 5–B
Cultural Consciousness Activities

1. Think about your own culture (specific to the geographic and familial environment in which you were raised) and list five rules or mores of your culture. (Examples: father is head of the house; church on Sunday is a must, etc.)

2. Thinking of your responses to Question 1, can you think of some cultures where the rules or mores are different?

3. Describe an ideal family in the culture of your childhood.

4. Describe the attitude of your culture toward disabilities.

5. Check the culturally linked attitudes and behaviors that are associated with your culture:

   ____ Punctuality

   ____ Elders have final authority

   ____ Informal child rearing (few rules)

   ____ Birthright inheritance

   ____ Assertiveness, directness

   ____ High expectations for child

   ____ Formality in family relationships

____ Nuclear family most important

____ Greater family (all relatives) most important; family cohesiveness

____ Independence valued

____ Religious family orientation

____ Respect for elderly

____ All older people considered as parents

____ Matriarchal family structure

____ Patriarchal family structure

____ Competition between siblings valued

____ Equality in family structure

____ Adults defined by occupation

____ Marriage affirmed by children

____ Divorce acceptable

____ Unmarried children should live with parents

____ Privacy valued

____ Freedom of opinion

____ Family democracy

____ Importance of tradition

____ Family above personal gain

CHAPTER 6

Health and Safety

Pei-Fang Hung

An ounce of prevention is worth a pound of cure.
—Benjamin Franklin
(scientist/inventor and Founding
Father of the United States)

The aim of this chapter is to describe various medical-related matters that a speech-language pathology assistant (SLPA) may encounter when working with clients in various clinical settings, such as child care centers, schools, community clinics, long-term care facilities, private homes, and hospital settings. The purpose is to provide an overview of common medical conditions related to your work as an SLPA and practical information to ensure a safe working environment for both you and the clients you serve. Infection control, standard precautions, first aid, cardiopulmonary resuscitation (CPR), common medical conditions, and precautions are each discussed.

INFECTION CONTROL AND STANDARD PRECAUTIONS

The purpose of infection control is to ensure the protection of individuals who are at risk of acquiring an infection in various settings, such as in the general community or while receiving health care treatment (Centers for Disease Control and Prevention [CDC], 2011). When receiving health care treatment, patients are vulnerable to health care–associated infections (HAIs). According to the U.S. CDC (2011), HAIs affect nearly 2 million individuals every year in the United States and contribute to approximately 80,000 deaths annually.

Infectious diseases are caused by microorganisms called pathogens, which infect their hosts (Signore, 2013). The most common pathogens are various bacteria, viruses, fungi, and protozoa (Signore, 2013). These microorganisms are transmitted via several routes, which can be direct or indirect. Direct transmission can either be direct contact or droplet spread. Indirect transmission can be airborne, vehicle-borne, or vector-borne (Box 6–1).

All health care providers, including SLPAs, are responsible for providing safe care to clients. According to the World Health Organization (WHO), infection control is the prevention of the spread of infection and ensures the protection of individuals who might be vulnerable to infection (WHO, 2009). The American Speech-Language-Hearing Association (ASHA) includes infection control within program operation in its policy docu-

ments: *Quality Indicators for Professional Service Programs in Audiology and Speech-Language Pathology: Section III. D. Physical Facilities, Equipment, and Program Environment* (ASHA, 2005).

SLPAs may be exposed to a variety of infectious diseases when performing their duties. As such, it is critical to protect yourself and your clients from the spread of disease in all forms. If you do not take effective precautions against infection, you are at high risk of becoming infected. Similarly, without effective protection, there is a high possibility that the infectious disease can further spread to your clients, colleagues, family members, and the community at large. Therefore, infection control is essential to all health care providers, including SLPAs.

Standard precautions (previously known as universal precautions) are "the minimum infection prevention practices that apply to all patient care, regardless of suspected or confirmed infection status of the patient, in any setting where healthcare is delivered" (CDC, 2011, Adhere to Standard Precautions, para. 1). Standard precautions are designed to protect health care providers and to prevent infections from being spread. Key standard precautions important to an SLPA include hand hygiene, use of personal protective equipment, safe handling of potentially contaminated equipment or surfaces, and respiratory hygiene/cough etiquette.

Hand Hygiene

Hand hygiene is the most important way to prevent infection and to reduce the risk of spreading infections (WHO, 2009). For a comprehensive review of hand hygiene, please refer to the *WHO Guidelines on Hand Hygiene in Health Care* (WHO, 2009).

Box 6–1. Modes of Transmission (CDC, 2012)

Contact Transmission

Contact transmission is divided into direct and indirect contact. Two examples of contact transmissible infectious agents include methicillin-resistant Staphylococcus aureus (MRSA) and vancomycin-resistant enterococcus (VRE).

- *Direct contact transmission* refers to the transfer of infectious agents through physical contact with an infected individual. An example of direct body-to-body physical contact includes touching an infectious person.
- *Indirect contact transmission* involves the transfer of infections agents by making physical contact with contaminated items and surfaces. Examples of indirect contact include touching contaminated doorknobs, computer keyboards, or handles.

Droplet Transmission

Droplets are produced when talking, coughing, or sneezing. Infectious droplets can travel through air but cannot remain suspended in the air because they are large particles (>10 micrometers). When these pathogens drop, they can contaminate the environment and cause indirect contact transmission.

Airborne Transmission

Airborne transmission occurs when very small particles (microorganisms <10 micrometers) containing infectious agents spread in the air and enter the respiratory tract to cause infection, such as tuberculosis (TB). Airborne transmission does not require face-to-face contact with an infected individual.

Vehicle–Borne Transmission

Vehicle-borne transmission is a type of indirect transmission of an infectious agent that occurs when microorganisms are transmitted by consuming or contacting contaminated items, such as food or water sources.

Vector–Borne Transmission

Vector-borne transmission occurs when pathogens are transmitted through vectors, such as mosquitoes, flies, or rats.

Good hand hygiene includes hand washing with water and soap and the use of alcohol-based hand rubs.

For SLPAs, hand hygiene should be performed in, but not limited to, the following conditions (WHO, 2009):

- Before and after treating a client
- After touching blood, body fluids, or any contaminated items even when gloves are worn
- Immediately after removing personal protective equipment, such as gloves
- Immediately if skin is contaminated or injury occurs
- After activities involving personal body functions, such as blowing one's nose.

Also, SLPAs should encourage clients to perform hand hygiene at the beginning of the therapy session, prior to handling task materials, or after activities involving personal body functions.

Table 6–1 summarizes the proper steps in hand washing and hand rubbing, as recommended by WHO (2009) and the CDC (2011).

Personal Protective Equipment

When there is a risk of coming in contact with non-intact skin, mucous membranes, or body fluids, personal protective equipment is required. According to the Occupational Safety and Health Administration (OSHA, 2003), personal protective equipment refers to equipment designed to protect the wearer from injury (CDC, 2011). Examples of personal protective equipment include gloves, goggles, helmets, and protective clothing. The most commonly worn personal protective equipment is gloves. Gloves act as a barrier between the skin and potentially hazardous agents and should be worn when there is a risk of coming in contact with non-intact skin, mucous membranes, or body fluids, but wearing gloves should not replace good hand hygiene. For SLPAs, the following common situations may require wearing gloves:

- Assisting with an oral peripheral examination or oral hygiene
- Handling dirty materials
- Working with clients who are immune compromised or when

Table 6–1. Steps for Proper Hand Washing and Hand Rubbing

Hand Washing	Hand Rubbing
1. Remove hand and arm jewelry.	1. Remove hand and arm jewelry.
2. Wet hands with warm water and apply soap.	2. Apply between one and two full pumps of alcohol-based hand sanitizer onto one palm.
3. Rub all aspects of hands for a minimum of 15 seconds, concentrating on the fingertips, between fingers, the back of hands, and the base of thumbs.	3. Spread product over all surfaces of both hands, concentrating on the fingertips, between fingers, the back of hands, and the base of thumbs.
4. Rinse and dry hands thoroughly with an air dryer or paper towel.	4. Rub hands until product is dry.
5. Turn off taps with paper towel.	

Source: CDC, 2011; Interorganizational Group for Speech Language Pathology and Audiology, 2010.

additional precaution is needed (e.g., clients with *Clostridium difficile* infection)
- Assisting with feeding and swallowing treatment activities
- When touching someone's body fluids (such as blood, respiratory secretions, vomit, urine, or feces), certain hazardous drugs, or potentially contaminated items

Using gloves correctly is essential (CDC, 2016). It is important to select the proper glove material. For example, vinyl gloves are designed for personal care and latex gloves are for sterile invasive procedures. Avoiding latex gloves should be considered to prevent latex allergies. Second, be sure to use the correct size of gloves and do not reuse single-use disposable gloves. Lastly, before touching a clean environment or when an activity or procedure is completed, remove gloves immediately. Some additional things to consider before using medical gloves (U.S. Food and Drug Administration, n.d.) include:

- Wash your hands before putting on gloves.
- Make sure your gloves fit properly and you can wear them comfortably during all patient care activities.
- Be aware that sharp objects can puncture medical gloves.
- Always change your gloves if they rip or tear.
- After removing gloves, wash your hands thoroughly with soap and water or alcohol-based hand rub.
- Never reuse medical gloves.
- Never wash or disinfect medical gloves.
- Never share medical gloves with other users.

- If you or your patient is allergic to natural rubber latex, choose gloves made from other synthetic materials, such as polyvinyl chloride (PVC), nitrile, or polyurethane.

To protect your eyes, nose, and mouth from the splash of a potentially infectious material or body fluids, you can use eye protectors (e.g., goggles), masks, and face shields (Siegel, Rhinehart, Jackson, Chiarello, & the Healthcare Infection Control Practices Advisory Committee, 2007). Preferred masks include the National Institute for Occupational Safety and Health (NIOSH)–certified N95 filtering facepiece respirators (Figure 6–1) or the P100 filtering facepiece respirators with the elastomeric facepiece seal (CDC, 2013a).

Safe Handling of Potentially Contaminated Equipment or Surfaces

As an SLPA, you may be asked to participate in cleaning and disinfecting treatment materials and the clinical environment.

Figure 6–1. 3M N95 Filtering facepiece respirators. Image courtesy of Wikimedia Commons.

Sterilization is not often required. Cleaning refers to the physical removal, of foreign material, such as dust, soil, or secretion by using water and detergents (CDC, 2008). High-traffic areas, such as furniture in the therapy room, should be cleaned frequently. Treatment materials should be placed on shelves and in bins after use. Shelves and bins should be kept clean and dust free.

Disinfection refers to the elimination of harmful microorganisms living on the surface of objects, but disinfection does not destroy all microorganisms, especially some bacterial spores (CDC, 2008). For low-level disinfection, SLPAs can apply an Environmental Protection Agency (EPA)-registered disinfectant on equipment or surfaces and let the solution sit for at least 1 minute before wiping (CDC, 2008). While using the disinfectant, wear rubber gloves to protect hands from irritation and wash hands immediately afterward. When EPA-registered disinfectant is not available, SLPAs may use a fresh chlorine bleach solution. The formula of diluted bleach solution is 1 tablespoon of bleach to 1 quart (4 cups) of water. The CDC and the Healthcare Infection Control Practices Advisory Committee (HICPAC) provide guidelines on environmental infection control measures. A copy of the cleaning and disinfection guidelines for schools is available in Appendix 6–A. Additional information on this topic can also be found on the CDC's website (http://www.cdc.gov/hai/).

Respiratory Hygiene/Cough Etiquette

According to the CDC (2012), respiratory etiquette should be implemented for all individuals with signs and symptoms of a respiratory infection. The following measures are used to contain respiratory secretions (Healthcare Infection Control Practices Advisory Committee, 2017):

- Use respiratory hygiene and cough etiquette to reduce the transmission of respiratory infections.
- Prompt patients with symptoms of respiratory infection to contain their respiratory secretions by providing tissues, masks, and hand hygiene supplies.
- Prompt patients with symptoms of respiratory infection to perform hand hygiene after contact with respiratory secretions.
- When space permits, separate patients with respiratory symptoms from others as soon as possible upon entry into the facility.

Additional information on this topic can be found on the CDC's website (http://www.cdc.gov/flu/professionals/infectioncontrol/resphygiene.htm).

FIRST AID AND CARDIOPULMONARY RESUSCITATION

In case of an emergency, an SLPA should be trained in first aid and CPR to respond appropriately. This section discusses the general rules for first aid and CPR use and how to get certified.

General Rules About First Aid

First aid refers to the initial care or management for an injury or illness (American

Red Cross, 2011). Most treatment settings have a first aid kit available, which contains items for use in the event of injury. In the United States, OSHA requires all job sites and workplaces to have a first aid kit available. The kit is typically stored in a place where it is easily accessible for adults but out of reach of children. As an SLPA you should know where this kit is and what items are in it.

Key items that should be included in a first aid kit (Cronan, 2010) include a first aid manual, sterile gauze pads, adhesive tape, adhesive bandages, antiseptic wipes, alcohol wipes, antibiotic ointment, antiseptic solution, pain killers, tweezers, scissors, safety pins, disposable instant cold packs, thermometers, plastic non-latex gloves, and a flashlight with extra batteries. The kit should be checked on a regular basis to replace low-stock items and medicines that may have expired and to check if the flashlight works properly and there are backup batteries available.

CPR/ Automated External Defibrillator (AED) Certification

According to American Heart Association (AHA, 2017), CPR is an emergency procedure that manually ensures blood can continue circulating in the body after an individual experiences cardiac arrest. All the cells in our body require oxygen and nutrients to survive, which are carried in the blood. When a cardiac arrest happens, the heart stops beating, blood stops circulating, and breathing ceases after a few minutes. A cardiac arrest can be caused a heart attack, other heart diseases, heart rhythm disturbance, drugs, blood loss, or head injury. CPR is an emergency procedure to keep the blood flowing in the body, but it cannot restart the heart. Fur-

ther measures, such as defibrillation, are needed to restart the heart.

In general, CPR involves chest compression and rescue breaths (AHA, 2017). Chest compressions manually pump the heart so blood continues flowing throughout the body. Rescue breaths supply air to the lungs and can be performed either by mouth-to-mouth resuscitation using a device. Early CPR is an integral part of providing lifesaving aid to people suffering sudden cardiac arrest. An automated external defibrillator (AED) is a computerized medical device that checks a person's heart rhythm. It can recognize a rhythm that requires a shock and advises a rescuer when a shock is needed. The AED uses voice prompts, lights, and text messages to tell a rescuer what steps to take. After the AED is attached and delivers a shock, most AEDs will prompt the operator to continue CPR while the device continues to monitor the victim.

CPR training is easy and it is extremely important for SLPAs to get CPR certification so they can react to emergency situations. It is also beneficial to get AED training and certification. The American Red Cross and AHA offer training and certification courses for first aid, CPR, and AED. For more information on CPR, visit the American Red Cross website (http://www.redcorss.org) and the AHA website (http://www.heart.org). Local fire departments also offer CPR training courses that are certified by the AHA.

COMMON MEDICAL CONDITIONS

When an SLPA is working with a client or patient, emergency medical situations can occur. This section covers several medical conditions that an SLPA might encounter when providing care or treatment. By understanding the causes and symptoms of these conditions, SLPAs can react to medical emergencies appropriately and seek medical attention immediately.

Stroke

According to the National Stroke Association (2013), stroke is the fourth leading cause of death in the United States. A stroke, also known as cerebrovascular accident (CVA), occurs when the blood supply to part of the brain is suddenly interrupted or when a blood vessel in the brain bursts, spilling blood into the brain or the spaces surrounding the brain. There are two kinds of stroke: ischemic stroke and hemorrhagic stroke. An ischemic stroke is caused by obstruction of a blood vessel that supplies blood to the brain. The obstruction can result from cerebral thrombosis or embolism. Cerebral thrombosis refers to the formation of a blood clot inside a blood vessel that blocks vascular circulation in the brain. A cerebral embolism happens when a clot breaks off from another part of body and travels to the brain, resulting in the obstruction of a blood vessel in the brain. A hemorrhagic stroke happens when a weakened blood vessel ruptures. Weakened blood vessels can result from a blood vessel malformation, such as arteriovenous malformation or a cerebral aneurysm.

When the vascular circulation in the brain is blocked or interrupted, neurons (brain cells) can no longer receive the oxygen and nutrients they need from the blood supply. This results in the death of neurons and the loss of abilities controlled by the brain area where circulation was interrupted. The effects of a stroke depend on where the stroke occurs in the brain and how much of the brain is damaged. For example, a small stroke may cause only minor weakness of an arm or leg, whereas a larger stroke can result in paralysis (total loss of muscle function) on one side of the body. A stroke can impair many important brain functions, such as speech, language, movement, vision, and memory. Stroke is one of the main causes of many acquired speech-language related disorders, such as aphasia, dysarthria, apraxia of speech, and other cognitive-linguistic disorders (ASHA, n.d.). Stroke is a medical emergency and prompt treatment is crucial. Box 6–2 summarizes possible signs and symptoms of a stroke. If a person is experiencing those symptoms,

---

Box 6–2. Common Symptoms and Signs of Stroke
(National Stroke Association, 2013)

- Sudden numbness or weakness of the face, arm, or leg, especially on one side of the body
- Sudden confusion, trouble speaking or understanding
- Sudden trouble seeing in one or both eyes
- Sudden trouble walking, dizziness, loss of balance or coordination
- Sudden severe headache with no known cause

an SLPA should immediately call 911 and get medical attention. Early intervention can minimize brain damage and potential complications.

Heart Attack

Similar to a stroke, a heart attack, also known as a myocardial infarction, happens when the blood vessels that supply blood to the heart become blocked (National Institutes of Health [NIH], 2013b). When the flow of oxygen-rich blood to a part of the heart is blocked or interrupted, the muscles of that section of the heart begin to die due to lack of oxygen and nutrients. Coronary heart disease (CHD) is the most common cause of a heart attack. CHD results from the buildup of plaque inside the coronary arteries, the major supplier of oxygen-rich blood to the heart.

If someone is experiencing symptoms of a heart attack you should get medical attention immediately by dialing 911 or a local emergency number. Box 6–3 lists the common symptoms of a heart attack. The chest pain may move from the chest to other parts of the body, such as shoulders, arms, back, or neck. Acting quickly when a

heart attack occurs can limit damage to the heart; according to the NIH (2013b), treatment for a heart attack works best when given right after the symptoms occur.

Traumatic Brain Injury (TBI)

Traumatic brain injury (TBI) is caused by a bump, blow, or jolt to the head that disrupts the normal function of the brain. TBI is a major cause of death and disability in the United States and contributes to about 30% of all injury deaths (CDC, 2017). Falls were the leading cause of TBI among children 0–14 years of age, and motor vehicle accidents were the leading cause for adolescents and adults 15–44 years of age (CDC, 2017). TBI can cause impairments in attention, memory, mobility, sensation, or emotion. Common symptoms include loss of consciousness, headache, blurry vision, nausea, dizziness, sensitivity to light, and lack of energy. People with TBI may also demonstrate difficulties in thinking, concentrating, and learning new information. They may also experience mood swings, emotional disturbances, and personality change (CDC, 2017).

When working with individuals with TBI, SLPAs should be aware of warning signs indicating a need for immediate medical attention. The warning signs are listed below (CDC, 2017):

- Loss of consciousness
- Headache that gets worse and does not go away
- Weakness, numbness, or decreased coordination
- Vomiting or nausea
- Slurred speech
- Very drowsy affect or inability to wake up
- Seizures

Box 6–3. Common Symptoms of Heart Attack (NIH, 2013b)

- Chest pain or discomfort (because the heart is not getting enough blood)
- Shortness of breath
- Fatigue with activity
- Sweating
- Nausea

- Increased confusion, restlessness, or agitation
- Other unusual behaviors

Airway Obstruction

Airway obstruction means a blockage in either the upper or lower airway. (NIH, 2013a). The upper airway includes the nasal cavity, pharynx, and larynx, and the lower airway refers to the trachea, bronchial tree, and lungs. Airway obstruction can prevent air from getting into the lungs (partially or totally). This can be fatal and requires immediate medical attention. Airway obstruction may be classified as chronic airway obstruction or acute airway obstruction.

Chronic airway obstruction takes a long time to develop. Examples of chronic airway obstruction are chronic obstructive pulmonary disorders (COPD), emphysema, and abscesses in the airway. Acute airway obstruction occurs quickly. The common causes of acute airway obstruction SLPAs might encounter include inhaling, swallowing, or choking on a foreign object, allergic reactions, or a small object lodged in the nose. Children are at higher risk of foreign object obstruction than are adults (American Society for Gastrointestinal Endoscopy, 2011). Therefore, make sure to keep small items away from children when working with them and constantly monitor them for any unsafe behaviors, such as trying to put small toys into the nose or mouth or swallowing large pieces of food without chewing.

The symptoms of airway obstruction depend on the location of obstruction; Box 6–4 lists common symptoms of airway obstruction. When any of these symptoms are noticed, get medical help immediately.

Box 6–4. Common Symptoms of an Airway Obstruction (NIH, 2013a)

- Difficulty breathing
- Wheezing breathing noise
- Change of skin color (bluish tinge)
- Panic
- Gasping for air

If trained personnel are available onsite, the Heimlich maneuver can be performed for someone choking on a foreign object and CPR can be used for someone who is not breathing.

Seizures

Seizures are caused by sudden disorganized and abnormal electrical activity in the brain, causing muscles to contract and relax repeatedly (U.S. National Library of Medicine, 2012). There are many different types of seizures. Seizures can occur suddenly and can result from many medical conditions, such as brain injury, stroke, brain tumor, liver or kidney failure, high fever, low blood sugar, or drug abuse. Specific symptoms of seizures depend on what part of the brain is involved Box 6–5 lists some common symptoms. Symptoms may stop after a few seconds or minutes, and usually last no longer than 10 to 15 minutes. Table 6–2 lists things that should be taken into consideration during and after a seizure.

Severe Allergic Reactions

Most of the time, people experience minor allergic symptoms when having allergic

---

Box 6–5. Common Symptoms of a Seizure
(U.S. National Library of Medicine, 2012)

- Brief blackout with confusion, drooling, eye movement, grunting, or snoring
- Sudden falling
- Uncontrollable muscle spasms with jerking limbs or shaking of the entire body
- During mild seizures, there may be no muscle contraction or body shaking, and the person may seem to be staring into space

---

Table 6–2. What to Do During and After a Seizure

During a Seizure	After a Seizure
• Stay calm and try to time the seizure.	• Make sure to check for any injuries or difficulty of breathing.
• If the person is pregnant or the seizure lasts longer than 3 minutes, call 911.	• Provide a safe area for the person to rest and do not offer anything to eat or drink until fully conscious and oriented.
• Remove objects that might hurt the person and provide postural support to prevent further injury.	
• If the person is on the ground, position him or her on his or her side to avoid saliva or vomit from entering the airway.	
• Do not attempt to open the mouth and put anything in the mouth; this could pose a choking hazard (O'Hara, 2007).	
• Do not attempt to give anything to drink or eat while the person is having a seizure (O'Hara, 2007).	

Source: Chillemi & Devinsky, 2011.

---

reactions. However, when a severe allergic reaction happens it can be rapid and potentially life threatening (NIH, 2013a). Allergic symptoms occur when a person's own immune system reacts to normally harmless substances. According to the NIH (2013a), the most common allergy triggers include certain foods, medications, pollen, dust mites, mold, insect stings, and latex. Mild allergic symptoms include mild eye irritation, localized skin rash, and congestion. Severe allergic reactions include generalized swelling, wheezing, nausea, vomiting, fast heartbeat, and difficulty breathing.

Before working with clients, an SLPA should review clients' medical history thoroughly to find out if they have any known allergies. Make sure to avoid exposing clients to common allergy triggers. Severe allergic reactions require immediate medical treatment. If someone starts to have a significant allergic reaction, such as difficulty breathing or increased heart rate, call 911 immediately, or go to the nearest emergency room.

SAFETY FOR CHILDREN WITH DISABILITIES

Safe Environment

Children who have limited ability to move, see, hear, or understand pain might not realize that something is unsafe or might have trouble getting away from something unsafe (CDC, n.d.). Always ensure that every area children can reach is safe. It is also important to make sure that therapy materials are safe based on the child's age and current level of function. Additionally, materials should be brought into the therapy room and properly without creating safety hazards.

Safety Equipment

Children with epilepsy may experience sudden drops or falls that can cause head injury. Therefore, having the child wearing a protective helmet may be helpful to minimize consequences of unexpected seizure episodes. As an SLPA, you should talk to your speech-language pathologist (SLP) supervisor to ensure the proper use of safety equipment during therapy.

Safety Talk

Children who have difficulty understating and communicating may have limited ability to learn about danger and safety. It is beneficial to keep instructions simple, model safe behaviors, and have the child practice safety drills on a regular basis. It is also critical to educate all individuals who work with the child about how to communicate with the child if there is any danger. Some simple phrases through

verbal production and augmentative and alternative communication (AAC) can also be taught, such as *"I am hurt," "I need help,"* and so forth.

ADDITIONAL THINGS TO CONSIDER: WORKING WITH CLIENTS WITH SPECIAL MEDICAL NEEDS

SLPAs might work with clients who have special medical needs. It is important to understand these specific needs and provide reasonable accommodation. This section discusses the precautions that SLPAs should be aware of when working with clients who have special medical needs.

Oxygen Use

SLPAs might work with clients who use oxygen. Oxygen is used for individuals who cannot keep appropriate oxygen levels in their blood. Oxygen is a prescribed drug that can improve respiration and decrease the work of heart (National Heart, Lung, and Blood Institute, 2011). Gaseous oxygen is delivered by an oxygen mask or a nasal cannula (Figure 6–2B). Common types of oxygen systems are oxygen concentrators (home and portable units), gas cylinders, and liquid oxygen systems (American Lung Association, 2018). Oxygen concentrators filter oxygen from the air and offer users an unlimited supply of oxygen. Larger units are made for the home (Figure 6–2A); portable oxygen concentrators are similar, but smaller in size making them better for travel. Oxygen cylinders are painted green, which is the universal color for medical oxygen cylinders. They come in many different sizes depending on the needs of

A   B

Figure 6–2. A. EverFlo oxygen concentrator (Respironics) and **B.** Nasal cannula. Images courtesy of Wikimedia Commons.

the patient or client. In general, they range from 2 to 6 feet in height. Once the gas cylinder is empty, it must be refilled by trained personnel. Liquid oxygen systems are large self-contained thermos-like reservoirs which store oxygen at a very cold temperature. When you need oxygen you turn the unit on to warm the oxygen, which turns to a gas as it leaves the reservoir. Liquid oxygen stored in the reservoir needs to be refilled by trained personnel, usually weekly (American Lung Association, 2018).

Although oxygen is nonflammable, it makes things burn much faster than usual. Thus, smoking is prohibited in any room where oxygen is in use. "NO SMOKING" signs are commonly placed in treatment rooms where oxygen is used. Make sure to keep oxygen 6 feet away from any heat sources, such as heat ducts, radiators, space heaters, fireplaces, matches, and lighters. If the client uses a gas cylinder, keep the tank in its stand to avoid rolling or falling—it can injure the client or persons nearby. Also, SLPAs should pay attention to the oxygen tubing because a client may get tangled in the tubing or trip over the tubes, which can interfere with oxygen circulation.

Dysphagia and Aspiration Precautions

Dysphagia is the medical term for swallowing difficulty. Individuals with dysphagia experience difficulty transmitting food or liquid from mouth to stomach due to the tongue, throat (pharynx and larynx), or esophagus not working properly (Groher & Crary, 2010). Dysphagia can result from numerous medical conditions, such as stroke; head injury; progressive neurodegenerative diseases (e.g., Parkinson disease); oral, pharyngeal, and esophageal cancers; and other esophageal diseases. Neurologic diseases can impair the nerves and muscles used for swallowing. Cancers can cause reduced movement of the tongue, pharynx, or larynx. Esophageal disorders can cause the esophagus to become narrower than usual so food

or liquid cannot travel along the esophagus smoothly. Common symptoms and signs of dysphagia are summarized in Box 6–6.

Individuals with dysphagia are at high risk of aspiration. Aspiration refers to the entry of food or liquid into the larynx or lungs. The chances of food or liquid entering the airway increase with dysphagia due to the difficulties transmitting food or liquid from the mouth to the stomach. Things that can be inhaled into the larynx or lungs include saliva, vomited stomach contents, and stomach acid, which can cause substantial damage to lungs and result in pneumonia, lung abscess (a collection of pus in the lungs), airway obstruction, and even death.

ASHA addresses dysphagia in its SLPA scope of practice document (2013, Responsibility Outside the Scope for SLPAs, para. 1), stating that SLPAs, may not:

■ perform procedures that require a high level of clinical acumen and technical skill (e.g., vocal

---

Box 6–6. Common Symptoms and Signs of Dysphagia
(Groher & Crary, 2010)

■ Increasing chewing time
■ Need to swallow multiple times
■ Drooling or liquids leaking through the nose
■ Difficulty or discomfort when swallowing
■ Coughing or choking when swallowing
■ Difficulty breathing during feeding
■ Feeling of food stuck in the throat
■ Frequent clearing of the throat
■ Vomiting swallowed food
■ Loss of appetite
■ Dehydration, malnutrition, or weight loss

tract prosthesis shaping or fitting, vocal tract imaging and oral pharyngeal swallow therapy with bolus material);
■ tabulate or interpret results and observations of feeding and swallowing evaluations performed by SLPs;
■ develop or determine the swallowing strategies or precautions for patients, family, or staff.

As a care provider though, it is important you maintain a safe environment for the individuals you serve. This means when working with individuals with dysphagia, you are aware of the risk of aspiration and follow any precautions recommended by the supervising SLP. Aspiration precautions typically involve one or more of the following:

■ Have the patient or client sit in an upright position when eating food or drinking liquid.
■ Only allow the patient or client to consume food and liquid at the recommended consistency, such as finely chopped food and thickened liquid.
■ Remind the patient or client to chew well and eat slowly.
■ Eliminate distractions, such as turning off the TV or radio.
■ Check the person's mouth after eating for any food residue.
■ Keep the patient or client sitting upright for 30 to 45 minutes after eating.

If the client shows significant symptoms or signs of dysphagia, such as coughing or difficulty breathing, ask her or him to stop eating or drinking immediately, seek medical attention, and notify your supervising SLP.

Tube Feeding

When individuals with dysphagia are at a high risk of aspiration, they can no longer consume an oral diet safely. Alternative feeding methods are implemented to meet their nutrition and hydration needs while continuing to treat their dysphagia. Feeding tubes are the most common approach of alterative feeding (Hanson et al., 2008). Different types of feeding tubes are available depending on the patient's condition and needs. Nasogastric (NG) tubes and percutaneous endoscopic gastrostomy (PEG) tubes are two frequently used types (Groher & Crary, 2010). NG tubes are plastic tubes inserted through the nose, which then pass the throat and go into the stomach. The placement of PEG tubes requires a small incision in the abdomen to insert the tube into the stomach. NG tubes are for short term use, whereas PEG tubes can be used for a longer time or even permanently (Gomes et al., 2010).

Feeding tubes do not prevent aspiration, so it is essential for SLPAs to follow aspiration precautions when working with individuals with dysphagia and feeding tubes. Remember to keep clients with aspiration precautions in an upright position as much as possible. It's very important they do not lay flat when they are getting continuous feeding; lying flat increases the risk of food regurgitation and can further result in aspiration. If there is any leakage or blockage of the feeding tubes, contact the individuals' caregiver(s) or trained personnel for further assistance.

Ventilator Use and Tracheotomy

According to the NIH (2013c), a ventilator is a machine that supports breathing for those who cannot breathe independently. They are mainly used in hospitals, though they can also be used in long-term care facilities or the long-term in the home. Ventilators push oxygen into the lungs, remove carbon dioxide from the body, helping the patient breathe more easily. Examples of diseases and conditions that can affect lung function and lead to the use of a ventilator include pneumonia, lung diseases, COPD, brain injury, stroke, or laryngeal injuries.

A tracheostomy is a surgical procedure that creates a hole through the front of the neck and into the trachea (NIH, 2013c). The hole can be temporary or permanent. After placing a tube through the hole to provide an airway, breathing occurs through the tube rather than through the nose and mouth (Figure 6–3). One common reason for having a tracheostomy is if a ventilator needs to be used for more than a few weeks. The ventilator can connect to the tracheostomy tube to support breathing. Another possible reason for a tracheostomy tube is to help clear mucus or secretion from the lungs.

Because air no longer passes through the vocal folds, individuals who have a tracheostomy cannot easily use their voice. There are many ways to assist individuals in producing sound for speech. Certain tracheostomy tubes and many different types of valves can redirect airflow to produce speech. Trained SLPs can recommend options for communication and provide training to clients in the use of different devices to meet their communication needs.

Figure 6–3. Diagram of a tracheostoma and tracheostomy tube. *Note.* 1 = vocal folds; 2 = thyroid cartilage; 3 = cricoid cartilage; 4 = tracheal cartilages; 5 = balloon cuff. Image courtesy of Wikimedia Commons.

REFERENCES

American Heart Association. (2017). *2017 AHA guidelines update for cardiopulmonary resuscitation (CPR) and emergency cardiovascular care (ECC)*. Retrieved from https://eccguidelines .heart.org/index.php/circulation/cpr-ecc-guidelines-2/

American Lung Association. (2018). *Oxygen therapy*. Retrieved from http://www.lung .org/lung-disease/copd/living-with-copd/ supplemental-oxygen.html

American Red Cross. (2011). *American Red Cross first aid/CPR/AED participant's manual* (5th ed.). St. Paul, MN: Staywell.

American Society for Gastrointestinal Endoscopy. (2011). Guideline: Management of ingested foreign bodies and food impactions. *Gastrointestinal Endoscopy, 73*(16), 1085–1091. doi:10.1016/j.gie.2010.11.010

American Speech-Language-Hearing Association (ASHA). (n.d.). *Aphasia.* Retrieved from https://www.asha.org/PRPSpecificTopic.aspx?folderid=8589934663&section=Assessment

American Speech-Language-Hearing Association. (2005). *Quality indicators for professional service programs in audiology and speech-language pathology.* doi:10.1044/policy.ST2005-00186

American Speech-Language-Hearing Association. (2013). *Speech-language pathology assistant scope of practice.* Retrieved from http://www.asha.org/policy

Centers for Disease Control and Prevention (CDC). (n.d.). *Child safety: Keeping children with disabilities safe.* Retrieved from https://www.cdc.gov/ncbddd/disabilityandsafety/child-safety.html

Centers for Disease Control and Prevention. (2008). *Guideline for disinfection and sterilization in healthcare facilities.* Retrieved from http://www.cdc.gov/hicpac/pdf/guidelines/disinfection_nov_2008.pdf

Centers for Disease Control and Prevention. (2011). *Guide to infection prevention for outpatient settings: Minimum expectations for safe care.* Retrieved from https://www.cdc.gov/hai/settings/outpatient/outpatient-care-guidelines.html

Centers for Disease Control and Prevention. (2012). *Respiratory hygiene/cough etiquette in healthcare settings.* Retrieved from http://www.cdc.gov/flu/professionals/infectioncontrol/resphygiene.htm

Centers for Disease Control and Prevention. (2013a). *NIOSH-approved particulate filtering facepiece respirators.* Retrieved from http://www.cdc.gov/niosh/npptl/topics/respirators/disp_part/default.html

Centers for Disease Control and Prevention. (2013b). *Protocol for hand hygiene and glove use observations.* Retrieved from http://www.cdc.gov/dialysis/prevention-tools/Protocol-hand-hygiene-glove-observations.html

Centers for Disease Control and Prevention (CDC). (2016). *Hand hygiene in healthcare settings.* Retrieved from https://www.cdc.gov/handhygiene/providers/index.html

Centers for Disease Control and Prevention (CDC). (2017). *TBI: Get the facts.* Retrieved from https://www.cdc.gov/traumaticbraininjury/get_the_facts.html

Chillemi, S., & Devinsky, O. (2011). Quick tips: What to do if someone has a seizure. *Neurology Now, 7*(2), 12.

Cronan, K. (2010). *First aid kit.* Retrieved from http://kidshealth.org/parent/firstaid_safe/home/firstaid_kit.html?tracking=83967_G#cat31

Gomes, C., Lustosa, S., Matos, D., Andriolo, R., Waisberg, D., & Waisberg, J. (2010). Percutaneous endoscopic gastrostomy versus nasogastric tube feeding for adults with swallowing disturbances. *Cochrane Database of Systematic Reviews, 10*(11), CD008096. doi:10.1002/14651858

Groher, M., & Crary, M. (2010). *Dysphagia: Clinical management in adults and children.* Maryland Heights, MO: Mosby Elsevier.

Hanson, L., Garrett, J., Lewis, C., Phifer, N., Jackman, A., & Carey, T. (2008). Physicians' expectations of benefit from tube feeding. *Journal of Palliative Medicine, 11*(8), 1130–1134. doi:10.1089/jpm.2008.0033

Healthcare Infection Control Practices Advisory Committee (HICPAC). (2017, March). *Core infection prevention and control practices for safe healthcare delivery in all settings recommendations.* Retrieved from https://www.cdc.gov/hicpac/recommendations/core-practices.html

National Heart, Lung, and Blood Institute. (2011). *Respiratory failure.* Retrieved from https://www.nhlbi.nih.gov/health-topics/respiratory-failure

National Institutes of Health. (2013a). *Why food allergy is a priority for NIAID.* Retrieved from https://www.niaid.nih.gov/diseases-conditions/food-allergy-priority-niaid

National Institutes of Health (NIH). (2013b). *What is a heart attack?* Retrieved from https://www.nia.nih.gov/health/what-heart-attack

National Institutes of Health (NIH). (2013c). *Ventilator/ventilator support.* Retrieved from https://www.nhlbi.nih.gov/health-topics/ventilatorventilator-support

National Stroke Association. (2013). *Stroke 101 fact sheet.* Retrieved from http://www.stroke.org/site/DocServer/STROKE_101_Fact_Sheet.pdf?docID=4541

Occupational Safety and Health Administration. (2003). *Personal protective equipment*. Retrieved from https://www.osha.gov/SLTC/personalprotectiveequipment/

O'Hara, K. A. (2007). First aid for seizures: The importance of education and appropriate response. *Journal of Child Neurology, 22,* 30S–37S.

Siegel, J., Rhinehart, E., Jackson, M., Chiarello, L., & the Healthcare Infection Control Practices Advisory Committee. (2007). *2007 Guideline for isolation precautions: Preventing transmission of infectious agents in healthcare settings*. Retrieved from http://www.cdc.gov/hicpac/pdf/isolation/Isolation2007.pdf

Signore, A. (2013). About inflammation and infection. *EJNMMI Research, 3*(8). doi:10.1186/2191-219X-3-8

U.S. National Library of Medicine, National Institutes of Health. (2012). *Seizures*. Retrieved from http://www.nlm.nih.gov/medlineplus/ency/article/003200.htm.

U.S. Food and Drug Administration. (n.d.). *General hospital devices and supplies: Medical gloves*. Retrieved from https://www.fda.gov/MedicalDevices/ProductsandMedicalProcedures/GeneralHospitalDevicesandSupplies/ucm056077.htm

World Health Organization (WHO). (2009). *WHO guidelines on hand hygiene in healthcare*. Retrieved from http://apps.who.int/iris/bitstream/handle/10665/44102/9789241597906_eng.pdf?sequence=1

APPENDIX 6–A
CDC Cleaning and Infection Guidelines (Schools)

HOW TO CLEAN AND DISINFECT SCHOOLS TO HELP SLOW THE SPREAD OF FLU

Cleaning and disinfecting are part of a broad approach to preventing infectious diseases in schools. To help slow the spread of influenza (flu), the first line of defense is getting vaccinated. Other measures include staying home when sick, covering coughs and sneezes, and frequent hand washing. Below are tips on how to slow the spread of flu specifically through cleaning and disinfecting.

1. Know the difference between cleaning, disinfecting, and sanitizing.

   Cleaning removes germs, dirt, and impurities from surfaces or objects Cleaning works by using soap (or detergent) and water to physically remove germs from surfaces. This process does not necessarily kill germs, but by removing them it lowers their numbers and the risk of spreading infection.

   Disinfecting kills germs on surfaces or objects. Disinfecting works by using chemicals to kill germs. This process does not necessarily clean dirty surfaces or remove germs, but killing germs on a surface after cleaning further lowers the risk of spreading infection.

   Sanitizing lowers the number of germs on surfaces or objects to a safe level, as judged by public health standards or requirements. This process **works by either cleaning or disinfecting** surfaces or objects to lower the risk of spreading infection.

2. Clean and disinfect surfaces and objects that are touched often.

   Follow your school's standard procedures for routine cleaning and disinfecting. Typically, this means daily sanitizing of surfaces and objects that are touched often, such as desks, countertops, doorknobs, computer keyboards, hands-on learning items, faucet handles, phones, and toys. Some schools may also require daily disinfecting these items. Standard procedures often call for disinfecting specific areas of the school, like bathrooms.

   Immediately clean surfaces and objects that are visibly soiled. If surfaces or objects are soiled with body fluids or blood, use gloves and other standard precautions to avoid coming into contact with the fluid. Remove the spill, and then clean and disinfect the surface.

3. Simply do routine cleaning and disinfecting.

   It is important to match your cleaning and disinfecting activities to the types of germs you want to remove or kill. Most studies have shown that the flu virus can live and potentially infect a person for up to 48 hours after being deposited on a surface. However, it is not necessary to close schools to clean or disinfect every surface in the building to slow the spread of flu. Also, if students and staff are dismissed because the school cannot function normally (e.g., high absenteeism during a flu outbreak), it is not necessary to do extra cleaning and disinfecting.

Flu viruses are relatively fragile, so standard cleaning and disinfecting practices are sufficient to remove or kill them. Special cleaning and disinfecting processes, including wiping down walls and ceilings, frequently using room air deodorizers, and fumigating, are not necessary or recommended. These processes can irritate eyes, noses, throats, and skin; aggravate asthma; and cause other serious side effects.

4. Clean and disinfect correctly.

   Always follow label directions on cleaning products and disinfectants. Wash surfaces with a general household cleaner to remove germs. Rinse with water, and follow with an EPA-registered disinfectant to kill germs. Read the label to make sure it states that the EPA has approved the product for effectiveness against influenza A virus.

   If a surface is not visibly dirty, you can clean it with an EPA-registered product that both cleans (removes germs) and disinfects (kills germs) instead. Be sure to read the label directions carefully, as there may be a separate procedure for using the product as a cleaner or as a disinfectant. Disinfection usually requires the product to remain on the surface for a certain period of time (e.g., letting it stand for 3 to 5 minutes).

   Use disinfecting wipes on electronic items that are often touched, such as phones and computers. Pay close attention to the directions for using disinfecting wipes. It may be necessary to use more than one wipe to keep the surface wet for the stated length of contact time. Make sure that the electronics can withstand the use of liquids for cleaning and disinfecting.

5. Use products safely.

   Pay close attention to hazard warnings and directions on product labels. Cleaning products and disinfectants often call for the use of gloves or eye protection. For example, gloves should always be worn to protect your hands when working with bleach solutions.

   Do not mix cleaners and disinfectants unless the labels indicate it is safe to do so. Combining certain products (such as chlorine bleach and ammonia cleaners) can result in serious injury or death.

   Ensure that custodial staff, teachers, and others who use cleaners and disinfectants read and understand all instruction labels and understand safe and appropriate use. This might require that instructional materials and training be provided in other languages.

6. Handle waste properly

Follow your school's standard procedures for handling waste, which may include wearing gloves. Place no-touch wastebaskets where they are easy to use. Throw disposable items used to clean surfaces and items in the trash immediately after use. Avoid touching used tissues and other waste when emptying wastebaskets. Wash your hands with soap and water after emptying wastebaskets and touching used tissues and similar waste.

Source: U.S. Department of Health and Human Services, Centers for Disease Control and Prevention. Available from http://www.cdc.gov/flu/school

PART II

Skills Development

CHAPTER 7

Deciphering Lesson Plans and Goals

Our goals can only be reached through a vehicle of a plan, in which we must fervently believe, and upon which we must vigorously act. There is no other route to success.

—Pablo Picasso (famous artist)

As discussed in Chapter 1, one of the job responsibilities within the scope of duties of a speech-language pathology assistant (SLPA) is to follow treatment plans and protocols developed by the speech-language pathologist (SLP; American Speech-Language-Hearing Association [ASHA], 2013a). Specifically, ASHA states that SLPAs may execute specific components of a treatment plan if (ASHA, n.d.-a, Key Issues, Scope of SLPAs, para. 1):

■ The goals and objectives listed on the treatment plan and implemented by the SLPA are only those within the SLPA's scope of practice and are tasks the SLP has determined the SLPA has the training and skill to perform.

■ The SLP provides at least the minimum specified level of supervision to ensure quality of care to all persons served.

The amount of supervision may vary and must depend on the complexity of the case and the experience of the assistant.

Before services can be implemented by an SLPA, it is the responsibility of the supervising SLP to develop an individualized treatment plan for each client. The first step in this process is an assessment (also known as an evaluation). Assessments are conducted solely by an SLP (ASHA, 2013b). If treatment is recommended, the SLP develops a treatment plan in which specific treatment goals are outlined. In some settings, assessment results and a treatment plan are summarized in a single document, and in other settings in separate documents. The appendices of this chapter contain sample reports from an educational setting, including an individualized education plan (IEP; Appendix 7–A), private practice (Appendix 7–B), and medical settings (Appendix 7–C). In some settings, these documents may be on paper and in other settings, information is stored and accessed electronically (Krebs, 2008).

As discussed in Chapter 3, in all settings, these documents and the specifics of a client's treatment are strictly confidential and not to be shared with unauthorized individuals (ASHA, 2013b). You may not bring these documents home to review, nor may you send them or discuss their content with anyone not authorized to access this information. As an SLPA, you should familiarize yourself with the form of documentation used in your setting and how to access it. If you are asked to provide services to a client, you should review the client's assessment report(s) and treatment plan in detail. Be sure to ask your supervising SLP if you have any questions about it.

LESSON PLANS

After a treatment plan is developed by your supervising SLP, the next step is to explore specific details on how to implement the plan for each individual client. How this information is conveyed to you will vary across settings and supervisors. In some settings, a lesson plan is used to outline additional information needed to implement treatment (ASHA, 2009). It may be that you are required to develop a draft of this plan for your supervisor to review, prior to implementing treatment. In other settings, this plan will be developed for you by your supervising SLP. In both instances, collaboration between you and your supervising SLP is required.

The concept of a lesson plan is borrowed from the field of education and was originally designed as a detailed description of the instruction to be provided by a teacher during a given class session (Karges-Bone, 2000). When applied to the field of speech-language pathology, lesson plans highlight important details and procedures for a single treatment session or to be provided over a short period (e.g., over 1 or 2 weeks; Hegde & Davis, 2010; Meyer, 2004). A lesson plan recommended by ASHA (2009) for use by SLPAs has several columns, including the core components of the treatment goals (Goals And Objectives), a description of the materials and equipment needed that session (Materials/Equipment), a description of the activity or task to be used (Activity/Task), and columns used to suggest modifications (Make It Easier/Make It More Difficult). Commonly, the column for modifications is also referred to as "Prompts/Modifications." Lesson plans can also include information on the client's performance (Data Collection), which may include a description of data to be collected that session and a summary of the client's actual performance during the session,.

Figure 7–1 is an example of a lesson plan containing these components. Depending on the setting, some or all of these categories are used. The companion website of this textbook has additional blank copies of lesson plans applicable for SLPA use. The following sections address each component of the plan in greater detail. It is important that you clearly understand each component before you have any contact with a client. The importance of this cannot be overemphasized. To understand it in detail, as the picture and title of this chapter suggests, you must decipher the information very carefully.

Goals and Objectives

The Goals and Objectives section of a lesson plan lists the goals and objectives to be targeted during the treatment session(s). Understanding goals and objectives can be very challenging for a new SLPA, as the language used is often unfamiliar and complex. Take heart, though: with time and exposure to this terminology, the process gets easier. Goals and objectives are important because they guide the selection of therapy materials, content, and procedures (Mager, 1997). They also serve as the basis for determining if a behavior has been accomplished and, importantly, provide those involved (including the client and the clinician) a full description of the desired outcome(s) of treatment (Mager, 1997). In some settings, they are also used directly for insurance reimbursement purposes (Cornett, 2010). Although SLPAs do not write or modify

goals, it is still valuable to review their format to help you to decipher them.

Defining Goals

Treatment goals are statements of an outcome to be obtained. Traditionally defined, goals describe a behavior to be accomplished over the course of treatment (Roth & Worthington, 2001). Goals may or may not state a terminal behavior to be accomplished but generally are targeted over months or often, as in the case of a school setting, within an academic term. For example, a traditionally defined goal might be, "The client will read at grade level." By their nature, goals are broad statements of behavior. However, increasingly, the term long-term goal is used to identify the behavior to be accomplished, additional measurable terms (e.g., increase, decrease, maintain), and an expected ending level of performance, such as, "The student will increase the number of conversational topics that he spontaneously initiates from one to four (with no verbal or other prompts) in a student-adult conversation" (Minneapolis Public Schools, 2009). In some settings, the terms *goal* and *long-term goal* are used interchangeably, and in other settings, a general goal is followed by a set of specific long-term goals. The term *annual goal* denotes a goal that is to be accomplished that year, such as "By (annual IEP date), [the student] will listen attentively in class by using appropriate eye contact, body language, and/or proximity during oral communication in [8 out of 10] opportunities" (Porter & Steffin, 2006, p. 13).

Defining Objectives

Objectives accompany goals and are a series of steps needed to accomplish the

Client Name: Joseph Jones					
SLPA: Sarah S. Assistant			Teacher/Room #: Wilson 12		
Session Date(s): Week of 2/18/2018			Supervising SLP: Samantha A. Supervisor		
Goal/Objective	Activity/Task	Materials/ Equipment	Make it Easier	Make it More Difficult	Data Collection
Joseph will produce /ʃ/ in the initial positions of words with 90% accuracy, across 10 attempts in 2 separate sessions.	**Go Fish:** Have Joseph ask for cards with words containing the /ʃ/ in the initial position (e.g., ship, shell, she). If he accurately produces the target, reinforce this by stating yes I have a ____, or, No I don't have a ____ (as applicable), emphasizing the /ʃ/ sound. If he inaccurately produces the target sound, model a correct version and an incorrect version and ask him to clarify by re-attempting (e.g., "did you want a ____ (/ʃ/ accurately produced) or a ____ (/ʃ/ distorted production?"	Go Fish cards containing CVC words with /ʃ/ in the initial position of words (e.g., ship, shell, she) Reminder card with picture of hand over lip to represent /ʃ/ Mirror	Point to the reminder card and/or model lip rounding before each production and after production error. Give him cards with the word written on it and the /ʃ/ underlined	Require him to have accurate production for the target word AND Go Fish When he lays down his pairs, reference it as "shelving" and have him name the pairs he obtained in the sentence, "I'll shelve 2 ____, with correct production of /ʃ/ in shelve and the target word.	+ = Accuracy (no cues/modification) +C = Accurate with cues. Note cues • M = verbal model • V = visual reminder • W = Written word CA = close approximation − = Inaccurate, Despite cues

Figure 7–1. Sample SLPA lesson plan.

goal's desired behavior. Objectives are also referred to as short-term objectives or, in some settings, are called *short-term goals* or *benchmarks*. Objectives use very precise and measurable language to state not only the behavior to be obtained but also at what level, by when, and under what conditions (Meyer, 2004; Roth & Paul, 2007; Roth & Worthington, 2001). Box 7–1 lists three key components of objectives: the performance (or do statement), the condition, and the *criterion* (singular) or *criteria* (plural; Meyer, 2004; Roth & Paul, 2007; Roth & Worthington, 2001).

Box 7–1. Key Components of Behavioral Objectives

Performance: States what a client is expected to do to demonstrate mastery of the objective, including the *quality*[1] and *nature*[1] of performance. This is sometimes referred to as the "do" statement (e.g., the client will . . .).[2]

Examples:

Independently say the names of primary colors

Legibly write the numbers 1 to 10

Spontaneously greet members of the social group

Accurately produce the phoneme /t/ in the final positions of words

Condition: States what the client will be provided with (or denied) when performing the behavior, including (as applicable) terms to define the location,[1] with whom,[1] and given what type of assistance.[1]

Examples:

In the community, with a typical peer

During a classroom group-reading activity, given a story starter

In a one-on-one setting, given a verbal model from the clinician

In response to a written command, without verbal cues to initiate

Criterion: States how the objective will be evaluated and in some cases a time frame in which the behavior will be accomplished, including as applicable the frequency, duration, accuracy, latency, speed, and intensity of a behavior.[1]

Examples:

With 80% accuracy, given at least 20 attempts

Within 2 minutes of a verbal prompt, in 8 of 10 opportunities

For 2 minutes on two separate occasions

Appendix 7–D contains examples of goals and objectives from real-world settings.

To decipher goals and objectives, ask yourself specific questions about what is written and what additional information is needed, such as the questions listed in Box 7–2. The performance statement needs to be something that you can actually observe, meaning you can see or hear it (Meyer, 2004; Roth & Paul, 2007). If the performance is not something observable, the objective cannot be implemented. For example, verbs that describe performance, such as *understand, analyze,* and *process,* are not something you can see or hear, and as such, without further clarification you would have no way of knowing if the cli-ent was performing the required task(s). Hence, in terms of the performance (or do) portion of an objective, ask yourself the following:

1. Is the performance stated?
2. What is the performance?
3. Is the performance observable (e.g., can I see it or hear it)?
4. What additional information is needed?

Similarly, a condition statement must be something that you as an SLPA can reproduce.

For example, in an objective targeting pragmatics, the condition of "when speaking with grade-level peers" cannot

---

Box 7–2. Deciphering Goals/Objectives: Questions to Ask

PERFORMANCE

Is the performance stated? ☐ YES ☐ NO

What is the performance required? _____

Can I observe the performance? ☐ YES ☐ NO

Additional information needed? ☐ YES ☐ NO

CONDITION

Is the condition stated? ☐ YES ☐ NO

What is the condition? _____

Can I replicate the condition? ☐ YES ☐ NO

Additional information needed? ☐ YES ☐ NO

CRITERION

Is the criterion stated? ☐ YES ☐ NO

What is the criterion? _____

Can I measure the criterion? ☐ YES ☐ NO

Additional information needed? ☐ YES ☐ NO

be replicated in a one-on-one session with the clinician. Similarly, if a fluency goal included a condition of "during episodes of blocking" but you do not know what an episode of blocking is, you would not be able to replicate that condition. As such, it is important to ask yourself the following:

1. Is the condition stated?
2. What is the condition?
3. Can I replicate the condition?
4. What additional information is needed?

Lastly, the criterion of an objective must be stated in a way that you can measure it. The information you record is often referred to as *data*. Data is the information that is typically listed under "Data Collection" in the lesson plan. In order for you to record the client's performance on a given task, the criterion portion of an objective must be something that you can effectively measure. For example, if a criterion states, "with fewer than one stuttered word," but you are not familiar with what to count as a stuttered word, you will not be able to record the client's performance accurately. Similarly, if the criterion calls for "80% accuracy" in the accurate production of /r/, but you cannot accurately distinguish between correct, partially correct, and incorrect production of /r/, you will not be accurate in recording information about the client's performance. It also is impossible to record data accurately if parts of the criterion are missing. As such, in deciphering the criterion of an objective, ask yourself the following:

1. Is the criterion stated?
2. What is the criterion?
3. Can I measure the criterion (e.g., collect data)?
4. What additional information is needed?

Any time you have a question or need additional clarification, be sure to ask your supervisor before you implement any treatment activity. The companion website of this textbook contains a sample worksheet with these questions. Appendix 7–D contains sample goals and objectives from real-world settings. The sample reports in Appendices 7–A to 7–C also contain samples of goals and objectives. A good way to develop your skills in deciphering goals and objectives is to use these examples and identify the performance, condition, and criterion, asking important questions about each.

Activity/Task

This section of a lesson plan contains information relative to the type of activity or task to be used during treatment in addressing a specific goal or objective. Although objectives are detailed in their format and language, they can often be addressed utilizing a variety of activities or tasks, selected based on the client's interests, age, and specific needs. For example, consider the objective, "The client will request objects by pointing to an icon in his AAC device, in 9 of 10 opportunities." If this is implemented with a 6-year-old boy with autism who likes trains, an activity to target this goal might be to have the client build a train track by requesting different colors and types of trains, track, and other building materials, using a train theme page from his AAC notebook. In contrast, if this same objective is implemented with an adult with aphasia who enjoys cooking, the activity may be to bake a cake following a recipe and requesting needed items from the cooking page on her voice output AAC device.

Your supervising SLP will assist you in determining the type of activity or task most appropriate for each client. The following chapters on play and literacy (Chapter 16), speech sound remediation (Chapter 13), and group therapy (Chapter 12) each provide some sample tasks and activities. A review of sample activities across all ages and disorders is beyond the scope of this book; however, here are a few suggestions that will help familiarize you with an activity/task prior to implementing treatment:

1. *Self-study.* Before you engage in treatment activities with a new client, review treatment information specific to the client's disorder and unique presentation. Many resources, both online and in traditional treatment textbooks for communicative disorders, provide both a general framework of treatment techniques and a list of sample activities/tasks to use with specific treatment objectives or approaches. If you are not familiar with how to access this information, ask your supervising SLP for assistance.

2. *Observe.* Observe your supervising SLP engaging in the activity/task prior to implementing it yourself. This is valuable in helping you understand nuances that are not easily conveyed in a written description. Be sure to take notes so that you can refer back to them prior to implementing treatment.

3. *Role-play.* Role-play the activity/task with your supervising SLP. This is also an excellent way to become comfortable with implementing an activity/task. Be sure to play the role of the therapist, as this is the role you will play when implementing treatment.

4. *Ask questions.* During supervisory conferences, be sure to clarify any questions you may have about a specific activity or task. Ask too, about the "whys" of the activity/task. This will help you understand the SLP's rationale for selecting that particular activity or task.

Materials/Equipment

This section of a lesson plan lists any materials or equipment needed to implement treatment. This could be wide ranging, including items specific to the activity or task itself, such as pictures, worksheets, toys and games, tokens for reinforcement. It may also include items needed to record a client's performance, such as a specific score sheet or audio recorder. Materials are used specifically to elicit a target response are referred to as *stimuli* (plural) or *stimulus* (singular), You should ensure you have these items ready and accessible before the treatment session begins. Be sure to review your materials and equipment well ahead of time to make sure they are in good working order. This ensures that no time is wasted locating, repairing, or troubleshooting missing items or malfunctioning equipment once the session begins. Chapter 10 provides some general principles for selecting appropriate stimuli, as do Chapters 12, 13, and 16. As discussed in Chapter 6, remember that all equipment and materials used must be properly cleaned for use in any treatment session.

Prompts and Modifications (Also Known as Make It Easier/ Make It More Difficult)

This section of an SLPA lesson plan includes any suggested modifications to the activity or task that could be used to reduce or increase task demands, including any recommended prompts or assistance appropriate to the task. Remember, treatment is a dynamic process. It may be that a given activity or task needs to be adjusted slightly to increase the client's participation and thereby address the desired objective. These modifications are not intended to alter the treatment goals or objectives, but rather to enhance participation in the designated activity or task. As with all aspects of a client's treatment, these should be discussed with the supervising SLP. Recognize as well that formats of a lesson plan vary across settings,

and not all supervising SLPs will use or require this information on a lesson plan. If not, discuss any needed modifications with your supervising SLP to ensure that you understand how to modify an activity or task appropriately so that it remains consistent with the SLP's treatment plan for that particular client. Chapter 10 provides information on prompts and cues, as well as a discussion on the use of reinforcement in shaping behaviors. These are an important part of task/activity modification. Box 7–3 has additional examples of techniques to modify an activity or task, by altering the time constraints, tasks demands, or reinforcement. Not all

---

Box 7–3. Potential Modifications in Activity/Task

1. Increase or decrease time constraints

   EXAMPLES

   - Give the client more time to respond (make it easier)
   - Require a quicker response (make it more difficult)
   - Give more breaks between responses (make it easier)
   - Require more responses in a shorter period (e.g., fewer breaks) (make it more difficult)

2. Increase or decrease the task demands

   EXAMPLES

   - Require a fully correct response (make it more difficult)
   - Accept a partially correct response (make it easier)
   - Require a shorter or less complex response (make it easier)
   - Require a longer or more complex response (make it more difficult)

3. Increase or decrease the reinforcement provided

   EXAMPLES

   - Provide reinforcement after every response (make it easier)
   - Provide intermittent reinforcement (make it more difficult)
   - Provide tangible reinforcement (make it easier)
   - Provide token reinforcement (make it more difficult)

modifications are equally applicable to all objectives, particularly if the modification changes the task sufficiently to alter a treatment objective's condition, performance, or criterion. That is not the purpose of modifications. For example, if the objective were, "The student will use present progressive tense when describing pictures not visible to the clinician in 18 of 20 attempts," but you made the task easier by requiring the client to say a list of 20 verbs in present progressive tense after you say them, the activity would no longer be targeting the desired objective. As an SLPA, you must not modify elements of a treatment activity or task in any way that alters the treatment plan (ASHA, 2013a).

Data Collection

Recording data about the client's performance is critical (Mowrer, 1982). Accurate data collection is particularly important in that, as an SLPA, you are the eyes and ears for your supervising SLP when you are implementing treatment and she or he is not present to observe the client's performance. The Data Collection section of a lesson plan might include a description of any specific or important aspects of information recorded that session. In some cases, the lesson plan itself may also have space to record the data from a specific session. In that case, it doubles as a data collection sheet. Chapter 8 discusses data collection in detail and Chapter 9 addresses how to summarize this information effectively in a note about treatment.

REFERENCES

American Speech-Language-Hearing Association. (n.d.-a). *Speech-language pathology assistants*. Retrieved from https://www.asha.org/Practice-Portal/Professional-Issues/Speech-Language-Pathology-Assistants/

American Speech-Language-Hearing Association (ASHA). (n.d.-b). *Writing measurable goals and objectives*. Retrieved from http://www.asha.org/uploadedFiles/Writing-Measurable-Goals-and-Objectives.pdf

American Speech-Language-Hearing Association (ASHA). (2009). *Practical tools and forms for supervising speech-language pathology assistants*. Rockville, MD: Author.

American Speech-Language-Hearing Association (ASHA). (2013a). *Speech-language pathology assistant scope of practice*. Retrieved from https://www.asha.org/policy/sp2013-00337/

American Speech-Language-Hearing Association (ASHA). (2013b). *Confidentiality*. Retrieved from https://www.asha.org/Practice/ethics/Confidentiality/

Cornett, B. S. (2010). Health care reform and speech-language pathology practice. *ASHA Leader, 15,* 14–17. doi:10.1044/leader.FTR2.15092010.14

Hegde, M. N., & Davis, D. (2010). *Clinical methods and practicum in speech-language pathology* (5th ed.). Clifton Park, NY: Delmar.

Karges-Bone, L. (2000). *Lesson planning: Long-range and short-range models for grades K–6.* Boston, MA: Allyn & Bacon.

Krebs, J. M. (2008). Paper, paper everywhere? How to go paperless in your private practice. *ASHA Leader, 13,* 20–22. doi:10.1044/leader.FTR3.13122008.20

Mager, R. F. (1997). *Preparing instructional objectives: A critical tool in the development of effective instruction.* Atlanta, GA: Center for Effective Performance Press.

Meyer, S. M. (2004). *Survival guide for beginning speech-language clinician* (2nd ed.). Austin, TX: Pro-Ed.

Minneapolis Public Schools. (2009). *Consensus points on language goals.* Retrieved from https://www.asha.org/uploadedFiles/Consensus-Points-on-Language-Goals.pdf

Mower, D. E. (1982). *Methods of modifying speech behaviors: Learning theory in speech pathology.* Prospect Heights, IL: Waveland.

Porter, J., & Steffin, B. (2006). *Speech-language pathology goals and objectives written to the California standards.* Retrieved from https://prakovic.edublogs.org/files/2015/06/SLPGoalsandObjectivesupdate-1plo8wj.pdf

Roth, F., & Paul, R. (2007). Communication intervention. In R. Paul & P. Cascella (Eds.), *Introduction to clinical methods in communication disorders* (pp. 157–178). Baltimore, MD: Paul H. Brookes.

Roth, F. P., & Worthington, C. K. (2001). *Treatment resource manual for speech-language pathologists* (2nd ed.). Albany, NY: Delmar.

CHAPTER ENDNOTES

1. ASHA (n.d.-b)
2. Roth & Paul (2007); Roth & Worthington (2001)

Educational Setting—Sample Reports

ABC School District

Initial Speech-Language Assessment Report

Student: XXXXXXX
DOB: XXXXXXX
Parents: XXXXXXX
Address: XXXXXXX
Assessment conducted by: XXXXXXX, CCC-SLP
Assessment dates: March 16, 2018, March 17, 2018, and March 18, 2018
Report date: April 2018

Reason for Referral:
This assessment was conducted at the request of the child's parents. Specifically, they reported that XXXXXX is difficult to understand without context, uses short utterances, and is easily frustrated. His parents indicated that XXXXXX's frustration is at least in part because he is unable to express his wants and needs.

Brief Background Information:
XXXXXX is a 2-year, 11-month-old boy whose primary language is English, although some French is spoken in the home. He resides with his parents and a younger sibling. There is no history of ear infections and no reported serious accidents or illnesses. The family receives private, in-home behavioral therapy to address XXXXXX's disruptive behavior and tantrums.

Behavioral Observations:
XXXXXX presented as a pleasant, inquisitive, and well-behaved child. Good rapport was established with this examiner after a brief "warming up" period. XXXXXX's father remained present during the assessment. XXXXXX participated fully in the assessment process and completed all necessary testing to obtain present levels of speech and language function. Testing took place over three sessions lasting approximately 1 hour each, and XXXXXX received snacks and breaks as needed.

Over the course of assessment, XXXXXX was easily distracted; however, when redirected, he was able to re-engage with this examiner and return to the task. He appeared to put forth his best effort during the course of testing and appeared to understand the directions presented by this examiner.

Assessment Results:

Assessment was conducted at a local elementary school in the speech-language therapy room. Test materials have been validated for the specific purposes for which they were used. Assessment results are considered a valid estimate of XXXXXX's current level of performance.

Assessments Administered:

Parent Interview

Informal Language Observation

Clinical Assessment of Articulation and Phonology (CAAP)

Receptive One-Word Picture Vocabulary Test (ROWPVT)

Expressive One-Word Picture Vocabulary Test (EOWPVT)

Preschool Language Scales-5 (PLS-5)

Language Sample

Oral-Peripheral Examination

Informal Observation (voice, fluency, and intelligibility)

(See Appendices at the end of the report for test validity statements and test score description)

Articulation:

Speech Production Abilities:

The Clinical Assessment of Articulation and Phonology (CAAP) was administered to assess XXXXXX's speech production. The CAAP is a norm-referenced assessment that measures articulation and phonology in preschool and school-age children ages 2 years, 6 months to 8 years, 11 months. The results of this assessment follow:

Consonant Inventory Score	55
Standard Score	64
Percentile	3

XXXXXX's standard score of 64 is significantly below average.

Performance Summary:

Single phonemes: As demonstrated in the following chart, which classifies phonemes by typical age of acquisition, XXXXXX's performance on the CAAP revealed the following specific articulation errors:

Typical Age of Mastery*	Phonemes	Misarticulated Sound/Location	Error Example
4 Years	/p/, /b/, /m/, /n/, /w/, /h/, /k/, /g/, /f/, /d/, /j/	/p/ final position /b/ final position /g/ final position /f/ final position	[shee] for /sheep/ [we] for /web/ [do] for /dog/ [kni] for /knife/
6 Years	/ŋ/, /t/, /l/, /r/	/ŋ/ final position /t/ initial and final position /l/ final position	[ki] for /king/ [ees] for /teeth/ [da] for /gate/ [heza] for /seal/
7 Years	/sh/, /ch/, /dg/, /th/	/ch/ final position /dg/ final position /th/ (voiceless) initial and final positions	[raw] for /watch/ [ka] for /cadge/ [fum] for /thumb/ [ees] for /teeth/
8 Years	/v/, /s/, /z/, /ð/	/v/ final position /s/ initial /z/ initial and final /th/ (voiced) initial and final positions	[hi] for /hive/ [heza] for /seal/ [do] for /zoo/ [chee] for /cheese/ [vem] for /them/ [ba] for /bathe/

Stimulability: XXXXXX was stimulable for several erred sounds including /gate/ and /star/, but was unable to produce /thumb/, /them/, or /clown/ given an immediate model.

Phonological Processes: Phonological processes are sound production patterns, or simplifications, that are different from typical adult pronunciations and are used by children as they develop their phonological system. A phonological process is considered active if it occurs 40% of the time or more in a given sample. XXXXXX demonstrated the following phonological processes:

Final Consonant Deletion (85%):   [pi] for /pig/

Cluster Reduction (70%):   [fwa] for /flag/

Vocalization (100%):   [koo] for /school/

As indicated above, phonological processes are normal in a child's early speech development, and the above processes, with the exception of vocalization, are found in the speech repertoire in typically developing children. The above noted errors significantly reduce XXXXXX's intelligibility.

Multisyllabic Words: In addition to assessment on single-syllable words, XXXXXX was assessed on multisyllabic words, which require additional sequencing, planning, and precision. The error patterns and phonological processes XXXXXX demonstrated on the single-syllable words were mirrored in the multisyllabic words.

Vocabulary Development:

The Receptive One-Word Picture Vocabulary Test (ROWPVT-4) was administered to assess XXXXXX's ability to comprehend age-level vocabulary items. For this assessment, XXXXXX was asked to point to objects, actions, and concepts pictured in a field of four illustrations. XXXXXX demonstrated receptive vocabulary skill within the average range. The results were as follows:

Results of ROWPVT-4

Raw Score	31
Standard Score	98
Percentile	45

The Expressive One-Word Picture Vocabulary Test (EOWPVT) was administered to assess XXXXXX's ability to name specific items (i.e., concepts, objects, and actions) pictured in a field of four illustrations. XXXXXX's ability to use a wide variety of vocabulary items falls in the average range. The results were as follows:

Results of EOWPVT-4

Raw Score	23
Standard Score	92
Percentile	30

Language Functioning:

The Preschool Language Scales-5 (PLS-5) was administered to gain insight into XXXXXX's comprehensive developmental language skills. This is an interactive play-based instrument and is designed for children from birth through age 7. Items assessed range from preverbal interactional skills to emergent language and early literacy. The results were as follows:

Modality	Standard Score	Percentile
Auditory Comprehension	87	19
Expressive Communication	85	16
Total Language Score	85	16

On the *Auditory Comprehension* portion of the assessment, XXXXXX responded correctly to the following:

- Identification of familiar items (i.e., block, cup, car)
- Understanding of object use (i.e., "show me what you use to drink water")
- Identification of colors (i.e., "show me the blue crayon")

Examples of items XXXXXX was unable to respond to correctly include:

- Recognizing actions in pictures (i.e., "show me the child who is washing")
- Understanding of spatial concepts (i.e., "put box on the table")

XXXXXX's performance on the Auditory Comprehension portion of the PLS-5 falls in the low average range.

On the *Expressive Communication* portion of the assessment, XXXXXX responded correctly to the following:

- Naming objects in photographs
- Using a variety of words (e.g., girl, kids, truck)
- Using words for a variety of functions (e.g., requesting objects, actions, assistance)

Examples of items XXXXXX was unable to respond to correctly include:

- Using different word combinations (i.e., verb + noun/pronoun)
- Using words more often than gestures to communicate

XXXXXX's performance on the Expressive Communication portion of the PLS-5 falls in the low average range.

Performance Summary:
XXXXXX's Total Language score on the PLS-5 falls in the low average range. While XXXXXX performed very comparably across the two modalities, he demonstrated a slight advantage in his ability to comprehend spoken language.

Language Sample
Language samples were obtained on March 16th and March 18th during the parent interview and during the psychological and speech-language assessments. During these sessions, XXXXXX generally played quietly and independently at a table with toys (i.e., cars, trucks, pencils). He interacted verbally with his father to a request (e.g., "cars!") and occasionally to comment (e.g., "the kids"). After some initial reticence, he responded verbally to questions and commands delivered by the school psychologist and this examiner, and demonstrated limited verbal interaction during play sequences with this examiner.

During these observations, XXXXXX did not demonstrate a significant number of spontaneous utterances; as such a formal language sample with a minimum of 50 utterances could not be obtained. However, XXXXXX's limited spontaneous language was analyzed, specifically his observed phrase length and his language form (e.g., inflectional markers, parts of speech). Overall, XXXXXX used one-word phrases, regular plurals, and negation. Examples of his spontaneous utterances follow:

- "The dogs!"
- "Car!"
- "Truck!"
- "Nana."
- "Boy."
- "No!"

While a formal language sample was not obtained, it can be inferred from his spontaneous language use that XXXXXX uses shorter phrases than would be expected based on criterion-referenced norms of utterance length, which suggest that a child 2 years, 11 months of age typically and consistently uses phrases that contain between 2.5 to 3.5 words.

During a play sequence scaffolded by this examiner (e.g., playing with cars), XXXXXX consistently produced two-word phrases appropriate to an accompanying action (e.g., "truck go," "truck stop," "truck crash!"). This ability to imitate the modeled language may be suggestive of an emerging expansion of phrase length.

Oral-Peripheral Examination:
The Oral-Peripheral Examination assesses physical structures organically and function for speech production adequacy. External structures and muscles of the face, lips, and jaw were judged to be within normal limits for speech production.

Voice and Fluency:
Voice quality was judged to be age and gender appropriate. No abnormal disfluencies were observed.

Intelligibility:
Per observation by this examiner, XXXXXX was 80% intelligible at the single-syllable, single-word level with context. At the short phrase level, he was 70% intelligible with context and 60% intelligible without context.

Summary and Impressions:
XXXXXX, at 2 years, 11 months of age, presents with a speech and language disorder, as evidenced by significant speech sound errors and impaired expressive communication abilities. Relative strengths are noted in XXXXXX's receptive language functioning, particularly in the area of receptive vocabulary development. Significant deficits and delays were noted in his speech sound development. These phonological delays are readily apparent and appear to affect all areas of expressive language development.

It can be inferred from these findings that XXXXXX's speech and language impairments present no indication of spontaneous recovery and may significantly attract adverse attention, adversely affect his educational performance, and interfere with his ability to communicate with others.

Recommendations:

Members of the Individualized Education Program team need to review the above information along with other pertinent information to determine the Least Restrictive Environment and the most appropriate education setting and interventions to meet the student's education needs.

_____

Speech-Language Pathologist

EFG School District

☐ Written Translation Requested
Language: English

Individualized Education Program

Last Name	XXXXXX
First Name	XXXXX
Student ID	XXXXX
IEP Date	4/14/2017
Next IEP	4/14/2018
Last Annual IEP	4/14/2018
Last Eval	4/14/2017
SPED Entry Date	4/15/2017

Purpose of Meeting: ☒ Initial ☐ Annual ☐ Triennial ☐ Transition ☐ Pre-expulsion ☐ Interim ☐ Expanded ☐ Other: _____

DOB: 11/9/2010 ☐ F ☒ M **Grade**: Kindergarten **Migrant:** ☐ Yes ☒ No

Home Language: English **EL:** ☐ Yes ☒ No ☐ Redesignated
Interpreter: ☐ Yes ☒ No

Residency: Parent or Legal Guardian
School Attending: ABC Elementary School

Parent/Guardian: XXXXX

District of Residence: EFG School District
School of Residence: ABC Elementary School

Ethnicity: 1. <u>WHITE</u> 2. _____ 3. _____ 4. _____

Primary Disability   Eligible for Special Education   ☒ Yes   ☐ No

☐ Autism (AUT)	☐ Hard of Hearing (HH)*	☐ Other Health Impairment (OHI)
☐ Deaf-Blindness (DB)*	☐ Mental Retardation (MR)	☒ Specific Learning Disability (SLD)
☐ Deafness (DEAF)*	☐ Multiple Disability (MD)	☐ Speech/Language Impairment (SLI)
☐ Emotional Disturbance (ED)	☐ None	☐ Traumatic Brain Injury (TBI)
☐ Established Medical Disability (EMD)	☐ Orthopedic Impairment (Ol)*	☐ Visual Impairment (Vl)*

Secondary Disability

☐ Autism (AUT)	☐ Hard of Hearing (HH)*	☐ Other Health Impairment (OHI)
☐ Deaf-Blindness (DB)*	☐ Mental Retardation (MR)	☒ Specific Learning Disability (SLD)
☐ Deafness (DEAF)*	☐ Multiple Disability (MD)	☐ Speech/Language Impairment (SLI)
☐ Emotional Disturbance (ED)	☐ None	☐ Traumatic Brain Injury (TBI)
☐ Established Medical Disability (EMD)	☐ Orthopedic Impairment (Ol)*	☐ Visual Impairment (Vl)*

*Low Incidence Disability

Eligibility Statement:
A severe discrepancy exists between intellectual ability and academic achievement in written expression and listening comprehension. XXXXXX evidences processing disorders in attention (the ability to sustain attention and concentrate on a task or activity) and a personal weakness in auditory processing (the ability to recognize, perceive, and interpret auditory stimuli).

Describe how the student's disability affects involvement and progress in the general curriculum (or, for preschoolers, participation in appropriate activities):
He will benefit from small group and individual specialized instruction that is not available in the general class.

For Initial Placement Only
Has the student received prereferral early intervening services in the past 2 years?

   ☒ Yes   ☐ No

Date of initial referral for special education services: 2/17/2017

Person initiating the referral for special education service: Student study/intervention team

Date district received parental consent: 2/17/2017

Date of initial meeting to determine eligibility: 4/14/2017

PRESENT LEVELS OF ACADEMIC ACHIEVEMENT/ FUNCTIONAL PERFORMANCE

Educational Strengths/Preferences/Interests
He tries to work in small groups. He enjoys working on the computer and uses the DS game at home.

Concerns of parent relevant to educational progress
Mom is concerned about his reading. Mom indicated he had 2 full years of pre-school. When he doesn't want to work, he stops working completely.

State Standards

English/Language Arts	☐ Adv.	☐ Proficient	☐ Basic	☐ Below Basic	☐ Far Below Basic
Mathematics	☐ Adv.	☐ Proficient	☐ Basic	☐ Below Basic	☐ Far Below Basic
Hist./Soc. Science	☐ Adv.	☐ Proficient	☐ Basic	☐ Below Basic	☐ Far Below Basic
Science	☐ Adv.	☐ Proficient	☐ Basic	☐ Below Basic	☐ Far Below Basic

Most Recent Scores

Listening _____ Speaking _____ Reading _____ Writing _____

Fitness/PE Test (Grades 5, 7, & 9 only) _____

Other Assessment Data (e.g., curriculum assessment, other district assessment)

DRA Level 1, knows 8 of 27 kindergarten sight words, almost all capital and lower case letters

Hearing _____ ☐ Pass ☐ Fail ☐ Other: _____
Vision_____ ☐ Pass ☐ Fail ☐ Other: _____

The **Brief Written Language**-<k.0; Spelling subtest-<k.0; requires the production of single letters and words in response to oral prompts; **Writing Samples** subtest-<k.0; measures the ability to convey ideas in writing; requires the production of meaningful written sentences in responses to a variety of task criteria.

The **Listening Comprehension** cluster provides a measure of achievements including understanding directions and comprehending oral language. XXXXXX's overall listening comprehension ability is within the low average range. His performances on the Understanding Directions and Oral Comprehension subtests were within the low range.

Cognitive Functioning

The assessments results indicate that XXXXXX meets eligibility criteria for SLD. A severe discrepancy exists between intellectual ability and academic achievement in the areas of written expression and listening comprehension. XXXXXX evidences processing disorders in the area(s) of *Attention* (the ability to sustain attention and concentrate on a task or activity) as well as a personal weakness in *Auditory Processing* (the ability to recognize, perceive, and interpret auditory stimuli).

Communication Development

XXXXXX continues to exhibit decreased speech intelligibility. He exhibits difficulty producing /v/ in all word positions and he produces a frontal distortion for /s/ and /z/ in all word positions. XXXXXX is stimulable for correct production of /v/ in all word positions when given a verbal model. Additionally, XXXXXX exhibits the phonological processes of gliding, and substituting [w] for /r/ and /l/ in all word positions. Both the SLP and classroom teacher reported that his expressive and receptive language skills appear to be within normal limits. The frontal distortion of /s/ and /z/ and substitution of [w] for /r/ and /I/ is appropriate for his age.

Gross/Fine Motor Development

Gross and fine motor development appear to be within normal limits.

Social Emotional/Behavioral

XXXXXX is social, affectionate, and talkative; however, he is easily distracted. He is respectful of adults and is learning social boundaries from his peers.

Health (including medication information)

XXXXXX has general good health and parents report his hearing and vision are within normal limits.

Vocational

XXX tries to be responsible and is beginning to read the calendar.

Self-Help

XXXXXX can get himself dressed and take care of his personal needs.

Area of need to be addressed in goals and objectives for student to receive educational benefit:

☐ Math Calculations ☐ Math Applications ☐ Reading Fluency ☐ Self-Help Skills

☐ Social Behavior ☐ Attendance ☐ Pre-vocational skills ☒ Writing

☒ Reading Comprehension ☒ Speech and Language ☐ Other: _____

SPECIAL FACTORS TO BE CONSIDERED

Does the student require assistive technology devices and/or services?
☒ No   ☐ Yes

Does the student require low incidence services, equipment, and/or materials to meet educational goals?   ☒ N/A   ☐ No   ☐ Yes

Considerations if the student is blind or visually impaired: ☒ N/A

Considerations if the student is deaf or hard of hearing: ☒ N/A

If the child is an English learner, consider the language needs of the child as those needs relate to the IEP: ☒ N/A

Does student's behavior impede learning of self or others?   ☒ No   ☐ Yes

☐ Behavior Support Plan (BSP) attached
☐ Behavior Intervention Plan (BIP) attached

Statewide Testing

Participation in Math
☒ Grade Exempt (before Grade 2/after Grade 11)

Participation in Science
☒ Grade Exempt

Participation in English Language Arts
☒ Grade Exempt (before Grade 2/after Grade 11)

Participation in History (8th grade)
☒ Grade Exempt

Participation in Writing (4th and 7th grade)
☒ Grade Exempt

ANNUAL GOALS

Area of Need: Pre-Academic/ Academic Reading	Measurable Annual Goal #1 By 4/14/18: In the resource room & in the general ed. class, XXX will use the pictures from a story to make predictions about its content with 80% correct each opportunity as measured by work samples & observation records.
Baseline: He has trouble blending words and remembering what he reads.	☒ Enables student to be involved/progress in general curriculum/state standard #C 0.2.2 ☒ Addresses other educational needs resulting from disability ☐ Linguistically appropriate ☒ Person(s) Responsible: *General Education Teacher & RSP*

Area of Need:	Measurable Annual Goal #2
Pre-Academic/ Academic Reading	By 4/14/18: In the resource room & in the general ed. class, XXXXXX will blend vowel-consonant sounds orally to make words or symbol with 80% correct each opportunity as measured by work samples & observation records.
Baseline: He knows sounds of words but he does not consistently blend the words in context or isolated.	☒ Enables student to be involved/progress in general curriculum/state standard #W 0.1.9 ☒ Addresses other educational needs resulting from disability ☐ Linguistically appropriate ☒ Person(s) Responsible: _General Education Teacher & RSP Parents_

Area of Need:	Measurable Annual Goal #3
Pre-Academic/ Academic Writing	By 4/14/18: In the resource room & in the general ed. Class, XXXXXX will determine a reasonable spelling, using pre-phonetic knowledge, letter sounds, and knowledge of letter names with 80% correct each opportunity as measured by work samples & observation records.
Baseline: He tries to write words to form a sentence. He can write a missing word for a sentence given a review of choice of words to write.	☒ Enables student to be involved/progress in general curriculum/state standard #C 0.1.2 ☒ Addresses other educational needs resulting from disability ☐ Linguistically appropriate ☒ Person(s) Responsible: _General Education Teacher & RSP Parents_

Area of Need:	Measurable Annual Goal #4
Language/ Communication	By 4/14/18, XXXXXX will independently produce /v/ in all word positions in sentences with 80% accuracy across 2 consecutive sessions.
Baseline: When on task, produces /v/ in all word positions with 30% accuracy with verbal models.	☐ Enables student to be involved/progress in general curriculum/state standard #_____ ☒ Addresses other educational needs resulting from disability ☒ Linguistically appropriate ☒ Person(s) Responsible: _Speech/Language Specialist General Education Teacher & Parents_

Area of Need:	Measurable Annual Goal #5
Language/ Communication	By 4/14/18, in the speech room, XXXXXX will produce sentences using the correct subjective pronoun to describe pictures and stories with 80% accuracy across two consecutive sessions.
Baseline: XXXXXX exhibits difficulty producing the appropriate subjective pronoun to describe stories and photographs. For example, XXXXXX frequently substitutes him for he and her for she, which detracts the reader from the message.	☒ Enables student to be involved/progress in general curriculum/state standard #S 3.1.4 ☒ Addresses other educational needs resulting from disability ☐ Linguistically appropriate ☒ Person(s) Responsible: _Speech/Language Specialist_ _General Education Teacher & Parents_

SERVICES

Service Options considered: ☒ General Education ☒ DIS ☒ RSP ☐ SDC ☐ NPS
☐ Other _____

Services		Provider	Start/ End Date	Frequency	Duration (Total Minutes)	Location
Specialized academic instruction	I/G	a District of service	4/15/17	(4×) Weekly	30	a Special Education Room
			4/15/18			
Speech & Language	I/G	a District of service	4/15/17	(4×) Weekly	30	a Special Education Room
			4/15/18			

Special Transportation: ☐ Yes ☒ No   **Extended School Year (ESY):** ☐ Yes ☒ No

Programs and services will be provided according to when student is in attendance and consistent with the public school calendar and scheduled services, excluding holidays, vacations, conference schedules, and non-instructional days.

PLACEMENT

Physical Education: ☐ General ☐ Specially Designed (describe) _____

   ☐ APE   ☐ High School PE Requirements (2 years): ☐ Met ☐ In Progress

Service District: <u>EFG School District</u>

School of Attendance: <u>ABC Elementary School</u>

School Type   <u>Public Day School</u>

Federal Setting: <u>Regular Classroom</u>

All special education services provided at student's home school: ☒ Yes ☐ No

Other Agency Services:

   ☐ California Children's Services (CCS)   ☐ Regional Center

   ☐ Probation   ☐ Department of Rehabilitation

   ☐ Dept. of Social Services (DSS)   ☐ Other _____

   ☐ County Mental Health (CMH)

Student Eligible for Mental Health Services under Chapter 26.5   ☐ Yes ☒ No

Mental Health Services Language Included on the IEP   ☐ Yes ☒ No

Transportation: ☐ None ☒ General ☐ Special Ed _____

Student Transition:

☒ N/A   ☐ PK to Elementary   ☐ Elementary to Middle School

☐ Middle to High School   ☐ High School to Adult Transition

☐ High School to Post Secondary   ☐ Other _____

GRADUATION PLAN
(Grade 8 and Higher)

Projected graduation date and/or secondary completion date _____

   ☒ Diploma

   ☐ Non-Diploma Certificate

APPENDIX 7–B
Private Practice—Sample Reports

 ABC Speech Services
Speech & Language Evaluation Report

Name: XXXXXXXXX   Date of Birth: 4/11/16

Address: XXXXXXXXXX   Chronological Age: 1.9-year-old (21 months)
         XXXXXXXXXX

Date of Report: 2/4/18

Telephone: XXXXXXXX   Assessment Date: 1/22/18

RCOC Service Coordinator: XXXXXXXXX

I. BACKGROUND INFORMATION:
   The reason for the referral is to determine XXXXX's level of functioning in
   the areas of speech and language. XXXXX is a 1.9-year-old boy who lives
   with his mother, father, and baby sister. He was diagnosed with autism by
   XXXXX at 16 months of age. At or during birth, XXXXX may have had
   a brain injury, which caused left-side weaknesses of his upper and lower
   extremities and left eye droop (ptosis). Vietnamese is his primary language.
   Per parent report, there is a family history of autism (two of XXXXX's cous-
   ins). He is currently receiving physical therapy 1 hour per week at XXXXXXX.
   In the past, he received feeding therapy at XXXXXXX and six sessions of
   speech therapy at XXXXX. He has constipation problems and takes Miralax
   daily. His mom reported some sensory problems such as rubbing objects on
   his mouth, grabbing her hand repeatedly to rub or lick, and rubbing his face.
   XXXXX passed his newborn hearing screening and there are no concerns
   with his hearing and vision at this time. Please refer to the Regional Center
   intake summary for further medical and developmental information.

II. ASSESSMENT RESULTS:
   XXXXX's speech, language, pragmatics, and informal cognitive/play skills
   were assessed using clinical observations, parent report, review of records,
   <u>Developmental Assessment of Young Children (DAYC)–Cognitive Subtest</u>,
   and <u>The Rossetti Infant-Toddler Language Scale</u>. The speech and language
   assessment was conducted in Vietnamese.

DAYC–Cognitive Subtest:

Age Equivalent:	23 months
Percentile:	70%ile
Standard Score:	108

The Rossetti Infant-Toddler Language Scale

Pragmatics:	3 months scattering to 9–12 months (86% delay)
Language Comprehension:	15 months with scattering to 33–36 mos. (29%delay)
Language Expression:	12 months with scattering to 33–36 mos. (43% delay)

A. RECEPTIVE LANGUAGE:

In the area of language comprehension, XXXXXX scored solidly at the 15-month level with scattered skills up to the 33- to 36-month level (29% delay). He is able to identify pictures, objects, action words, and body parts upon request. Also, XXXXXX follows one-step commands, recognizes family member names, understands the prepositions "in, on," and responds to simple questions. He does not identify objects by category, understand 50 words, and follow related two-step commands.

B. EXPRESSIVE LANGUAGE:

In the area of language expression, XXXXXX scored solidly at the 12-month level with scattered skills up to the 33- to 36-month level (43% delay). Although he uses up to four-word sentences to communicate wants and needs, his language is mostly scripted. As a result, his language is highly restricted. He does not spontaneously combine novel utterances. He demonstrates both immediate and delayed echolalia. XXXXXX is often off topic and will say random words out of context. If joint attention is established, then he is able to ask and answer simple questions. He is inconsistent with imitating words. Despite talking a lot, XXXXXX does not engage in a back-and-forth conversation and rarely initiates conversation with others.

C. SPEECH:

Oral structures appear adequate for speech production. XXXXXX used the age-appropriate consonants /p, b, m, w, t, d, n, h/ during the assessment. Speech intelligibility was judged to be 90% to 100%.

D. COGNITIVE/PLAY SKILLS:

According to the Rossetti, XXXXXX's pragmatics skills are at the 3-month level with scattered skills up to the 9- to 12-month level, which is considered significantly below the average range (86% delay). During play, he demonstrates limited interactions, rarely initiates play acts, and has to be prompted to maintain play. He is object oriented and his play is rigid and repetitive. He sees shapes and letters in objects and gets fixated by them. He is not able to maintain eye contact, vocalize to gain attention, consistently respond to his name, initiate turn-taking routines, or imitate other children. Results of the DAYC cognitive subtest indicated he is at the 70th percentile, which places him in the average range. He spontaneously names objects, uses pretend objects in play, counts 1 to 20, matches objects by color and shape, and stacks at least six blocks.

III. OBSERVATIONS:

XXXXXX participated in most of the test tasks and activities. His mom sat in during the testing and served as informant. He demonstrates fleeting eye contact, inconsistent joint attention, and flat affect. When excited, XXXXXX exhibits awkward arm and leg movements (e.g., when he got to play with the shape sorter). Per parent report, XXXXXX has compliance issues and tantrums at home (e.g., when there is a change in routine). When around peers, he would look at what the peers are doing but never interact with them.

IV. SUMMARY & RECOMMENDATIONS:

XXXXXX demonstrates an 86% delay in pragmatics (solid at 3 months), a 29% delay in receptive language skills (solid at 15 months), and a 43% delay in expressive language (solid at 12 months). It is recommended that XXXXXX receive 2 hours per week of speech therapy. Per parent report, there are some sensory and behavioral problems at home. It is recommended that XXXXXX receive an OT and ABA evaluation to determine if therapy is warranted.

V. GOALS:

1. XXXXXX will follow related two-step verbal directions with 80% accuracy.
2. XXXXXX will spontaneously produce novel utterances to communicate his wants and needs with 80% accuracy.
3. XXXXXX will consistently imitate words upon request with 80% accuracy.
4. XXXXXX will initiate one-step play acts during pretend play with 80% accuracy.
5. XXXXXX will initiate one to three comments and/or questions during pretend play with 80% accuracy.
6. XXXXXX will appropriately use words to get someone's attention with 80% accuracy.
7. XXXXXX will initiate turn-taking games with 80% accuracy.

XXXXXXXXXX
Speech-Language Pathologist

ABC Speech Services

Speech & Language Evaluation Report

Name: XXXXXX

Address: XXXXXXXXXX
          XXXXXXXXXX

Telephone: XXXXXXXX

Date of Birth: 1/08/2005

Chronological Age: 12.1-year-old

Date of Report: 2/16/2017

I. BACKGROUND INFORMATION:

XXXXXX is a 12.1-year-old girl who is currently home-schooled through XXXXXX Charter School. She is in the sixth grade. She has been receiving speech and language therapy since she was 2¾ years old. She no longer receives occupational therapy. Her hearing and vision are within normal limits. She lives with both of her parents and an older sister. This assessment is for XXXXXX's triennial review.

II. ASSESSMENT RESULTS:

XXXXXX was assessed on 2/6/17 and 2/9/17 for a total of 2.75 hours. Based upon observations, she gave good effort on all of the test items. XXXXXX's speech and language skills were assessed using clinical observations, parent report, records review, Comprehensive Assessment of Spoken Language (CASL), and CELF-4 Pragmatics Profile.

A. LANGUAGE:

Comprehensive Assessment of Spoken Language (CASL):

	Standard Score	Percentile
Nonliteral language	120	91%ile
Meaning from context	117	87%ile
Inference	111	77%ile
Ambiguous sentences	114	82%ile
Pragmatic judgment	107	68%ile

Based upon parent report and observations, XXXXXX tends to perform well on standardized language tests but has difficulty using and generalizing what she knows with different people and across different situations and settings. XXXXXX scored within average range on all subtests. On the nonliteral language subtest, she had to explain the meaning behind the nonliteral language that was given. For example, When Mother heard about the accident, the ground started shifting beneath her feet. What does this mean? XXXXXX responded, "Mother was worried." On the meaning from context subtest, XXXXXX was asked to figure out the meaning of an unusual word from listening to a sentence. For example, Sara got tired of moving her head up and down to follow the saltations of the Russian dancers. Explain what saltations means. XXXXXX said, "Jumping." On the inference subtest, she had to listen to a story and make an inference to figure out clues in the story. For example, Darrell and Todd waited patiently in line for a chance to buy two of the remaining tickets for the rock concert. They left the ticket window without tickets. Why? XXXXXX responded, "The tickets were sold out." On the ambiguous sentences subtest, she had to explain two different meanings for an ambiguous sentence. For example, The man followed the tracks for three miles, and then exhaustion overcame him. XXXXXX answered, "Animal tracks and railroad tracks." On the pragmatic judgment subtest, the therapist described some events and XXXXXX had to explain the best thing to say or do in the given situation. For example, It is a hot summer day. MayLee's friend is wearing a heavy jacket. What does MayLee ask her friend? XXXXXX responded, "Why are you wearing a heavy jacket when it's hot outside?"

CELF-4 Pragmatics Profile:
Per parent report, she had a raw score of 99, but her criterion score for her age should be >142 (below average). Some test items that her mom rated as "never" include the following: initiates greetings, introduces others, and apologizes appropriately. Examples of test items that her mom rated as "sometimes" are as follows: asks for clarification during conversations; tells/understands jokes; agrees and disagrees using appropriate language; uses appropriate facial expressions, tone of voice, and body language; and uses nonverbal cues appropriate to the situation.

Clinical observations (social skills group):
During therapy, XXXXXX is able to engage in long reciprocal conversations about preferred topics (e.g., animals, books) with adults and peers. She tends to talk about preferred topics and does not realize that other people might not be interested. However, she is only able to maintain non-preferred topics (e.g., shopping, arts & crafts) with peers by making two to eight conversational exchanges. She offers significantly more comments than questions. She needs to work on asking more questions to show the listener that she is interested in what he or she is saying. Also, XXXXXX needs to practice selecting appropriate topics of conversation and play choices based on what she already knows about the other person's likes and dislikes. During conversations with people she knows, she is able to maintain eye contact. However, she avoids eye contact and does not initiate greetings or conversation with new people. XXXXXX reported that she only talks to people she knows and feels that she is too shy and does not know what to say to new people. When we go on field trips (e.g., shopping at the mall, Color Me Mine), XXXXXX demonstrates limited interactions and needs maximum prompting in order for her to talk to her friends.

Also, she tends to avoid talking to other people. For example, she needed to throw away trash at Color Me Mine. She asked me where the trash can was located and I told her to ask the store clerk. Instead of asking the store clerk, XXXXX just held on to her trash.

In the area of nonverbal communication, XXXXX is aware of other people's facial expressions, tone of voice, and hand and body gestures. During structured activities, she is able to read the nonverbal cues and figure out what to do or say when given different social situations with 80% accuracy. However, she continues to have difficulty reading nonverbal cues and responding appropriately to them in real-life situations. In role playing activities, XXXXX correctly displays nonverbal cues appropriate to the social situation with 80% accuracy. However, she demonstrates limited range of facial expression (mostly smiling or neutral facial expression) and tone of voice in real-life situations. She rarely uses hand gestures while she is talking. Generalization of learned skills to different people, situations, and settings continues to be difficult for XXXXX.

Perspective taking (theory of mind concepts) is another area of difficulty. It is difficult for her to take someone else's perspective and infer what the other person might be thinking and/or feeling. As a result, it is difficult for her to alter her verbal and nonverbal language to accommodate to the person or situation. XXXXX struggles with flexibility in her thinking and assumes that other people think the same way as she doesso it is difficult for her to see multiple interpretations. Despite being in multiple group activities (e.g., church, sailing, horseback riding), XXXXX rarely interacts with her peers. She expresses a desire to have friends but does not know how to go about it. When asked who her friends are, she named her dog and her sister. XXXXX also named acquaintances at church, in her neighborhood, and after-school activities. She mostly plays with boys who are younger than her (limited talking required). The play choices (e.g., tag, hide & seek) are immature for her age (limited talking required). Her mom reported that XXXXX has the awareness of what it takes to make friends because she is very bright. She also is willing to integrate with peers but has significant difficulty applying what she knows to real-life situations. Parental concerns include: as social demands increase, XXXXX will have a harder time making and keeping friends and XXXXX might be depressed in the future if she does not have true friendships with her peers.

B. SPEECH:
Oral structures and functions are adequate for speech production. XXXXX is able to correctly produce all of her sounds in all word positions at the conversational level and no longer needs articulation therapy.

III. SUMMARY & RECOMMENDATIONS:
XXXXX demonstrates delays in the area of social skills and pragmatics. She would benefit from intervention to improve her social language skills and

interactions with her peers. It is recommended that XXXXXX receive individual speech therapy for .5 hour per week and social skills group for 1 hour per week. It is also recommended that she receive 3 hours total of speech ESY.

IV. NEW GOALS:

1. XXXXXX will appropriately initiate greetings and conversation with new people during structured activities such as school events and after-school activities with 80% accuracy as measured by clinical observations, therapy notes, and parent report across three consecutive sessions.

2. XXXXXX will state appropriate topics of conversation and play choices depending on who she is talking to (e.g., 6 years old vs. 13 years old, boys vs. girls), with 80% accuracy as measured by clinical observations and therapy notes across three consecutive sessions.

3. XXXXXX will maintain the topic of conversation by making at least eight exchanges (emphasis on asking more questions than making comments) with non-preferred topics with adults and peers with 80% accuracy as measured by clinical observations and therapy notes across three consecutive sessions.

4. XXXXXX will appropriately use a total of five different body gestures, hand gestures, facial expressions, and/or tones of voice per conversation with 80% accuracy as measured by clinical observations and therapy notes across three consecutive sessions.

5. XXXXXX will take someone's perspective and make an inference about what he or she likes or is thinking with 80% accuracy as measured by clinical observations and therapy notes across three consecutive sessions.

6. XXXXXX will problem solve by stating two things that you should do or say and explain the consequences for each solution when given different social situations and/or conflicts with 80% accuracy as measured by clinical observations and therapy notes across three consecutive sessions.

_____

XXXXXXXXXX
Speech-Language Pathologist

Medical Setting—Sample Reports

XYX Medical Facility
Patient ID: XXXXXX

Pt. was seen in the speech clinic for a cognitive evaluation on 01/28/17 sec. to pt. c/o memory problems. Patient is a 25 y/o Army Combat Veteran who was deployed to Afghanistan from 2009–2010 and to Iraq from 2012–2013. Pt. reported that he fell on his head and neck, with LOC for unknown period of time, and was treated in the ER. Pt endorses left-side numbness and neck spasms. Records also indicate subjective complaints of right-side weakness. Pt also reported a syncopal incident after his fingers were cut off in a noncombat accident in the military (see psychosocial hx for details). Pt did not endorse any other hx of head trauma prior to, or during the military.

Pt. endorsed problems with memory and attention. Pt. reported that he has difficulty remembering details of readings, how to complete math problems, new learning in school, dates, events, and tasks. Pt. also reported misplacing important items.

Pt. stated that he is sleeping approximately 3 hours per night without medication and 4–5 hours (broken) with medication. Pt. eats 2 meals per day. Pt. reported that he drinks ETOH 1× per week (usually four beers). Pt. drinks ½ cup of coffee every other day. Pt. denied smoking or recreational drugs.

Pt. is currently compensating for memory difficulties by using his Blackberry smartphone; pt. utilizes the calendar application but not the task application. Pt. is currently enrolled in college; however, he is considering withdrawing from school sec. to panic attacks and difficulty learning. Pt. is unsure of goals at this time; pt. reported "living day-to-day." Pt's goals for therapy are to learn tips for memory.

I. Global Positioning System (GPS) Questionnaire:
"Are you having difficulty driving at this time?" and/or "Are you having any difficulty following directions while driving?"

[ ] NO = GPS not indicated. Discontinue assessment.
[x] YES

Comments: Pt. reported zoning out while driving. Pt. owns a GPS but he doesn't use it consistently. SLP encouraged pt. to use the GPS while driving to both familiar and unfamiliar destinations. GPS is not medically indicated.

II. Rivermead Behavioral Memory Test (RBMT-3):
SLP administered the Rivermead Behavioral Memory Test (RBMT-3). The RBMT provides a systematic method of assessing cognitive deficits associated with

nonprogressive brain injury and monitoring change over time. This test was standardized on 333 people (172 females, 161 males) ranging in age from 16 to 89. RBMT-3 subtests are converted to subtest scaled scores with a mean of 10 and a standard deviation of 3. In addition to providing scaled scores for the RBMT-3 subtests, a General Memory Index (GMI), representing overall memory performance, was also used. The GMI has a mean of 100 and a standard deviation of 15.

Subtest	Scaled Score
First and Second Names—Delayed Recall	2
Belongings—Delayed Recall	5
Appointments—Delayed Recall	8
Picture Recognition—Delayed Recognition	1
Story—Immediate Recall	4
Story—Delayed Recall	4
Face Recognition—Delayed Recognition	4
Route—Immediate Recall	7
Route—Delayed Recall	7
Messages—Immediate Recall	11
Messages—Delayed Recall	11
Orientation and Date	7
Novel Task—Immediate Recall	7
Novel Task—Delayed Recall	5

Sum of Scaled Scores: 83
General Memory Index: 64 (2.4 SD below mean)
Percentile Rank: 0.8

IMPRESSION: Pt. presented with moderate-to-severe memory deficits. Suspect pt.'s adjustment issues, lack of sleep, and dx. of PTSD are largely contributing to his cognitive deficits. Neuropsych assessment found similar results. Pt. has begun MH services and was encouraged to continue actively treating PTSD. Pt. would benefit from training to use his smartphone as a memory aid and organizational tool. Will defer cognitive therapy at this time until mental health issues are better controlled. Pt. might benefit from the College Connection program if he decides to withdraw from school this semester.

RECOMMENDATIONS: (1) SLP scheduled a f/u appt. to review test results and recommendations. (2) If pt. is agreeable, SLP will schedule 1–2 sessions to train pt. to use his Blackberry to improve organization and time management. (3) Pt. was encouraged to use the GPS while driving to both familiar and unfamiliar destinations. (4) SLP encouraged pt. to continue actively treating PTSD.

XYX Medical Facility
Patient ID: XXXXXX

Pt. was seen in the speech clinic on 04/23/18 for continued assessment to determine most appropriate treatment plan. Pt. was alert and an active participant in the evaluation. Pt. was fully cooperative with all assessment tasks with no frustration noted. Results are as follows:

SLP administered portions of the Boston Naming Test. Pt. responded accurately to 42% of stimuli presented (14/33 spontaneous responses); 7 of the 14 correct responses were self-corrections. Pt's incorrect responses were typically characterized by phonemic errors (e.g., holipotter for helicopter, mushumber for mushroom). Perseverations of paraphasias were typical; each attempt/repetition was closer to the correct word. Pt. was provided with semantic and phonemic cues; however, pt. was unable to accurately respond following cues. Pt. presented with reduced awareness of phonemic paraphasias; pt. showed potential to improve awareness. SLP verbally provided pt. with the correct response and incorrect response containing a phonemic error. Pt. was able to identify if the word was correct vs. incorrect 75% of the time. Pt. also spontaneously utilized compensatory strategies to improve verbal expression such as gestures, circumlocutions, or substituting the word.

SLP administered the ACLC, which is an assessment of auditory comprehension; normative data are not available for this test. Pt. correctly identified a pictured object/action/adjective from a field of 5 with 78% accuracy (39/50 trials). Pt. identified two-critical elements from a field of four with 50% accuracy (5/10 trials). Pt. identified three-critical elements with 70% accuracy. Suspect improvement with the more complex task is sec. to pt.'s increased use of strategy of asking for repeats.

IMPRESSIONS: Pt. would benefit from speech therapy to improve auditory comprehension, self-awareness/self-monitoring, and verbal expression. Pt. is motivated to improve communication skills and is stimulable to implement compensatory strategies. Pt. would highly benefit from intensive therapy 5 days per week; unsure if goals can be accomplished as an outpatient. Pt. might also benefit from occupational therapy to address cognitive skills given his high level of functioning prior to injury.

PLAN: SLP will schedule speech and language therapy 5 days per week for a minimum of 4 weeks with goals as follows:

Auditory Comprehension

STG 1a: Pt. will correctly identify a pictured object from a field of 4 at 90% accuracy while using compensatory strategies for improved auditory comprehension as needed (e.g., ask for repeat of message, ask for a written cue) across 30 trials and 2 consecutive sessions.

STG 1b: Pt. will correctly identify a pictured object from a field of 6 at 90% accuracy while using compensatory strategies for improved auditory comprehension as needed (e.g., ask for repeat of message, ask for a written cue) across 30 trials and 2 consecutive sessions.

STG 1c: Pt. will correctly identify a sequence of 2 pictures from a field of 6 at 90% accuracy while using compensatory strategies for improved auditory comprehension as needed (e.g., ask for repeat of message, ask for a written cue) across 30 trials and 2 consecutive sessions.

STG 1d: Pt. will correctly identify a sequence of 2 pictures from a field of 8 at 90% accuracy while using compensatory strategies for improved auditory comprehension as needed (e.g., ask for repeat of message, ask for a written cue) across 30 trials and 2 consecutive sessions.

Self–Awareness/Self–Monitoring

STG 2a: Pt. will reduce his perseverative errors to no more than 2 repetitions per word during a picture-naming task with 90% accuracy across 30 trials and 2 sessions.

STG 2b: Pt. will reduce his perseverative errors to no more than two repetitions per word during a phrase-level picture description task with 90% accuracy across 30 trials and two sessions.

STG 2c: Pt. will reduce his perseverative errors to no more than two repetitions per word during a sentence-level picture-description task with 90% accuracy across 30 trials and two sessions.

Self–Awareness/Self–Monitoring

STG 3a: Pt. will judge the SLP's verbal productions as correct vs. incorrect during a picture-naming task with 90% accuracy across 30 trials and two consecutive sessions.

STG 3b: Pt. will judge his verbal productions as correct vs. incorrect during a picture-naming task with 90% accuracy across 30 trials and two consecutive sessions.

STG 3c: Pt. will judge his verbal productions as correct vs. incorrect during a phrase-level picture-description task with 90% accuracy across 30 trials and two consecutive sessions.

STG 3d: Pt. will judge his verbal productions as correct vs. incorrect during a sentence-level picture-description task with 90% accuracy across 30 trials and two consecutive sessions.

Verbal Expression

STG 4a: To improve verbal expression, pt. will implement appropriate compensatory strategies (e.g., pause to plan, circumlocution, word substitution, use of gestures, writing word) during a picture-naming task in 90% of relevant instances across two consecutive sessions.

STG 4b: Pt. will implement appropriate compensatory strategies to improve verbal expression (e.g., pause to plan, circumlocution, word substitution, use of gestures, writing word) during a phrase-level picture-description task in 90% of relevant instances across two consecutive sessions.

STG 4c: To improve verbal expression, pt. will implement appropriate compensatory strategies (e.g., pause to plan, circumlocution, word substitution, use of gestures, writing word) during a sentence-level picture-description task in 90% of relevant instances across 2 consecutive sessions.

Long-Term Goals

LTG 1: To improve auditory comprehension, pt. will correctly identify a sequence of 3 pictures from a field of 8 at 90% accuracy, while using compensatory strategies as needed (e.g., ask for repeat of message, ask for a written cue), across 30 trials and 2 consecutive sessions.

LTG 2: Pt. will reduce his perseverative errors to no more than 2 repetitions per word during a wh-question response task with 90% accuracy across 30 trials and 2 sessions.

LTG 3: Pt. will judge his verbal productions as correct vs. incorrect during a wh-question response task with 90% accuracy across 30 trials and 2 consecutive sessions.

LTG 4: Pt. will implement appropriate compensatory strategies to improve verbal expression (e.g., pause to plan, circumlocution, word substitution, use of gestures, writing word) during a wh-question response task in 90% of relevant instances across 2 consecutive sessions.

XYZ Children's Hospital
Department of Pediatric Rehabilitation
Speech and Language Evaluation Report

RELATED DIAGNOSIS
Ependymoma (*ICD-9-CM:* 191.9)

BACKGROUND INFORMATION
Referral Concerns
XXXXXX was referred for a speech and language evaluation by Dr. Y due to concerns regarding mild cognitive communication deficits. His mother reported no concerns with regards to XXXXXX's speech and language, but she expressed concerns about his attention and memory.

Developmental History
XXXXXX reportedly reached all of his developmental milestones at an age-appropriate time, including gross and fine motor skills, and speech and language.

Social History
XXXXXX lives in an English-speaking home in Utah with his two siblings, parents, and grandparents. He enjoys hanging out with his friends, riding his bike, reading, and playing chess with his older brother.

Educational History
XXXXXX is currently in sixth grade at a local school district. XXXXXX has an active individualized educational program (IEP); he is in a special day class and has recently been placed into a higher reading and language arts class. XXXXXX is reportedly a good student across subjects, and receives good grades. Per parent report, prior to the ependymoma diagnosis, he performed well in school. When not at school, XXXXXX is cared for by his parents and grandparents.

Feeding History
XXXXXX's mother expressed no concerns regarding feeding and feeding history is unremarkable.

MEDICAL HISTORY
Medical history was obtained from a review of his chart. XXXXXX was initially diagnosed with an ependymoma in 2012. At that time, XXXXXX underwent surgical resection followed by radiation. He was not treated with chemotherapy at that time. He was followed continually over the next several years. In January 2015, scans revealed tumor recurrence. At that time he again underwent surgical resection followed by chemotherapy consisting of but not limited to Cisplatin, Vincristine, Cytoxan, and Etopiside. Chemotherapy was completed in June 2015.

In response to his mother reporting frequent episodes of falling, a stat MRI was ordered in July 2015, but no evidence of any abnormal enhancement to suggest tumor recurrence. Per parent report, XXXXXX has a significant visual impairment in his left eye.

EVALUATION

Information for this evaluation was obtained through parent/patient interview, elicitation of behaviors, and clinical observation of skills. The outpatient evaluation took place in a quiet therapy room located at the Pediatric Rehabilitation Department. The following people were present at various points during the evaluation: XXXXXX, his grandmother, his mother, and a speech-language pathologist. The evaluation was completed in English. Due to XXXXXX's visual impairment, when there was a visual stimulus in an assessment, a brightly colored (pink) piece of paper was placed to the left of the page to encourage XXXXXX to make a complete visual scan.

Formal Assessment
Tests Administered
Clinical Evaluation of Language Fundamentals (CELF-4)
The *CELF-4* is a flexible and multiperspective assessment that examines a child's language and communication strengths and weaknesses from ages 5 to 21 years and 11 months old. Areas assessed include vocabulary, syntax, morphology, pragmatics, memory, comprehension, and expression. XXXXXX's results are detailed below and are gauged to be an accurate reflection of his current skills.

Three subtests from the *Clinical Evaluation of Language Fundamentals, 4th Edition (CELF-4)* were administered to assess XXXXXX's language and cognitive skills as they compare to typical peers; Word Classes (Expressive), Word Classes (Receptive), and Concepts and Following Directions,

CELF-4 4/7/18

Subtest	Raw Score	Scaled Score	Percentile	Interpretation
Word Classes, Expressive:	7	7	16th	*Mild*
Word Classes, Receptive:	11	7	16th	*Mild*
Word Classes, Total:	18	9	37th	*Mild*
Concepts and Following Directions	54	13	84th	*High Average*

For these assessments, the mean scaled score for is 10 and the standard deviation is 3. Typical performance ranges between 7 and 13.

Word Classes, Expressive & Receptive:
This subtest examines the child's ability to hold a list of four words in working memory, identify the two words that are most closely related, and then describe their relationship. **For both expressive and receptive language, XXXXXX scored in the mild range compared to his same-age peers.**

Concepts and Following Directions:
This subtest requires the student to identify pictures of geometric shapes in response to orally presented directions. The student must wait for the entire set of directions and then follow the directions in the order that the items were presented. **XXXXXX scored in the high average range compared to his same-age peers.**

Ross Information Processing Assessment–Primary (RIPA-P)

The *Ross Information Processing Assessment–Primary* (*RIPA-P*) assesses impairments in information-processing skills in children from 5 to 12 years of age who have experienced neuropathologies that may affect these skills. Due to time constraints, only selected subtests from the *RIPA-P* were administered for this evaluation.

XXXXXX's results are detailed below and are gauged to be an accurate reflection of his current skills. On the individual subtests, XXXXXX's performance ranged between "within normal limits" and "moderate impairment." However, when the subtests were grouped by composite quotient, his performance fell within normal limits. His strongest performance was in his ability to remember the immediate past and his spatial orientation (e.g., the location of United States with respect to the Mexico). He was most challenged when asked to recall general information (e.g., the name of a famous American).

The RIPA-P was standardized on individuals with traumatic brain injury. As such, standard measurements of performance, such as standard scores, are not used to represent "average function."

RIPA-P 4/7/18

Subtest	Raw Score	Standard Score	Percentile	Interpretation
Immediate Memory	69	16	98	*Within Normal Limits*
Recent Memory	75	13	84	*Mild*
Recall of General Information	56	10	50	*Moderate*
Spatial Orientation	75	17	99	*Within Normal Limits*
Temporal Orientation	63	12	75	*Mild*
Organization	67	13	84	*Mild*
Problem Solving	69	12	75	*Mild*

Composite Quotients	Sum of Standard Score	Percentile	Quotient	Interpretation
Memory Quotient	39	90	119	*Within Normal Limits*
Orientation Quotient	29	97	127	*Within Normal Limits*

Immediate Memory:
This subtest requires the child to repeat numbers, words, and sentences of increasing length and complexity. Items are presented auditorily. XXXXXX's performance on this subtest can be interpreted to be within normal limits.

Recent Memory:
This subtest requires the child to recall specific new acquired information relative to his or her environment and daily activities. XXXXXX's performance on this subtest reflects a mild impairment.

Recall of General Information:
This subtest requires the child to recall general information in remote memory. The stimuli represent information that is acquired between the ages of 5 and 12. XXXXXX's performance on this subtest reflects a moderate impairment.

Spatial Orientation:
This subtest requires the child to answer questions related to spatial concepts and orientation. XXXXXX's performance on this subtest can be interpreted to be within normal limits.

<u>Temporal Orientation:</u>
This subtest requires the child to answer questions related to time-based information. XXXXXX's performance on this subtest reflects a mild impairment.

<u>Organization:</u>
This subtest requires the child to recall category members within a 1-minute time limit and recall a category type given three category members. XXXXXX's performance on this subtest reflects a mild impairment.

<u>Problem Solving:</u>
This subtest requires the child to respond to stimulus items containing day-to-day problems. XXXXXX's performance on this subtest reflects a mild impairment.

Test of Narrative Language (TNL)
The Test of Narrative Language (TNL) measures a child's ability to answer literal and inferential comprehension questions. It also is a good measure of how well children use language in narrative discourse. There are three narrative formats: no picture cues, sequence picture cues, and single picture cues. Narrative language abilities require the integration of semantic, syntactic, and pragmatic language for the construction of form—meaning relationships at the sentence and text level. Children who score below 90 on the Narrative Language Ability Index may demonstrate deficits in vocabulary and difficulty with recall, general language comprehension, and syntax. Scores in this range may also be indicative of challenges with social and academic language.

XXXXXX's results are detailed below and are gauged to be an accurate reflection of his current skills. On Narrative Comprehension, XXXXXX answered questions about a story that had been read to him. He performed within the average range on these tasks. On Oral Narration, XXXXXX was expected to retell two stories and create one of his own. He performed within the average range on these tasks. His strongest performance was in his ability to answer familiar, concrete questions about a story (e.g., remembering character names) and in his creativity in the creation of his own fictional story (e.g., the aliens wanted the two kids to take them to see the President of the United States).

TNL 4/7/18

	Raw Score	Standard Score	Interpretation
Narrative Comprehension	31	9	*Average*
Oral Narration	68	13	*Average*
Narrative Language Ability Index	22	65	*Average*

Informal Assessment Administered

Divided Attention Activity Worksheet

This worksheet required XXXXXX to maintain his focus on a task with competing requirements; he had to follow a pattern and trace a line from one target to the next in sequential order (i.e., moving from A–1–B–2–C–3, etc.). XXXXXX was able to complete this worksheet with 95% accuracy. During the task, XXXXXX repeatedly reviewed the written instructions provided on the worksheet to check his accuracy. During one of the reviews, he spotted an error, erased the line in error, and redrew the line correctly. This strategy of review was very effective on this task and may help him with homework assignments that present a greater than average challenge for him.

SKILLS RELATED TO COMMUNICATION

Attention/Behavior

Attention is a key component for developing language. To function appropriately at home and within the classroom, children are expected to focus and attend to a speaker, listen to what is being said, and then utilize and act upon information given (usually instructions or rules).

During the assessment, XXXXXX was able to sustain attention and focus on tasks at hand; he required no repetitions for directions. For example, during one of the narrative tasks, his grandmother entered the room. Although her entry caused a distraction, XXXXXX was able to continue with the task without requiring a review of the information. Further, when asked between assessments if he needed a break, he replied that he did not and continued for another 30 minutes.

Overall, XXXXXX demonstrated appropriate attention and was polite and interacted appropriately with his grandmother, mother, and the speech-language pathologist.

Memory

Memory involves encoding, storing, and retrieving information. These memory skills are important within the classroom and at home because they are required every day when teachers/parents ask their students/children to follow directions related to lessons, assignments, and activities as well as when taking notes and learning vocabulary.

Encoding/Storing/Retrieving for auditory and visual stimuli: On the Concepts and Following Directions subtest, XXXXXX was able to recall directions that increased in length and complexity (e.g., "point to the small orange car" and "point to the small black fish after you point to the big fish and then point to the shoe and ball"). Further, at the end of the session, XXXXXX was able to recall the spelling of the word *bueno* that the speech-language pathologist had talked about early in the session. His performance on this assessment is reflective of his current level of academic performance.

In general, XXXXXX demonstrates appropriate skills with regard to memory.

Executive Functions

Executive functions refer to the ability to initiate and stop actions, monitor and change behavior as needed, and plan future behavior when faced with new tasks and situations. Executive functions allow us to anticipate outcomes and adapt to changing situations. The ability to form concepts and think abstractly is often considered a component of executive function.

Per parent report, XXXXXX is very independent and helpful around the house; he is very involved with his siblings and participates in daily chores in addition to his schoolwork. He has demonstrated no problems with his homework. XXXXXX's performance on the Divided Attention Task is reflective of effective executive function.

Within this evaluation and as reported by his family, XXXXXX demonstrates appropriate executive function as evidenced in the results of the individual formal and informal assessments.

Play Skills
Play skills were not evaluated.

COMMUNICATION

Receptive Language
Receptive language refers to XXXXXX's ability to comprehend and process what others are saying. In general, XXXXXX is able to respond appropriately to questions and comments addressed to him. The Word Classes–Receptive subtest of the CELF-4 was administered to assess his receptive language skills in depth. XXXXXX was significantly more challenged by multiple-syllable words (e.g., catastrophe, latitude, and permanent) than by single-syllable words (e.g., joined and sun).

In general, XXXXXX presents with receptive language skills reflective of a mild impairment.

Expressive Language
Expressive Language refers to XXXXXX's ability to communicate and express his wants, needs, thoughts, and ideas to those around him. In general, XXXXXX is able to express himself appropriately during his daily activities. The Word Classes–Expressive subtest of the CELF-4 and the TNL were administered to obtain an in-depth understanding of XXXXXX's expressive language skills. XXXXXX was able to find relationships between words that were part of his daily life (e.g., pillow/blanket and window/glass) and struggled with words that were more abstract (e.g., connected/joined and achieving/accomplishing).

In general, XXXXXX presents with expressive language skills reflective of a mild impairment.

Oral Motor/Articulation
XXXXXX demonstrated appropriate articulation and motor speech skills.

Voice
Based on informal observations during conversational speech, XXXXXX exhibits appropriate vocal characteristics at this time, including pitch and loudness, which do not impact his overall ability to communicate with others.

Fluency
No abnormal dysfluencies were noted in running speech.

Social Communication/Pragmatics
Pragmatics refers to the way that language is used to communicate with others (the social use of language). Throughout this assessment, and as reported by his family, XXXXXX exhibited appropriate social communication.

In general, XXXXXX presents with appropriate social communication skills. He was polite and respectful during the evaluation. He willingly and actively engaged in conversation with the speech-language pathologist. Per parent report, he is well liked and respected by his peers and teachers.

SUMMARY
XXXXXX is a polite, well-behaved adolescent boy who was referred for a speech and language evaluation due to concerns regarding attention and memory. Results of this assessment indicate that both attention and memory are appropriate for his age and his recovery from an ependymoma.

Per parent report, he is receiving effective support through his IEP and the academic structure of the special day class. Based on these results, it is recommended that XXXXXX continue with his current support system through his school. If he exhibits a change in his academic performance or demonstrates any status changes in speech, language, attention, or memory, it is recommended that he be evaluated again.

Thank you for the opportunity to participate in the assessment of XXXXXX. Please feel free to contact me should you have any questions or concerns regarding the content of this report.

_____
Speech-Language Pathologist

Cc: family, (MD Name) ***, insurance

XYZ REHABILITATION HOSPITAL
COMMUNICATIVE DISORDERS SERVICE

Medical Diagnosis: Stroke

Date of Onset: April 2016   **Date of Report:** 6/12/2016

Speech/Language Pathologist: XXXXXXXXX

Referring Physician: XXXXX   **Report:** Initial: _X_ Final: _X_

1. **BACKGROUND INFORMATION/PROGRESS REPORT:**

   37 y/o male, well known to speech clinician from previous LBMMC visit rehab center admit. Pt initially presented with altered LDC, nausea, and vomiting, having been out drinking with friends the previous night. Initially nonverbal and unable to sit up. Paramedics were called and reported CGS 1-5-1 and alcohol odor. Pt taken to LB Community Hospital, where a head CT was initially read as a bleed, then re-read as negative. Pt c/o chest pain or palpitations in ER. PMHx: headaches, anxiety, HTN, hyperlipidemia. Follow-up CT revealed occluded **L** internal carotid artery. Pt was d/c'd with residual mod-severe receptive aphasia and severe expressive aphasia, and **R** hemiplegia. SOHx: Pt lives with wife and 4-year-old daughter; with other family members involved.

2. **SPEECH/LANGUAGE/COGNITIVE DIAGNOSIS:** Pt was evaluated in clinic office with his wife present. Portions of the Boston Diagnostic Aphasia Exam (BDAE), the Boston Naming Test, and the Reading Comprehension Battery for Aphasia (RCBA) were given. The following results were obtained:

   Cognition: Difficult to fully assess all areas secondary to expressive language. However, immediate recall of short paragraph was 100% accurate for y/no responses. Problem solving during functional activities is at min assist-to-supervised.

   Speech: Verbal attempts were 100% accurate during non-structured tasks, such as picture description of "cookie theft" from BDAE. Pt was 20% accurate for verbal attempts in response to automatic phrases in structured task. Imitations of short sentences, verbally presented, were 30% accurate, with apraxic distortions. Pt was 100% accurate for automatics (i.e., counting, days, months).

   Lang.: Pt was 75% to 100% accurate for y/no responses to questions regarding complex ideational material, verbally presented. Pt was 40% accurate reading sentences and pointing to printed pictures from field of 3.

3. **PROGNOSIS:** ____ Excellent _X_ Good _X_ Fair ____ Guarded ____ Poor

   Secondary to: above results and pt.'s progress over time

4. **RECOMMENDATIONS:**
   Speech/Language/Cognitive therapy <u>3×</u> times weekly for <u>4</u> weeks.

5. **GOALS:**
   <u>Patient/Family</u>: To talk.   **Discharge Goals Met:** ____ Yes ____ No

   <u>Treatment:</u>

   ↑ reading comprehension of survival words/signs to min assist
   (75%–80% acc.).

   ↑ automatic speech thru melodic intonation therapy to mod assist.

   ↑ naming of family members & common household items to mod assist.

Thank you for referring this patient.

                                    NAME: XXXXXX
                                    M.D.: XXXXXX
                                    MMC NO.: XXXXXX   AGE: <u>37</u>

_____

Speech-Language Pathologist

APPENDIX 7-D
Sample Goals and Objectives

ADULT LANGUAGE DISORDERS

Target Area: Spoken Language Expression

Objective 1: Given a visual prompt (e.g., picture) and not more than three cues (e.g., written, semantic, phonemic), the patient will say the names of familiar <u>people</u>, in 7 of 10 opportunities.

Objective 2: Given a visual prompt (e.g., picture) and not more than three cues (e.g., semantic, phonemic) in a clinic setting, the patient will say the names of 10 familiar <u>places</u> in 7 of 10 opportunities.

Objective 3: Given a visual prompt (e.g., picture) and not more than three cues (e.g., semantic, phonemic) in a clinic setting, the patient will say the names of 10 familiar <u>objects</u> in 7 of 10 opportunities.

Objective 4: Given a visual prompt (e.g., picture) and not more than three cues (e.g., semantic, phonemic) in a clinic setting, the patient will say the names of 10 familiar <u>activities</u> in 7 of 10 opportunities.

Target Area: Multimodality Communication

Goal: To improve communicative effectiveness, XXXXXX will switch communication modalities to writing, drawing, or description when word retrieval difficulties occur in conversation.

Objective 1: In response to word retrieval difficulties, XXXXXX will switch communication modalities to writing, drawing, or description during picture description in 8 of 10 opportunities.

Objective 2: In response to word retrieval difficulties, XXXXXX will switch communication modalities to writing, drawing, or description during conversation in 8 of 10 opportunities.

Target Area: Auditory Comprehension

STG 1a: Pt. will correctly identify a pictured object from a field of four at 90% accuracy while using compensatory strategies for improved auditory comprehension as needed (e.g., ask for repeat of message, ask for a written cue) across 30 trials and two consecutive sessions.

STG 1b: Pt. will correctly identify a pictured object from a field of six at 90% accuracy while using compensatory strategies for improved auditory comprehension as needed (e.g., ask for repeat of message, ask for a written cue) across 30 trials and two consecutive sessions.

STG 1c: Pt. will correctly identify a sequence of two pictures from a field of six at 90% accuracy while using compensatory strategies for improved auditory comprehension as needed (e.g., ask for repeat of message, ask for a written cue) across 30 trials and two consecutive sessions.

STG 1d: Pt. will correctly identify a sequence of two pictures from a field of eight at 90% accuracy while using compensatory strategies for improved auditory comprehension as needed (e.g., ask for repeat of message, ask for a written cue) across 30 trials and two consecutive sessions.

AUGMENTATIVE AND ALTERNATIVE COMMUNICATION

Target Area: AAC Use

Goal: The student will access his *Proloquo2go* app on his iPad to make requests during speech therapy sessions.

>*Objective 1:* When verbally prompted once (e.g., "Turn on your iPad."), the student will follow visual instructions to turn on his iPad and open the *Proloquo2go* app, in four of five opportunities, during speech therapy sessions.

>*Objective 2:* When verbally prompted once (e.g., "What should we do next?"), the student will access his *Proloquo2go* app on his iPad to make requests, in four of five opportunities, during speech therapy sessions.

Target Area: Functional/Expressive Communication

By May 2014, during daily activities and routines, XXXXXX will use her AAC device for functional communication (e.g., protesting, requesting, stating opin-

ions), given visual supports in four of five opportunities across 3 trial days, as measured by observation and data collection.

Target Area: Receptive Language

By May 2014, during daily activities and routines, XXXXXX will use her AAC device to answer familiar yes/no questions, given visual supports in four of five trials across 3 trial days as measured by observation and data collection.

By May 2014, during daily activities and routines, XXXXXX will use her AAC device to answer familiar "who" and "what" questions given visual supports in four of five trials across 3 trial days as measured by observation and data collection.

By May 2014, during structured speech-language activities, XXXXXX will use her AAC device to answer basic "wh" comprehension questions (i.e., who, what doing, where, when) related to a short passage/story, given visual supports as needed in four of five trials over three consecutive sessions as measured by observation and data collection.

AUTISM SPECTRUM DISORDERS

Target Area: Play

Goal: The client will perform sequences of common play scripts (e.g., restaurant, store, library), in response to a video self-model in the clinic setting.

>*Objective 1:* The client will imitate a minimum of four actions and four verbalizations of imaginative play sequences of common play scripts (e.g., restaurant, store, library), following a video self-model, in at

least two play scripts, in the clinic setting.

Target Area: Social Skills

Goal: To improve social skills, the client will demonstrate appropriate use of social rules in conversations with familiar and unfamiliar communication partners.

Objective 1: When presented with a visual stimulus (i.e., video modeling), the client will demonstrate appropriate use of social rules (e.g., greetings, introductions, and asking questions) given moderate (3–5) verbal cues and gestures, in three of five opportunities with the clinician in the clinic setting.

Objective 2: When presented with a visual stimulus (i.e., video modeling), the client will demonstrate appropriate use of social rules (e.g., greetings, introductions, and asking questions) given minimal (1–2) verbal cues and gestures, in four of five opportunities with the clinician in the clinic setting.

Target Area: Language

By December 2018, during naturalistic activities (e.g., play, snack, library), given no more than two prompts (e.g., visual, phonemic, questioning), XXXXXX will produce semantic relations within the modifier + object category, using at least two-word utterances, with 70% accuracy.

By December 2018, during two of three naturalistic activities (e.g., play, snack, library), with no more than two prompts (e.g.,

visual, phonemic, questioning), XXXXXX will produce semantic relations within the negation + object category, using at least two-word utterances, with 70% accuracy.

CHILD LANGUAGE DISORDERS

Target Area: Auditory Comprehension

Goal: The student will follow one- to two-step instructions with verbal prompts.

Objective 1: The student will follow one- to two-step instructions in 40% of opportunities with verbal and visual prompts.

Objective 2: The student will follow one- to two-step instructions in 50% of opportunities with verbal and visual prompts.

Objective 3: The student will follow one- to two-step instructions in 50% of opportunities with verbal prompts.

Target Area: Preliteracy / Phonology

Goal: To improve preliteracy skills, the client will demonstrate increased phonological awareness by segmenting monosyllabic words.

Objective 1: To improve preliteracy skills, the client will demonstrate increased phonological awareness by categorizing (e.g., Which one begins with a different sound: *feet, five, soup, fat*?) in response to print and verbal cues in 7 of 10 opportunities.

Objective 2: To improve preliteracy skills, the client will demonstrate increased phonological awareness by deletion (e.g., Say *trip* without the /t/) in response to print and verbal cues in 7 of 10 opportunities.

Objective 3: To improve preliteracy skills, the client will demonstrate increased phonological awareness by substitution (e.g., Replace the /m/ in *man* with /f/) in response to print and verbal cues in 7 of 10 opportunities.

Objective 4: To improve preliteracy skills, the client will demonstrate increased phonological awareness by manipulation (e.g., Say the word *stop*. Now move the /s/ to the end of the word and say it again) in response to print and verbal cues in 7 of 10 opportunities.

Target Area: Morphology

By May 2016, during pretend play activities, following therapist recasts, XXXXXX will produce -*ing* verbs (e.g., children are singing) in at least 10 utterances across three sessions.

By May 2016, during pretend play activities, XXXXXX will complete cloze procedures to produce -*ing* verbs (e.g., we are . . .) in at least 10 utterances across three sessions.

By May 2016, during pretend play activities, the client will spontaneously produce -*ing* verbs (e.g., puppy jumping) in at least 10 utterances across three sessions.

Target Area: Pragmatics

Goal: The client will produce appropriate sentences for a variety of social functions (e.g., requesting, turn-taking, repairing conversational breakdowns).

Objective 1: The client will produce an appropriate sentence for a

variety of social functions (e.g., requesting, turn-taking, repairing conversational breakdowns) when given moderate prompting (e.g., verbal and/or visual prompts), with 80% accuracy across 10 trials as measured by recorded data.

MOTOR SPEECH

Target Area: Voice

Objective 1: The patient will demonstrate controlled exhalation by sustaining phonation of the vowel /a/ for 10 seconds or longer, in 80% of trials, across two consecutive therapy sessions.

Objective 2: The patient will demonstrate controlled exhalation by sustaining phonation of the vowel /a/ for 20 seconds or longer, in 80% of trials, across two consecutive therapy sessions.

Target Area: Fluency

Goal: The client will increase fluency in response to token reinforcement (response cost) in structured play therapy.

Objective 1: The client will demonstrate increased fluency in response to token reinforcement (response cost) with no more than 30 dysfluencies during 5 minutes of structured play therapy.

Objective 2: The client will demonstrate increased fluency in response to token reinforcement (response cost) with no more than 20 dysfluencies during 5 minutes of structured play therapy.

Objective 3: The client will demonstrate increased fluency in response to token reinforcement (response cost) with no more than 10 dysfluencies during 5 minutes of structured play therapy.

PHONOLOGY

Target Area: Phonological Awareness

Goal: The client will demonstrate phonological awareness skills by identifying initial and final sounds in CVC, CV, and VC words.

Objective 1: Given a visual cue and verbal prompts, the client will match the beginning sounds of words with 70% accuracy as measured by clinician observation, other informal assessments, and data collection.

Objective 2: Given a visual cue and verbal prompts, the client will identify the beginning sounds of words with 70% accuracy as measured by clinician observation, other informal assessments, and data collection.

Objective 3: Given a visual cue and verbal prompts, the client will match the ending sounds of words with 70% accuracy as measured by clinician observation, other informal assessments, and data collection.

Objective 4: Given a visual cue and verbal prompts, the client will match the ending sounds of words with 70% accuracy as measured by clinician observation, other informal assessments, and data collection.

Target Area: Articulation

Goal: XXXXXX will produce /s/ in the initial and final position at the word level 50% of the time.

Objective 1: Given pictures, a model, and a verbal prompt, XXXXXX will produce /s/ in the initial and final position, at the word level, with 20% accuracy.

Objective 2: Given pictures, a model, and a verbal prompt, XXXXXX will produce /s/ in the initial and final position at the word level with 40% accuracy.

Target Area: Articulation

Goal: The client will produce the phonemes /r/, /l/, /s/, and /z/ in all positions in one-syllable words.

Objective 1: With no more than one prompt, the student will produce the phonemes /r/, /l/, /s/, and /z/ in CV and VC syllables with 80% accuracy.

Objective 2: The student will produce the phonemes /r/, /l/, /s/, and /z/ in the initial position of one-syllable words with 70% accuracy.

Objective 3: The student will produce the phonemes /r/, /l/, /s/, and /z/ in the final position of one-syllable words with 70% accuracy.

CHAPTER 8

Data Collection

Accuracy of observation is the equivalent of accuracy of thinking.
—Wallace Stevens
(Pulitzer Prize–winning poet)

The terms *data* (plural) and *datum* (singular) refer to "factual information (as measurements or statistics) used as a basis for reasoning, discussion, or calculation" (Merriam-Webster, 2003). Hence, data collection is the process of obtaining this information. In the field of speech-language pathology, collecting, analyzing, and summarizing data is a vital part of decision-making and documentation. As a speech-language pathology assistant (SLPA), you will learn about evidence-based practice (EBP), which is the "integration of clinical expertise, best current evidence, and client values to provide high-quality services reflecting the interests, values, needs, and choices of those we serve" (Rao, 2011, para. 4). Data collection is an integral part of EBP (Boswell, 2005; Epstein, 2008; Lemoncello & Fanning, 2011) and as such, is a very important aspect of what speech-language pathologists (SLPs) and, in turn, SLPAs do. Box 8–1 lists some of the job responsibilities of an SLPA that may involve data collection.

Clinically, data collection begins during assessment when the SLP analyzes information about communicative or swallowing behaviors. Although an SLPA does not conduct assessment or interpret any data collected (ASHA, 2013), as an SLPA you may be asked to assist during screening or assessment. This could include data collection, such as tallying or recording specific behaviors, transcribing a language sample, making phonetic notations, calculating percentages, transferring data onto standardized protocols, or creating graphs or charts to display assessment or screening data.

Data collection about a client continues during and may continue after treatment. These data are also critical because they allow the SLP to monitor the client's progress from session to session and to document the efficacy of a given treatment strategy (Mowrer, 1982; Roth & Worthington, 2001). This, too, may be an area where an SLPA can assist, as it also involves tasks such as tallying or recording specific behaviors, making phonetic notations, calculating percentages, and preparing charts or graphs about treatment data. As discussed in Chapter 7, treatment objectives include information about the types of data needed to establish if a client has met a given objective. This information is present in the "criterion" portion of behavioral objectives.

As an SLPA, your role in accurately collecting data is crucial, since inaccurate data will negatively influence clinical decisions. The sections that follow discuss methods for observing and recording data, including ideas for ways to record specific types of data. Chapter 9 discusses ways to summarize these data in note for-

---

Box 8–1. Examples of SLPA Duties Involving Data
(American Speech-Language and Hearing Association, ASHA, 2013)[1]

a. Assist the SLP with speech, language, and hearing screenings **without** clinical interpretation.
b. Assist the SLP during assessment of students, patients, and clients exclusive of administration and interpretation.
c. Follow documented treatment plans or protocols developed by the supervising SLP.
d. Provide guidance and treatment via telepractice to students, patients, and clients who are selected by the supervising SLP as appropriate for that service delivery model.
e. Document student, patient, and client performance (e.g., tallying data for the SLP to use; preparing charts, records, and graphs) and report this information to the supervising SLP.

mat. The companion website associated with this book contains samples of score sheets that can be used for charting data.

RECORDING AND DESCRIBING BEHAVIOR

There are many different methods for observing, recording, and describing communication behaviors. At the heart of each is careful observation, meaning that you actively and directly see and listen to the client, taking care to accurately record what you observe (Kawulich, 2005; Taylor-Powell& Steele, n.d.). Careful observation requires understanding the behaviors to be observed, the type of data to be collected, and the method for summarizing the information.

Some methods for recording data in the field of speech-language pathology include frequency counts and tallies, response analysis, and transcription and narration.

Frequency Counts and Tallies

Frequency counts and tallies determine if a behavior is present (and at what rate) during a specific period (Moore & Pearson, 2003; Mowrer, 1982; Roth & Paul, 2007). These methods are also referred to as simple enumeration (Mowrer, 1982). In these techniques, the objective is to record the presence of a specific behavior, such as a client interacting with a peer, asking a question, saying a specific sound or type of word, and so forth. To record this type of data, you must know which specific behavior to observe, how long to watch for the behavior, and during which activity you need to observe the behavior. You would then record the number of times that behavior occurred in that specified period (e.g., two times in 1 minute, 10 times in 2 minutes, etc.) during the specified activity. Tallies, hash marks, checks, and other symbols can be used to record this information. Figure 8–1 shows an example of a chart that could be used to record this type of information.

Response Rate

Response rate is a variant of frequency counts and tallies whereby a specific behavior is counted and the number is converted to a value that denotes responses per unit of time. Words per minute (WPM) is a common measurement that uses this technique (Shipley & McAfee, 2009). In this instance, the behavior is the number of words produced in a minute. To record WPM you would count the number of words produced and divided that number by the number of minutes the person was spoke. Syllables per minute (SPM) is another measure calculated in this fashion, but the count would denote the number of syllables produced per minute (Mowrer, 1982).

Checklists

A checklist is another variant of frequency counts and tallies. This technique denotes the presence of a list of behaviors (Moore & Pearson, 2003; Roth & Paul, 2007). It could be a checklist specifically created by your supervising SLP for a specific client (or group of clients), or it may be a modified version of an existing checklist. Figure 8–2 shows an example of a checklist specifically created to track behaviors in a group setting.

Client: Scott Smith (Mrs. Smith's Classroom)

Behavior/Time/Activity	Count
Behavior: Whole-word repetition Length of Time: 10 minutes Activity: Story retell Date: 12/15/17 Clinician: Sarah S. Assistant	✓ ✓ ✓ ✓ ✓ (5 in 12 min.)
Behavior: Final consonant deletion Length of Time: 10 minutes Activity: Story retell Date: 12/15/17 Clinician: Sarah S. Assistant	|||| || (7 in 12 min.)

Figure 8–1. Sample Frequency Count/Tally Data Sheet.

Client: John Jones

Activity: Aphasia Support Group – Thursday Session

SLPA: Sarah S. Assistant

Date: 1/3/18

Behavior	Note Y for *Yes* or N for *No*
Greets fellow group members upon entering room	Y
Finds name tag	N – located table, but needs assistance from group facilitator in locating name tag.
Finds designated seat	Y
Initiates small talk with a fellow group member	Y
Responds to a question posed by group facilitator	N
Comments during group discussion	Y – states "Like pizza" when discussing favorite foods

Figure 8–2. Sample Checklist Data Sheet.

The important thing about recording behaviors using frequency counts and tallies, response rate, and checklists is that you are very clear about the behavior to be counted. For instance, in Figure 8-1, if you did not know what a whole-word repetition was or how it differs from a part-word repetition, you could not accurately record its occurrence and, in turn, would be sharing inaccurate information about the frequency of the behavior with your supervising SLP. Thus, you should always confirm that you understand the exact parameters of the behavior to be counted and ask your supervising SLP if you have any questions.

Screening. In some settings, you may be asked to assist with speech, language, or hearing screenings (ASHA, 2013). A screening "involves the collection of data to decide whether there is a strong likelihood that an individual does or does not have a problem that will require more in-depth assessment" (Kennedy, 2007, p. 42). Screenings are not diagnostic in nature. Rather, they are used to determine if further testing is needed. Screenings use a predetermined cutoff or expected performance level to determine if a client either passes or fails the screening. Your supervising SLP may use a setting-specific instrument or one of many commercially available screening tools.

In some cases, screenings used are similar to checklists in that specific behaviors are listed and the screener denotes the presence or absence of each behavior in a specific context. In other cases, a screener gives the client a specific task and denotes the presence or absence of a required response. For example, in a hearing screening the screener tells clients to raise their hand in response to a series of tones, presented at different frequencies and loudness levels. The screener presents the tones and then notes whether clients raised their hand (presence of required response) or did not raise their hand (absence of required response) for each tone. Similarly, in a kindergarten speech and language screening, a student may be asked to count from 1 to 10. The screener then notes whether the student counted from 1 to 10 (presence of required

response) or did not count from 1 to 10 (absence of required response). In these instances, the screener uses a fully correct response as the criterion for the presence of a behavior. Any other response is noted as the absence of the required behavior. No interpretation of the meaning behind why clients did not raise their hand or count from 1 to 10 is made.

In most cases, screeners require the use a binary score, such as yes/no, absent/present, or correct/incorrect. In addition, some speech and language screeners require errors to be transcribed using the International Phonetic Alphabet (IPA) or written verbatim. A list of IPA symbols is available in Appendix 4–B in Chapter 4. The comments section of many screeners often ask them to note any special circumstances related to the screening that may have influenced the results, such as if the client was not paying attention during a task or did not appear to understand the directions. This type of additional information can be used by the SLP to interpret the results of the screening.

Conducting screenings requires specific training on the screening tool to be used. Administration of hearing screenings also requires that you learn how to operate an audiometer.

SLPA Roles: Caution. A word of caution is in order about checklists and screenings and their use by SLPAs. Many checklists and, in some cases, commercially available screeners, are used by SLPs to assess specific behaviors. These should not be confused with checklists and screenings designed for implementation by an SLPA. In cases where interpretation or diagnosis is required or implied, that is the sole domain of an SLP. For example, a common assessment tool utilized by an SLP is an oral peripheral examination, used to "identify or rule out structural or functional factors that relate to a communicative disorder or dysphagia" (Shipley & McAfee, 2009, p. 158). There are a number of checklists or forms available for use by SLPs for this purpose, most of which include some interpretative or diagnostic aspect. For example, Figure 8–3 contains an excerpt from the Oral-Facial Examination Form (Shipley & McAfee, 2009). In addition, some checklists contain rating scales that require the respondent to classify or rate the severity of a behavior, which is also diagnostic and interpretative in nature. Figure 8–4 is an excerpt from the Checklist for the Assessment of Clients with Clefts (Shipley & McAfee, 2009).

A diagnosis is "a concise technical description" (Merriam-Webster, 2003). The examples from Figures 8–3 and 8–4 both require interpretation and precise description. ASHA (2013) states that SLPAs may not "perform standardized or nonstandardized diagnostic tests, formal or informal evaluations, or swallowing screenings/checklists" (Responsibilities Outside the Scope of an SLPA, para.1). In addition, ASHA specifically highlights the

---

Evaluation of tongue

_____ Surface color: normal/abnormal (specify)_____
_____ Abnormal movements: absent/jerky/spasms/writhing/fasiculations_____
_____ Size: normal/small/large_____
_____ Frenum: normal/short _____

Tell the client to protrude the tongue.
_____ Excursion: normal/deviates to right/deviates to left _____
_____ Range of motion: normal/reduced_____
_____ Speed of motion: normal/reduced_____

(Shipley & McAfee, 2009, p. 196)

Figure 8–3. Excerpt from Oral-Facial Examination Form.

Assessment of Voice

Instructions: Evaluate the client's voice, paying particular attend to possible cleft-related problems. Check the deficits that are present and indicate severity. Record additional notes in the right-hand margin.

1 = Mild
2 = Moderate
3 = Severe

_____ Pitch variation is reduced_____
_____ Vocal intensity is reduced_____
_____ Vocal quality is hoarse/harsh/breathy (circle)_____

(Shipley & McAfee, 2009, p. 574)

Figure 8–4. Excerpt from Checklist for the Assessment of Clients with Clefts.

use of checklists for dysphagia (interpretative or otherwise) as outside the scope of responsibilities of an SLPA, stating that SLPAs "may not use a checklist or tabulate results of feeding or swallowing evaluations" (Responsibilities Outside the Scope of an SLPA, para. 1). As an SLPA, it is important that you maintain these boundaries for the benefit and safety of the clients you serve. There could be legal and ethical ramifications if you go beyond your scope of responsibilities as an SLPA.

Response Analysis

Response analysis is a type of data analysis beyond counting or denoting the presence of a behavior. Response analysis techniques look at the dimensions of correctness (response accuracy), delay (response latency), and assistance needed (response independence) to further quantify behavior. Appendix 7–D in Chapter 7 contains samples of treatment goals and objectives across a variety of response categories. After you read the sections that follow, see if you can identify what type of response analysis is used and what data collection methods you might use to record these behaviors.

Response Accuracy

To record response accuracy, you would be told about a behavior and details about what constitutes an accurate response (Mowrer, 1982). You would then count the number of correct responses and the total number of opportunities for that behavior to occur. An example of this is percent correct (Mowrer, 1982). In this method, you would divide the total number of correct responses by the total number of opportunities. This result could then be converted

to a percentage of correct responses, which is helpful because it denotes if the behavior occurred, and also what portion of the time it was accurate. For example, in charting accuracy in producing /s/ in the initial position of words, you would count the number of times the client produced the /s/ correctly in the initial position of words (total correct) and divide by the total number of opportunities the client had to say words with /s/ in the initial position (total opportunities). To convert this number to a percentage, you would then multiply by 100, as follows:

5	÷	10	× 100 =	50%
Total Correct		*Total Opportunities*		*Percent Correct*

An example data collection sheet for this task may look similar to the one listed in Figure 8–5. Figure 8–6 contains a similar

Client: Tina Thomas
SLPA: Sarah S. Assistant
Date: 1/15/18

Target: /s/ initial/single words

Key: + = correct/ – = incorrect

Word	Response
Sew	–
Say	+
Soup	+
Suit	–
Sock	–
Sub	–
Soap	+
Set	+
Sun	–
Sit	+

Score: 5/10 = 50%

Figure 8–5. Sample Percent Correct Data Sheet (Targets Noted).

Client: Tina Thomas

Date: 1/15/18

SLPA: Sarah S. Assistant

Objective: /s/ initial/single words

										Score
/	/	/	X	X	/	X	X	X	/	50%

Key: X = correct   / = incorrect

Figure 8–6. Sample Percent Correct Data Sheet (No Targets).

way to record these same data. You can see that in both of these examples, the client had 10 opportunities to say a word with /s/ in the initial position and did so accurately five times, resulting in a percent correct of 50%.

In Figure 8–5 the opportunities, as well as the words themselves, are recorded as a reference and the score sheet includes a key to denote that a "+" indicates times when the client produced /s/ in the initial position correctly, while a "−" indicates times when /s/ in the initial position of a word was not produced accurately. In Figure 8–6, no individual words are recorded, but an accurate production is noted with an X and an inaccurate production is noted with a /.

Another common technique that uses the concept of percent correct is a dysfluency index (Shipley & McAfee, 2009). This method counts the total number of syllables (total opportunities) and the total number of disfluencies. A percentage is then calculated, either as a measure of all types of disfluencies (e.g., % Total Disfluency) or for certain types of disfluencies (e.g., % Repetitions, % Prolongations). A similar calculation is used to determine Percent Syllables Stuttered (% SS) as follows (Jones, Onslow, Packman, & Gebski, 2006):

$$\textit{Syllables Stuttered/Total Syllables} \times 100 = SS\%$$

Response accuracy can also be described using an opportunity statement. In this method, correct responses and total opportunities are recorded, but the information is not displayed as a percentage. Rather, this information is summarized in a written statement, such as, "3 of 4 opportunities," "in 8 of 10 instances," or "given 20 of 25 attempts." The following objectives have criteria that use response accuracy:

- Given a verbal label of a category, the client will name three items that belong to that category in <u>8 of 10 opportunities</u>.
- With a visual cue or gesture prompt, Johnny will respond to a teacher-directed question by touching an appropriate symbol on his augmentative and alternative communication (AAC) device, in <u>three of</u>

four opportunities, over three consecutive sessions.

■ The student will correctly use present progressive tense to describe 15 of 20 pictures not visible to the clinician.

Response accuracy can be used for almost any type of behavior, using either percent correct or an opportunity statement. In fact, response accuracy is a common measure used by SLPs in the criterion portion of treatment objectives.

The key to collecting response accuracy is understanding what constitutes a correct or an accurate response and noting how many opportunities the individual had to produce a correct response. Keep in mind that a correct response may not necessarily be synonymous with a perfect response. There are instances when a close approximation or a partly correct response may be determined by your supervising SLP as correct. This information can be noted as the client's goal. If not, you can check with your supervising SLP to confirm that you understand the parameters that constitute "correct."

Response Latency

Response latency is a method for analyzing a response, given how long it took to produce a behavior (Mowrer, 1982). This type of data collection is less common than response accuracy in the field of speech-language pathology. To calculate response latency, you would need to count the length of time between presentation of a "stimulus" and when the client responded. This is typically calculated in seconds and measured with a stopwatch. A stimulus is basically an opportunity to respond. For example, when you ask a client to name something, like a picture of a train, a line drawing of a bed, or a real object like a cup, each of these items (the train, the line drawing, and the cup) is a stimulus. A question or command, such as, "Is grass green?" "What sound does a cow make?" or "Give me your hand," is also a stimulus as each is an opportunity for the client to respond. Figure 8–7 is an example of a data collection sheet for recording response latency. As you can see, in this instance the task is for the client to point to a picture described by

Client: Tim Thomas

SLPA: Sarah S. Assistant

Target: Point to picture described by clinician in <5 seconds

Measurement: Start – End of Questions/Stop – Points to a Picture

											Average Time
Items in field: 2	5.3	4.3	2.5	3.6	6.7	3.3	11.9	3.1	4.5	3.4	
Date: 2/7/18	–	–	+	+	–	–	–	+	+	+	
Items in field: Date:											
Items in field: Date:											

Figure 8–7. Sample Response Latency Data Sheet (Timed).

the clinician in less than 5 seconds. Data collection sheets can be very basic in this case, but the key to collecting this type of data is timing precision. In most cases, a timer is started at the end of stimulus presentation, such as at the end of a question or command, or once the picture or object stimulus is in full view. The timer is stopped at the onset of a response, although in some cases, time may be stopped once the response is completed. When collecting data on response latency, you should familiarize yourself with the timer to be used and also confirm with your supervising SLP the intended start and stop times.

In some instances, a rating scale may be used to denote an immediate or delayed response. This may eliminate the need for a stopwatch, but it still requires you to monitor if the client responded right away after the stimulus was presented (immediate) or if there was a delay in responding (delayed). An example of a score sheet that uses this type of rating scale for charting response latency is shown in Figure 8–8.

Note that for both the score sheets discussed above (Figures 8–7 and 8–8), each has a mechanism for recording response accuracy in addition to response latency. For example, in Figure 8–7, response accuracy is represented with a "+" under items that were correct and produced within the required length of time (less than 5 seconds), and a "–" for items that were either incorrect or were correct but not produced in less than 5 seconds. In Figure 8–8, response accuracy is noted with a "+" next to items named correctly. Often, potential exists to collect more than one form of data simultaneously. This can add important details to your data collection.

Client: Jessica Jones

SLPA: Sarah S. Assistant

Date: 8/14/18

Target: Name familiar, real objects

Key: 1 = Immediate response
       2 = Delayed response (greater than 3 second
       NR = No response

Object	Response
Comb	1
Key	NR
Knife	1+
Cup	1+
Phone	1+
Fork	1
Pen	2
Shoe	NR
Sock	1
Book	2+

Figure 8–8. Sample Response Latency Data Sheet (Rating Scale).

Response Independence

Response independence is another version of response analysis, fairly common in the field of speech-language pathology, particularly when clinicians use some type of assistance or prompt to achieve a desired response. Chapter 10 provides an overview of common prompts used in treatment.

In measuring response independence, you would be given details about a desired or accurate response, as well as the levels or types of assistance you can provide to help the client produce the response. You would then record if assistance was needed and, if so, what type of assistance was provided. For example, in targeting the production of prepositions, the desired or correct behavior maybe for the client to say one of four types of prepositions (e.g., *in, on, over,* or *under*) in response to a question such as, "Where is the kitten?" In this case, the desired response could be a short phrase (e.g., *in the box*) or a single word (e.g., *in*). An example of a task is using a stuffed toy kitten and a basket, eliciting different descriptions as the client moves the toy kitten to different locations (e.g., kitten in the basket, under the basket).

In terms of assistance, some options are to give the client a gestural cue, such as a hand motion representing the preposition; a phoneme cue, such as the initial sound of the appropriate preposition; or even a verbal model. Figure 8–9 shows a sample data collection sheet representing this task. As you can see, there is a code that represents three dimensions of assistance: gestural assistance, represented by a *G*; a phoneme cue, represented by a *P*; and a verbal model, represented by an *M*. This example also has notation for accurate production, represented with a ✓. Inaccurate production is represented with a 0, which indicates that despite assistance, the client was not able to produce the desired response. In the example provided, consistent cues were needed to obtain an accurate response. There are, of course, a variety of other ways to record this same task in terms of response independence, including the data collection sample depicted in Figure 8–10.

The key to recording response independence is to understand what constitutes an accurate response, the types of

Client: Florence Flower   SLPA: Sarah S. Assistant
Objective: Produce prepositions in, on, over and under

0 GPM	0 GPM	✓ G	✓ G	0 GPM	✓	✓ GPM	✓ G	✓ GP	✓ GPM	Date/Score
										Date: 7/22/18 No Cue = 10% G = 30% GP = 10% GPM = 20%
										Date:
										Date:

Key: ✓ = correct 0 = incorrect   CUES: G = Gesture P = Phoneme Cue M = Model

Figure 8–9. Sample Response Independence Score Sheet (Key Code).

Client: Florence Flower   SLPA: Sarah S. Assistant

Date: 5/18/18   Objective: Produce prepositions in, on, over and under

No Assist	Gesture	Phoneme Cue	Model	Preposition
–	–	–	–	Over
–	–	–	–	Under
–	+			In
–	+			On
–	–	–	–	Over
+				In
–	–	–	+	Under
–	+			In
–	–	+		On
–	–	–	+	Under

Figure 8–10. Sample Response Independence Score Sheet (Column Tally).

assistance that are appropriate, and to have a method for recording when assistance is provided. Of note as well, as with response latency, in both the examples you can also determine response accuracy. This combination of response accuracy and response independence within a single data collection method can be highly valuable to provide very detailed information to your supervising SLP. Furthermore, collecting data with this level of detail means that, if needed, you can categorize or summarize the client's performance based on what your supervising SLP indicates is an acceptable level of cues. For instance, in the example above, if the supervising SLP indicated that an accurate response was only a correct response produced with no additional assistance or cues, then the client's accuracy is 10%, since in only 1 of 10 attempts was a preposition accurately produced without any assistance. However, if the supervising SLP deemed that an accurate response could include the provision of

a gestural cue, then the client's response accuracy would be 40%, since she accurately produced a preposition one time without assistance and three times with only a gestural cue.

Narration/Transcription— Speech and Language Sample

The last area of data collection we will discuss is a speech and language sample. Speech and language samples are commonly used in the field of speech-language pathology (Haynes & Pindzola, 1998; Owens, 2004). Box 8–2 lists several potential uses for a speech and language sample (Shipley & McAfee, 2009). Research documents many potential advantages of speech and language samples, including ecological validity (e.g., how well it relates to real-life skills), its use in outcome and intervention measures, and sensitivity in assessment, particularly for individuals who find standardized assess-

> ### Box 8–2. Potential Uses of a Speech and Language Sample
> #### (Shipley and McAfee, 2009)[2]
>
> ■ Identify speech sound errors.
> ■ Evaluate rate of speech, fluency, and voice.
> ■ Determine speech intelligibility.
> ■ Compare errors in structured tasks with those of connected speech.
> ■ Analyze language, including skills in the areas of semantics, phonology, morphology, syntax, and pragmatics.
> ■ Determine mean length of utterance (MLU) and type token ratio (TTR).
> ■ Identify dysarthria and apraxia.

ment difficult (Costanza-Smith, 2010). A disadvantage, however, is that a speech and language sample is only as good as the sample collected and the skill of the person transcribing and summarizing the sample. In addition, speech and language samples can be time-consuming to record, transcribe, and analyze (Costanza-Smith, 2010). SLPAs can play an important role in collecting a speech and language sample and performing initial calculations of the sample for their supervising SLP. What follows is a discussion of ways to collect and analyze a speech and language sample.

Collecting the Sample

If your supervising SLP asks you to collect a speech and language sample, it is important that you do so in a way that is both reliable and valid. Reliable means the sample can be replicated (e.g., someone else could obtain a similar sample), and valid means the sample is a reasonable reflection of the client's actual speech and language abilities (Shipley & McAfee, 2009).

The first step in collecting a speech and language sample is asking your supervisor where, when, and what type of sample is needed. Audio recording is required for in-depth analysis and transcription. Videotaping is possible, but only if good audio quality is also available. Generally, digital audio files that can be stored and viewed on a computer-based program are preferred (Bunta, Ingram, & Ingram, 2003). The advantage of this method is that specific segments of the sample (e.g., sounds, words, phrases) can be reviewed more easily than with a traditional analog recording, such as a tape recorder. Samples of the digital audio files can also be embedded within a transcription for future reference.

A word of caution is in order regarding audio or video recordings. First, it requires consent from the client or the client's guardian, typically in writing. Never audio or videotape a client without his or her knowledge and expressed consent. Second, if audio or visual information is collected, this information becomes part of the client's official records and is protected by the same confidentiality regulations discussed in Chapter 3.

In general, a sample of at least 50 words is needed, but 100 to 200 words are recommended (Constanza-Smith, 2010;

Shipley & McAfee, 2009). Samples should be collected in a variety of communication contexts (i.e., a variety of communication activities). A general rule is to collect both a conversational sample and a narrative sample (Price, Hendricks, & Cook, 2010), but of course this depends on the instructions of your SLP supervisor. When collecting a sample, it is important that you help the client become comfortable interacting with you. This is particularly true with children, as the sample collected may not be a good reflection of their skills if you dominate the conversation or the client feels shy or nervous about communicating with you. Establishing a positive relationship before you collect the sample is very important (Shipley & McAfee, 2009). For young children, this may mean engaging in play before you begin collecting the sample; for older children or adults, this may mean engaging in small talk on a topic of interest. Box 8–3 contains additional recommendations for collecting a reliable and valid sample.

Conversation Sample. If you are working with adult clients or older children, you can collect a conversation sample by ask-

ing open-ended questions, such as, "Tell me about . . . " (Shipley & McAfee, 2009). Box 8–4 contains a list of additional conversation starters. For young children, incorporating pictures that depict the topic starter or pictures showing a scene with a variety of activities, such as a carnival or playground, may also be a good topic starter (Shipley & McAfee, 2009). Try to avoid, though, having the client name items in the picture. Rather, attempt to engage the client in natural conversation, with open-ended and topic-continuing statements, such as, "Tell me more about that" (Costanza-Smith, 2010; Shipley & McAfee, 2009).

Narrative Sample. A narrative is a story (Merriam-Webster, 2003). Producing a narrative requires more planning and organization than a conversation (Price et al., 2010; Shipley & McAfee, 2009). One common method for collecting a narrative sample is story retelling (Price et al., 2010; Shipley & McAfee, 2009). For example, you could read the client a story and then ask him or her to retell the story to you. You could also ask if the client can recall a familiar story, such as *Goldilocks and the*

Box 8–3. Recommendations for Collecting a Speech and Language Sample (Shipley and McAfee, 2009)[3]

- Minimize interruptions and distractions.
- Be willing to wait for the client to talk.
- Do not talk to fill silence.
- Preselect materials and topics of interest.
- Follow the client's lead.
- Vary the subject matter.
- Limit the use of yes/no questions.
- Ask questions to elicit longer responses (e.g., Tell me about _____. What happened then? Why?).
- Make natural contributions to the conversation.

> ## Box 8–4. Sample Conversation Starters
> (Shipley and McAfee, 2009)[4]
>
> ■ Tell me about what you would do if you won a million dollars (you had super-powers, or you _____)?
> ■ Have you ever been to a hospital (airport, or _____)? Tell me about it.
> ■ Do you like video games (movies, or _____)? Tell me about your favorite one.
> ■ Pretend I've never had a pizza (ice cream, or _____) before. Describe it to me.
> ■ What is your dream vacation (home, or _____)? Describe it to me.
> ■ Do you have a pet (brother, sister, or children)? Tell me about him/her/them.

Three Bears or *Little Red Riding Hood*, and ask them to tell you the story. Alternatively, you could show them a wordless storybook and ask them to tell you the story depicted, or give them several pictures depicting the elements of a story and ask them to place them in order and tell you the story they depict.

Sample Transcription/Analysis

To transcribe something is to make a written copy (Merriam-Webster, 2003). The first step in transcribing a speech and language sample is to listen to the audio recording and write (or type) everything said by the client and any conversation partners.

You should label who is speaking (e.g., P: _____ [Partner], C: _____ [Child], Cl: _____ [Clinician]). The initial(s) you assign to each person should be something easily recognized. Start a new line each time a new person speaks. Number the utterances and place a / at the end of each utterance. IPA symbols can be used to transcribe errors; however, for the

sake of time, use IPA symbols only with errors in production rather than transcribing the entire sample using IPA symbols (Shipley & McAfee, 2009). Unintelligible utterances can be marked with a – (e.g., I like to play –). Be sure to record everything said, including repeated words and phrases (e.g., "because he [he] doesn't like me"), filler (e.g., "the girl likes [um] strawberry ice cream with [uh] sprinkles"), and revisions ("the cat has [had] a string on her tail"; Price et al., 2010). Listen carefully. Remember that our minds are specifically tuned to make sense of what we hear. As such, although a word may make sense, you need to write down what was actually produced. For example, in the sentence, "I go to bed," you may understand in the context of the conversation that the client meant that he "went" to bed. You should write *go* though, because this is exactly what was said. Similarly, if a client produced a distorted production of the /r/ in the word *rabbit*, even though you may have understood the word to be *rabbit* despite this distortion, you would note the distorted production. In fact, that is a perfect example of an opportunity to use IPA symbols so that you can note exactly what the client said.

Once you have transcribed the sample accurately, the next step is to perform an analysis of the content. Your supervising SLP will instruct you on what type of analysis to perform. As discussed, there are many ways that a speech and language sample can be used, spanning the areas of phonology, morphology, syntax, semantics, and pragmatics. Although an extensive review of these methods is beyond the scope of this textbook, calculating MLU as a measure of morphological complexity, and calculating lexical diversity using TTR, are discussed in the sections that follow, as these are fairly common analyses.

Lastly, as technology advances, computer-aided language sample analysis (CLSA) is also available and may be used by your supervising SLP. With CLSA, information from a client's language sample is entered into specialized software designed to perform a wide variety of in-depth analyses. The use of CLSA requires specialized training. For readers interested in learning more about it, Price et al. (2010) provide a helpful tutorial on the topic of CLSA in clinical practice.

Mean Length of Utterance (MLU). MLU is the average number of morphemes (or of words) produced per utterance (Shipley & McAfee, 2009). A morpheme is "a minimal meaningful unit of language" (Paul, Tentnowski, & Reuler, 2007, p. 121). For example, in the sentence, "The cats are brown," there are five morphemes, as follows:

1. the
2. cat

3. -s (to denote the meaning of more than one)
4. are
5. brown

To calculate the MLU based on morphemes (MLUm), you first count the total number of morphemes (total morphemes) and then divide by the total number of utterances (total utterances). For example:

200 morphemes (total morphemes)/ 43 utterances (total utterances) = 4.6 MLUm

SLPs use MLU as a general indicator of language development, which corresponds to a child's chronological age in young children (Brown, 1973; Klee, Schaffer, May, Membrino, & Mougey, 1989; Miller & Chapman, 1981). SLPAs do not interpret MLUs, but as a general reference, Appendix 8–A contains information about MLUs relative to chronological age and the age of acquisition of common morphological features. Box 8–5 contains additional recommendations for counting morphemes.

Some SLPs prefer to calculate MLU using words (MLUw). In this case, you count the total number of words (total words) and divide by the total number of utterances (total utterances), as follows:

115 words (total words)/41 utterances (total utterances) = 2.8 MLUw

Type Token Ratio (TTR). TTR, developed by Johnson (1944), is a ratio of the different words (or *types*) compared with the total words produced (or *tokens*). SLPs use this information to assess the semantic aspects of a speech and language sample from children (Hess, Haug, & Landry, 1989; Owen

---

> ### Box 8–5. Recommendations for Counting Morphemes
> (Lund & Duchan, 1993; Paul et al., 2007)
>
> 1. Only use intelligible utterances.
> 2. Count the morphemes in the first 50 consecutive utterances.
> 3. Do not count
>   a. Imitations
>   b. Rote passages, such as nursery rhymes and songs that have been memorized
>   c. Noises (unless they are integrated into meaningful verbal utterances)
>   d. Utterances identical to those already said by the client; In this case, the utterance is counted only on its first occurrence and not on subsequent attempts.
>   e. Counting or other sequences of enumeration (e.g., "blue, green, yellow, red, purple")
>   f. Fillers (e.g., um, well, oh)
> 4. Count each of the following as one morpheme:
>   a. Compound words (e.g., birthday, somebody)
>   b. Proper names (e.g., Mickey Mouse)
>   c. Ritualized reduplication (e.g., choo-choo, night-night)
>   d. Diminutive forms (e.g., doggie, daddy)
>   e. Catenatives (e.g., gonna, wanna)
>   f. Auxiliary verbs (contracted and noncontracted forms; e.g., he is and he's)
>   g. Inflections (e.g., possessives, plural *s*, regular past *–ed*)

& Leonard, 2002). In the sentence, "Me go go go dance" there are three types (me, go, and dance), whereas in the sentence, "I like to go dancing" there are five types (I, like, to, go, dancing). Both sentences have the same number of tokens (five). TTRs closer to one represent a sample with a greater number of word types. To calculate TTR, count the total number of different words (types) and divide by the total number of words (tokens). For example:

32 different words (types)/
65 total words (tokens) = .49 TTR

EFFICIENCY/ACCURACY IN DATA COLLECTION

Each of the above sections about data collection stressed the importance of accuracy in data collection and what you can do to ensure you understand and can implement data collection that meets the needs of your supervising SLP. One additional factor, which applies to all types of data collection, is efficiency; that is, your ability to quickly (and accurately) collect data under a variety of circumstances.

Hopefully, as you read about these techniques, they will make sense to you and seem manageable. However, remember that you will be collecting data while you are implementing treatment and performing other tasks. In other words, you will need to multitask! You may also be collecting data in a variety of positions and locations and, in some cases, as discussed in Chapter 12, on more than one client at a time. Depending on the client, you may have only a small window of time between tasks to record data. In addition, your data collection may be a distraction or negatively affect your client's performance in some cases. With time, you will refine your methods for collecting data and you improve, but this is an area that will always benefit from refinement. Data collection is not easy, but as the introduction to this chapter suggests, it is critical. The following are tips for enhancing the efficiency of data collection, regardless of the situation:

1. *Plan in advance:* Review what is needed in advance. Make sure you have a data collection sheet ready in advance of data collection. Fill in any details you can in advance, including things like the client's name, date, and goals.

2. *Make notes or cheat sheets:* If you are using different symbols or notations to represent levels of cues (e.g., S = semantic cue, P = phoneme cue), record these symbols either at the top of your data collection sheet or in a location you can easily reference. Similarly, if you are addressing more than one goal or objective, or collecting different types of data, make a note or two in a convenient location to remind you of these important details.

3. *Do not wait to summarize:* As much as possible, summarize your data and make important notes right after the session ends.

4. *Be discrete:* Use symbols or coded scoring, such as O/Xs or A/B for correct/incorrect instead of +/−; this may be needed for some clients, particularly if you are working with a client who may be distracted by your data collection or concerned about errors in performance. Chapter 10 discusses additional techniques for positioning your data collection sheets so that they are accessible to you but out of view of your clients.

5. *Get creative:* Sometimes it is necessary to get creative with where you place your score sheet and what type of data collection sheet you use. For example, while engaging in a play activity on the floor with a group of preschoolers, it is not convenient to have a full sheet of paper located on a table in the room. Instead, try making tally marks or notes on a sticky note placed in a strategic location among the clients and the toys. Each client will be different, but think creatively about the circumstances and ways that you can improve efficiency with alternative solutions.

6. *Employ continuous quality improvement:* Data collection is not easy. It takes time to develop skills. Take every opportunity to learn from your mistakes. Talk to your supervising SLP about the quality of your data collection. If data collection is an area to improve, use the techniques suggested in Chapter 4 for self-assessment to evaluate your skills and find ways to improve.

REFERENCES

American Speech-Language-Hearing Association (ASHA). (2013). *Speech-language pathol-*

ogy assistant scope of practice. Retrieved from http://www.asha.org/policy

Boswell, S. (2005, September 27). Show me the data: Finding the evidence for school-based clinical decision making. *ASHA Leader.*

Brown, R. (1973). *A first language.* Cambridge, MA: Harvard University Press.

Bunta, F., Ingram, K., & Ingram, D. (2003). Bridging the digital divide: aspects of computerized data collection and analysis for language professionals. *Clinical Linguistics and Phonetics, 17*(3), 217–240.

Costanza-Smith, A. (2010). The clinical utility of language samples. *Perspectives on Language Learning and Education, 17*(1), 9–15.

Epstein, L. (2008). Clinical therapy data as learning process: The first year of clinical training and beyond. *Topic in Language Disorders, 28*(3), 274–285.

Haynes, W. O., & Pindzola, R. H. (1998). *Diagnosis and evaluation in speech pathology* (5th ed.). Boston, MA: Allyn & Bacon.

Hess, C. W., Haug, H. T., & Landry, R. G. (1989). The reliability of type-token ratios for the oral language of school-age children. *Journal of Speech and Hearing Research, 32*, 536–540.

Johnson, W. (1944). A program of research: Studies in language behavior. *Psychological Monographs, 56*, 1–15.

Jones, M., Onslow, M., Packman, A., & Gebski, V. (2006). Guidelines for statistical analysis of percentage of syllables stuttered data. *Journal of Speech, Language, and Hearing Research, 49*, 867–878.

Kawulich, B. B. (2005). Participant observation as a data collection method. *Forum: Qualitative Social Research, 6*(2). Retrieved from http://www.qualitative-research.net/index.php/fqs/article/view/466/996

Kennedy, M. (2007). Communication intervention. In R. Paul & P. Cascella (Eds.), *Introduction to clinical methods in communication disorders* (pp. 157–178). Baltimore, MD: Paul H. Brookes.

Klee, T., Schaffer, M., May, S., Membrino, I., & Mougey, K. (1989). A comparison of the age MLU relation in normal and specifically language-impaired preschool children. *Journal of Speech and Hearing Disorders, 54*, 226–233.

Lemoncello, R., & Fanning, J. L. (2011, November). *Practice-based evidence: Strategies for generating your own evidence.* Presented at the 2011 ASHA Convention, San Diego, CA.

Lund, N. J., & Dunchan, J. F. (1993). *Assessing children's language in naturalistic contexts.* (3rd ed.). Englewood Cliffs, NJ: Prentice-Hall.

Merriam-Webster. (2003). *Merriam-Webster's collegiate dictionary* (11th ed.). Springfield, MA: Author.

Miller, J., & Chapman, R. (1981). The relation between age and mean length of utterance in morphemes. *Journal of Speech and Hearing Research, 24*, 154–161.

Moore, S. M., & Pearson, L. (2003). Intervention. In *Speech-language pathology assistants* (pp. 449–461). Clifton Park, NY: Thomson Delmar Learning.

Mowrer, D. E. (1982). *Methods of modifying speech behaviors: Learning theory in speech pathology.* Prospect Heights, IL: Waveland.

Owen, A. J., & Leonard, L. B. (2002). Lexical diversity in the spontaneous speech of children with specific language impairment: Application of D. *Journal of Speech Language and Hearing Research, 45*, 927–937.

Owens, R. E., Jr. (2004). *Language disorders: A functional approach to assessment and intervention* (4th ed.). Boston, MA: Allyn & Bacon.

Paul, R., Tentnowski, J., & Reuler, E. (2007). Communication sampling procedures. In R. Paul & P. Cascella (Eds.), *Introduction to clinical methods in communication disorders* (pp. 111–156). Baltimore, MD: Paul H. Brookes.

Price, L. H., Hendricks, S., & Cook, C. (2010). Incorporating computer-aided language sample analysis into clinical practice. *Language, Speech, and Hearing Services in Schools, 41*, 206–222.

Rao, P. R. (2011, June 7). From the president: Evidence-based practice: The coin of the realm in CSD. *ASHA Leader.*

Roth, F., & Paul, R. (2007). Communication intervention. In R. Paul & P. Cascella (Eds.), *Introduction to clinical methods in communication disorders* (pp. 1–18). Baltimore, MD: Paul H. Brookes.

Roth, F. R., & Worthington, C. K. (2001). *Treatment resource manual for speech-language pathology.* Albany, NY: Delmar.

Shipley, K. G., & McAfee, J. G. (2009). *Assessment in speech-language pathology: A resource manual.* Clifton Park, NY: Delmar Cengage Learning.

Taylor-Powell, E., & Steele, S. (n.d.). *Collecting evaluation date: Direct observation.* Program Development and Evaluation: University of Washington, Cooperative Learning. Retrieved from http://learningstore.uwex.edu/assets/pdfs/G3658-5.PDF

Williamson, G. (2009). *Mean length of utterance.* Retrieved from http://www.sltinfo.com/downloads/mean-length-ofutterance.pdf

CHAPTER ENDNOTES

1. American Speech-Language-Hearing Association. (2013). *Speech-language pathology assistant scope of practice.* Available from http://www.asha.org/policy. © Copyright 2013 American Speech-Language-Hearing Association. All rights reserved. Reprinted with permission.
2. Adapted from Shipley and McAfee (2009).
3. Adapted from Shipley and McAfee (2009, pp. 161–162).
4. Adapted from Shipley and McAfee (2009, p. 163).

APPENDIX 8-A
Mean Length of Utterance (MLU) and Age Equivalent

MLU	Age Equivalent (Within 1 Month)
1.31	18 months
1.62	21 months
1.92	24 months
2.54	30 months
2.85	33 months
3.16	36 months
3.47	39 months
3.78	42 months
4.09	45 months
4.40	48 months
4.71	51 months
5.02	54 months
5.32	57 months
5.63	60 months

Source: Miller, 1981, as cited in Williamson, 2009.

APPENDIX 8–B
Common Morphological Features and Age of Mastery

Rank	Morphological Feature	Example	Age of Mastery (months
1	present progressive -*ing*	daddy sing<u>ing</u>, mummy play<u>ing</u>	19–28
2	in	key <u>in</u> cup, ball <u>in</u> box	27–30
3	on	ball <u>on</u> bed, cup <u>on</u> table	27–33
4	regular plural -*s*	two cat<u>s</u>, three dog<u>s</u>	27–33
5	irregular past tense	mummy <u>fell</u>, daddy <u>went</u>	25–46
6	possessive -*'s*	mummy<u>'s</u> hat, daddy<u>'s</u> car	26–40
7	uncontractible copula	she <u>is</u> (response to who is happy?)	28–46
8	articles	mummy got <u>a</u> dog, <u>the</u> ball	28–46
9	regular past tense -*ed*	daddy walk<u>ed</u>, a car crash<u>ed</u>	26–48
10	regular third person -*s*	mummy walk<u>s</u>, daddy play<u>s</u>	28–50
11	irregular third person	mummy <u>does</u>, daddy <u>has</u> a ball	28–50
12	uncontractible auxiliary	she <u>is</u> (response to *who is coming?*)	29–48
13	contractible copula	he<u>'s</u> happy (cf. *he is happy*)	29–49
14	contractible auxiliary	mummy<u>'s</u> playing (cf. *mummy is playing*)	30–50

Source: Brown, 1973; Miller, 1981, as cited in Williamson, 2009.

CHAPTER 9

Note Writing

*Observe, record, tabulate, communicate. Use your five
senses. Learn to see, learn to hear, learn to feel, learn to smell,
and know that by practice alone you can become expert.*

—William Osler
(one of the fathers of modern medicine)

As mentioned in Chapter 1, speech-language pathology assistants (SLPAs) may be asked to assist their supervising speech-language pathologist (SLP) in providing treatment or screening and data collection for individuals with communication disorders (American Speech-Language-Hearing Association [ASHA], 2013). In some cases, this may be with your supervisor present. In other cases, you may provide these services when your supervising SLP is not physically present in the room, but has given you specific instructions. In either case, as Chapters 7 and 8 suggest, it is critical that you perform these tasks as instructed and that you accurately record important aspects of the client's performance. It is equally important that you effectively summarize and consolidate this information, both as formal documentation of the services you provided, and as a means of conveying important information to other professionals, including your supervisor. Writing a clinical note is often used for this purpose. The format of these notes can vary across settings and with the mechanism(s) for reimbursement of services (ASHA, n.d.-a, n.d.-b; Sutherland Cornett, 2006). In addition, as an SLPA, how often you write a note for a client will be directed by your supervisor. Depending on the setting, notes are written after every encounter with the client, on a weekly basis, or as needed, given the specific type of interaction.

A common format in the field of speech-language pathology for writing notes is a SOAP note (Moon-Meyer, 2004; Roth & Worthington, 2001; Shipley & McAfee, 2009). SOAP is an acronym for the following: subjective (S), objective (O), assessment (A), and plan (P) (Shipley & McAfee, 2009). SOAP notes are often used in medical settings (Roth & Worthington, 2001) but can be modified in form and content to fit the needs of an educational setting. Understanding the SOAP format and how to convey information effectively in a clinical note in your setting is an important skill for an SLPA. However, as will be discussed, specific aspects of the SOAP note format are not consistently applicable to an SLPA's role or scope of services. The sections that follow discuss each aspect of a SOAP note from the perspective of an SLPA. The companion website of this textbook contains a blank version of an SLPA-applicable SOAP note for your use.

SUBJECTIVE (S)

The subjective (S) portion of a SOAP note contains "non-measurable and historical information" important for understanding the client's performance (Shipley & McAfee, 2009, p. 138). This portion of the note provides context to help the reader interpret what will follow in the remaining portions of the note. The dictionary defines *subjective* as "arising out of or identified by means of one's perception" (Merriam-Webster, 2003). The definition fits well, as the subjective portion of a SOAP note contains your opinions, observations, and information reported to you by others.

Key areas to include in the subjective section of a SOAP note (Moon-Meyer, 2004; Roth & Worthington, 2001; Shipley & McAfee, 2009) and corresponding examples are as follows:

Your observations about the client's mood:

- The client smiled and laughed frequently throughout the session.
- The patient was tearful today.
- Melissa greeted the clinician in the waiting area with a hug and was eager to begin the session.

Statements about clients' behavior or their current status, from the perspective of the client, family member(s), or others involved in the client's care (e.g., teachers, nurses, aides):

- Johnny's mother indicated that he has been remembering to close his mouth while breathing.
- The client indicated that he was successful with his homework

and felt it helped him recall the relaxation techniques, which he used during his classroom science fair presentation.

■ The patient's wife indicated that the patient is talking more at home and is regaining movement of his right arm.

■ Mrs. Smith reported that Susan experienced three seizures this week, with one resulting in admittance to the emergency room.

A description of the client's level of cooperation and participation:

■ Rebecca appeared reluctant to engage with her peers during the group reading activity, often averting her eyes or looking away when asked questions by her peers.

■ The client was cooperative and participated fully with all tasks.

■ The client refused to participate in the oral reading task.

■ Steven appeared distracted by the noise from the playground during screening. He frequently turned to look at the window and asked several times to be excused from the session.

A description of any factors in the environment, or other relevant conditions, that may have influenced the client's performance:

■ Due to a fire drill, screening was interrupted for 10 minutes while the SLPA and the client evacuated the building. Screening resumed after the drill.

■ The client's wife, Susan, was present during treatment.

■ Henry arrived 15 minutes late for the session, due to an assembly during the home period.

In this section of the note, you should describe what you see and not simply label the behavior. For example, if the client appeared happy to you, rather than saying, "Johnny was happy," describe the behaviors that you think lead you to that opinion, such as, "Johnny smiled and laughed frequently during the session." When you are reporting information shared with you, be sure to identify the source of this information in your statement. For example, instead of saying, "The patient was tired as he did not sleep well last night," report instead, "The nurse on duty indicated that the patient did not sleep well last night," or "The patient reported that he felt tired from not sleeping well the night before." Remember too, that your verb choice in this section and the objective (O) section (below) should be past tense, as you are describing something that already occurred.

Lastly, note that in the examples provided, the client is sometimes referred to by first name and other times by "the client" or "the patient." This will apply to all other sections of the note as well and will depend on the setting. In most hospital and clinical settings, the client's name is not used within the body of the medical records, in SOAP notes, or other reports. As such, in those settings, "the client" or "the patient" is the preferred term. In most educational settings, however, the client is referred to by first name. You should check with your supervising SLP to confirm which form is appropriate for your setting.

OBJECTIVE (O)

The objective (O) section of the SOAP note contains facts and measurable findings about the session (Moon-Meyer, 2004; Roth & Worthington, 2001; Shipley & McAfee, 2009). Typically, data collected during the session (see Chapter 8) are reported in this section. As the definition of *objective* suggests, this section contains observable and measurable information about the client's performance during that session (in contrast to subjective opinions, or reports from others).

This section typically begins with a brief summary of what occurred during the session. If screening was performed, state the name of the screener used or describe the screening methods. Describe any other forms of data collected as instructed by your supervising SLP. If this was a treatment session, state the goal(s) or objective(s) targeted during that session. Follow the summary with the actual data collected. Examples from objective (O) sections of SOAP notes are as follows:

- John's AAC goals were targeted today. For Objective 3 (requesting an activity using eye gaze), Johnny requested Bingo and Candy Land using eye gaze when the SLPA presented a field of two icon choices. For Objective 5 (switch activation), Johnny answered 10 yes/no questions accurately using his yes/no voice output device.
- Objective 1a (word opposites): 15 of 20 (75%) using picture cards.
- Fluency count was performed during morning story time in David's classroom (Figure 9–1).

Target Behavior:	√√√√√
Whole-word repetition	(5 in 12 min.)
Length of Time: 10 minutes	

Figure 9–1. Sample frequency count table for objective (O) section of a SOAP note.

- Goal: The client will correctly produce the /r/ phoneme in all positions of a word with 100% accuracy. Performance: The client was 75% accurate for this task during a Go Fish activity requiring the client to request cards containing one- and two-syllable words with /r/ in the initial, medial, and final position of the word.
- Prepositions (Objective 5) (Figure 9–2).

In some of the examples provided, the information is very brief, and in others, more detail is provided. In some instances, the information is provided in text format, and in others, tables and charts are used. The level of detail needed, and the actual format of this section, varies from setting to setting and depends on your supervisor's needs and her or his instructions. In some settings, the content of a SOAP note is incorporated within the actual data collection sheets used to record client performance (Appendix 9–A). In that case, an additional SOAP note may not be required. The companion website of this textbook contains a blank version of the form for your use. In preparation for writing a SOAP note, you should review typical notes in your setting and discuss

No Assistance	Gestural Cue	Sound Cue	Modeled Production	Preposition
-	-	-	-	Over
-	-	-	-	Under
-	+			In
-	+			On
-	-	-	-	Over
+				In
-	-	-	+	Under
-	+			In
-	-	+		On
-	-	-	+	Under
TOTALS: 1/10 (10%)	3/10 (30%)	1/10 (10%)	2/10 (20%)	

Figure 9–2. Sample cue record table for objective (O) section of a SOAP note.

with your supervisor the depth, format, and type of information she or he needs in each section .

Note that in some of the examples provided, the third-person personal pronoun is used to describe the SLPA's actions (e.g., "when *the SLPA* presented a field of two icons to choose from" in the first example). Third-person pronoun use is common in professional writing in the field of speech-language pathology and may be the preferred form in your setting. If that is the case, instead of saying, "I gave the client paragraphs to read," which uses a first-person pronoun (*I*), you would reword the note and refer to yourself as *the SLPA*, as in "*The SLPA* gave the client paragraphs to read." You should model your style of writing to match acceptable standards for your setting.

ANALYZE (AZ)

This section of the SOAP note and the one that follows (P) require modification for SLPA use as they differ substantively from the forms suggested for use by SLPs. In most references about SOAP notes the "A" portion of the note refers to "assessment" (Moon-Meyer, 2004; Roth & Worthington, 2001; Shipley & McAfee, 2009). As discussed in Chapters 1 and 2, SLPAs are not to perform any type of formal or informal assessment (ASHA, 2013). As such, changes in content and wording of this section are required to align with the duties and responsibilities of an SLPA. Revision of this section to reference *analyze* (Az) brings it in line with the scope and responsibilities of an SLPA. It is appropriate, and within the scope of an SLPA to analyze the session itself given: (1) an objective summary of the client's current performance compared with a previous session(s) (statement of performance), and/or (2) a description of whether the prescribed task, stimulus, or reinforcement was easy or difficult to implement during that session (description, task, stimulus, reinforcement).

In terms of a statement of performance, Table 9–1 contains a comparison of an "A" (assessment) that an SLP may write regarding the client's performance versus an "Az" (analysis), appropriate for an SLPA to write.

As you can see in the table, for the SLPA Az section, there is no interpretation of information regarding progress made toward achieving goals, or in relation to the client's current status. Appropriate SLPA format in this section limits the discussion to a summary of objective information from today's session as it relates to a previous session(s).

Also, it is appropriate for the SLPA to comment in the Az section on the tasks, materials, and reinforcement that were easy or difficult to implement (description of task, stimulus, reinforcement). This may be helpful to your supervising SLP in planning future sessions or understanding the objective data in more detail. Table 9–2 shows a comparison of a description of

Table 9–1. Assessment Versus Analyze (Statement of Performance)

Assessment (A) Appropriate for an SLP	Analyze (Az) Appropriate for an SLPA
Susan has made good progress in achieving Goal 2 (Objective 5). Her production for /s/ initial sounds has increased in accuracy from initial sessions, with some generalization noted for nontarget positions (e.g., /s/ final production). She is stimulable for /s/ final position sounds and was noted on one occasion during today's session to produce an /s/ initial word accurately in a conversational context.	Susan's performance on Goal 2 (Objective 5—/s/ in initial position of words) was 70%. During the previous session, her performance was 50% on this same objective.
The client remains with significant aphasia and significant difficulty verbally naming pictured items; however, he has improved in his use of multiple modalities, such as gestures, drawing, and writing. His performance on Objective 3 (use of gestures) indicates an increase in performance from the previous sessions.	This session, the client's scores on Objective 3 (use of gestures) increased from a score of 1 of 10 during last week's session to a score of 5 of 10 during today's session.

Table 9–2. Assessment Versus Analyze (Description of Task, Stimulus, Reinforcement)

Assessment (A) Appropriate for an SLP	Analyze (Az) Appropriate for an SLPA
The client continues to need cues to employ communication strategies during a group context and may benefit from a written reminder or one-on-one training in the scripted language needed to initiate questions or to ask for clarification/assistance in group contexts.	During the barrier communication task (Objective 5), the client needed several reminders (5) to *describe* the picture to fellow group members and to ask group members for questions if he did not understand their descriptions. (*Task*)
Jane's participation during speech sessions has increased with the use of personally relevant stimuli and given treatment activities using social structure and reinforcement. She may also benefit from treatment during small group sessions with peers.	Jane appeared to enjoy using the Sponge Bob cartoons to elicit the /s/ sound. She requested additional turns in making sentences with these cards. (*Stimulus*)
Steven benefits from the use of token reinforcement to increase on-task behaviors during speech sessions. This may be an area to discuss with his classroom teacher for increasing on-task participation during classroom activities as well.	Steven began following directions and participating more fully when tokens were provided for on-task behaviors. (*Reinforcement*)

tasks, stimuli, or reinforcement A (assessment) that an SLP may write, versus an Az (analysis), appropriate for an SLPA for this type of information.

Note that for each of the examples in Table 9–2, the information under Az for an SLPA is limited to a description of some aspect of the task itself, the stimulus or materials used, or the reinforcement. It does not extend to interpreting what this information means or generalizing what was observed to a statement about the client's overall performance or status. That is limited to the scope of an SLP (ASHA, 2013).

MY PLAN (PM)

The final section of a SOAP note is indicated by the letter "P." Similar to the "A" portion of a SOAP note, this section requires modification compared with the version that would be written by an

SLP. Traditional textbooks on the topic of SOAPs, written for SLPs, state that the "P" portion of a SOAP note consists of the plan for the future course of treatment (Moon-Meyer, 2004; Paul & Cascella, 2007; Roth & Worthington, 2001; Shipley & McAfee, 2009). Developing, modifying, or altering a client's plan of treatment from that specifically prescribed by an SLP is not within the scope of an SLPA (ASHA, 2013). As such, discussing the future course of treatment for a client in the "P" section of a note is outside the scope of practice for an SLPA. A reasonable modification, however, would be to include a plan of action specific to the needs of the SLPA, using "Pm," to indicate "my" plan (as an SLPA).

An excellent use of the Pm section of an SLPA note is to relay any specific concerns or requests conveyed to you by the client, family members, or other team members involved in the client's case. Counseling or the provision of "interpretative information to the student, patient, client, family, or others regarding the patient or client status or service" is outside the scope of duties of an SLPA (ASHA, 2013, Responsibilities Outside the Scope of an SLPA, para. 2). For example, if a client or family member expresses a concern or request for information about services, SLPAs should first inform the client or family member that they will relay this information directly to their supervising SLP. In most cases, this information should be given verbally, and immediately, to your supervising SLP. The Pm portion of your note is a place to document this information, as in the following examples:

- The client requested additional information about options for additional days of service.
- Alice's mothers asked to speak with the supervising SLP about Alice's performance in the classroom and impending individualized educational plan (IEP) meeting.
- Stephen's teacher (Mr. Collings) requested information about the client's treatment goals and progress.
- The client indicated he is concerned that his speech is not improving with treatment. He indicated that he fears he will not improve further.
- Mrs. Smith asked about developmental milestones and if Susan's language and speech have met them.

You should also check with your supervising SLP to confirm her or his preference as to the location of this information. Some supervisors may prefer this information go in the S section of the note.

As in the S section, when you are reporting information shared with you, be sure to identify the source of in your statement. Be sure to also indicate how you responded to the request or concern, such as, "The SLPA indicated she would ask her supervising SLP to contact the client's mother immediately with these details," or "The SLPA informed the client that this information was not within her scope of duties to discuss but that she would convey his concerns directly to her supervisor," or "The SLPA provided Mr. Collings with the SLP's direct phone number and indicated that she would relay this request directly to her as well."

The Pm section is also used to request additional information, assistance, or resources from your supervising SLP. In this respect, statements in the Pm section would start with, "Plan to discuss with supervisor . . . ," or like the following examples:

- Plan to discuss with supervisor Johnny's distraction during treatment tasks and ways to increase his participation during group activities.
- Plan to discuss with supervisor how the client's AAC system should be used during reading activities.
- Plan to clarify what would be classified as a whole-word repetition during Stephen's conversational speech.
- Plan to request additional information about facilitating techniques referenced in Scott's treatment plan.
- Plan to review with supervisor current data collection methods to ensure accuracy in recording information requested.

Lastly, the Pm section of an SLPA note can be used to detail any specific preparation you need before the next session with this client, such as the following:

- Plan to place game choices under the table before beginning a session so they are not a source of distraction during the group treatment session.
- Plan to presort stimulus cards into three piles (sounds, words, phrases) to facilitate easy access while targeting Objective 5.
- Plan to code data collection sheet ahead of time with required scoring parameters to make data collection more efficient and effective during the treatment session.
- Plan to use timer to ensure treatment activities end with enough time to review assigned homework activities.
- Plan to start next treatment with a review of good listening rules.

These statements would most likely begin with "Plan to . . . " They may be preparations you have already identified as applicable to a future session. If not, you can list them as an area to discuss with your supervising SLP. However, consistent with an SLPA scope of practice, any plan of action outlined by an SLPA must not be related to the client's course of treatment, such as, "Plan to target short-term Goal 5," or "Plan to discharge Goal 3 due to achievement," or "Plan to modify literacy objective to include sound letter correspondence training." Each of those statements is the specific domain of the supervising SLP (ASHA, 2013).

As discussed in Chapter 4, the use of a reflection journal to document your per-

formance during a clinical session may be a good source of information to include in the Pm section of an SLPA note. The companion website of this textbook has a blank reflection journal sheet for your use and Box 9–1 shows the sample reflection journal entry provided in Chapter 4. The bolded sections are examples of items that may carry over into a Pm note for a particular session, such as the following:

- Plan to discuss with supervisor methods for effective data collection.
- Plan to rearrange position of table in treatment room, facing away from the window to ensure students are not distracted during treatment.
- Plan to change instruction and procedures for group activity, including preselecting order of activities and assigning turns for who goes first in each activity.

TIPS FOR EFFECTIVE NOTE WRITING

Appendix 9–B has sample SLPA notes written following the format described above. Note that they vary in length and complexity, but all roughly follow an S, O, Az, Pm format. It is valuable to review examples of notes in your setting to ensure your notes are consistent with setting-specific expectations. Keep in mind that many of the tips on professional writing discussed in Chapter 4 also apply to writing a clinical note. Specific to clinical notes, Figure 9–3 contains a checklist of tips to make your note writing effective in any setting. This information is also available in a checklist on the companion website of this chapter.

Box 9–1. Reflection Journal Entry

Date: *2/14/2018*
Task: *10:00 a.m. Small Group Session (JL, AS, TM)*

Successes:
JL and AS participated fully and had high levels of accuracy for target sounds. The session ended on time. The students appeared to enjoy the session and were eager to begin. I felt relaxed and was able to stay focused on each student's targets during the session.

Difficulties:
TM was distracted during the session. He left the table several times to look out the window. I wasn't sure how to shape this behavior, other than reminding him that he needed to participate. I had difficulty keeping track of errors and the number and type of cues I gave for sound production. When I listened to the audio recording of the session, I provided many more models than I had noted on my data sheet. I also said "okay" twice when JL's target sound was not correct. The time spent on preparing for the session's activities took too long (10 minutes). The students argued about which activity to do first and who would start in each activity.

Areas to Improve:
1. *Increase structure of the session at the onset.* **Make sure to briefly instruct the students in the rules of the activity. Don't allow them to choose the order of the activities. Rotate who goes first per session or have them draw from a deck of cards and whoever gets the highest card goes first.**
2. *Improve data collection methods. Collect additional examples of data collection sheets used for group sessions.* **Check with supervisor about her methods for effectively and quickly noting both errors and cues in group settings.** *Possibly rearrange data collection sheet in advance with a column to place an X under each type of cue. Place a sticky note reminder on my data collection sheet for next time, reminding me not to say "okay." Listen to the audio recording from next week's session and record the number of "okays."*
3. *Close the blinds in the room or* **move the table so the students aren't distracted by the things happening outside the window.**

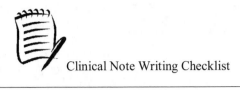

Clinical Note Writing Checklist

____ Note is dated.

____ Note is free of spelling errors.

____ Note is free of grammatical errors.

____ Note is free of any interpretation, assessment, or recommendation about a specific

course of treatment.

____ Note is free of slang and colloquialism

____ Note uses standard forms of medical abbreviation and phonetic notation

____ As applicable, third person personal pronoun is used to describe your actions (e.g., "The SLPA . . . ")

____ Setting specific terms are used to reference the client (e.g., referring to the client by his first name, full name, or by using the terms "the client" or "the patient").

____ Information conveyed to you by others is referenced as such (e.g., The client's family reports . . . , Susan stated . . . , etc.)

____ Note uses language that describes a behavior observed and does not label or diagnosis the behavior.

____ Note contains a description of what was done.

____ Note states specific treatment goals and objective targeted

____ Note states specific tools or procedures used

____ Note contains a summary of the client's performance in objective terms (e.g.,

percentages, frequency counts, etc.).

____ Note uses past tense in applicable sections (typically O and S, and sometimes Az section)

____ Note uses future tense in the Pm section.

Figure 9–3. Clinical Note Writing Checklist.

REFERENCES

American Speech-Language-Hearing Association. (n.d.-a). *Documentation in school settings: Frequently asked questions.* Retrieved from http://www.asha.org/SLP/Documentation-in-Schools-FAQs

American Speech-Language-Hearing Association (ASHA). (n.d.-b). *Private health plans frequently asked questions: Speech-language pathology.* Retrieved from http://www.asha.org/practice/reimbursement/private-plans/php_faqs_slp.htm#7

American Speech-Language-Hearing Association (ASHA). (2013). *Speech-language pathology assistant scope of practice.* Retrieved from https://www.asha.org/policy/sp2013-00337/#sec1.6.2

Merriam-Webster. (2003). *Merriam-Webster's collegiate dictionary* (11th ed.). Springfield, MA: Author.

Moon-Meyer, S. (2004). *Survival guide for the beginning speech-language clinician.* Austin, TX: Pro-Ed.

Paul, R., & Cascella, P. W. (2007). *Introduction to clinical methods in communication disorders* (2nd ed.). Baltimore, MD: Paul H. Brookes.

Roth, F. R., & Worthington, C. K. (2001). *Treatment resource manual for speech-language pathology.* Albany, NY: Delmar.

Shipley, K. G., & McAfee, J. G. (2009). *Assessment in speech-language pathology: A resource manual.* Clifton Park, NY: Delmar.

Sutherland Cornett, B. (2006). Clinical documentation in speech-language pathology: Essential information for successful practice. *ASHA Leader, 11* 8–25. doi:10.1044/leader.FTR3.11122006.8

APPENDIX 9–A
Data Sheet Incorporating SOAP Format

Student: _____ **Teacher:** _____ **Room #:** _____

Date: _____ (Length of Session: _____)

Session goal(s)	Comments (S)	Data (O)	Plan
		Results (A)	

Date: _____ (Length of Session: _____)

Session goal(s)	Comments (S)	Data (O)	Plan
		Results (A)	

Date: _____ (Length of Session: _____)

Session goal(s)	Comments (S)	Data (O)	Plan
		Results (A)	

APPENDIX 9–B
Sample SOAP Notes

SOAP NOTE EXAMPLE 1

S:/ The patient's wife indicated that the patient is talking more at home and is regaining movement of his right arm. The patient greeted group members with a smile as he entered the treatment room.

O:/ Target Goal 2a (in response to word-finding difficulties during group conversation, the patient will independently use a related gesture in three of five opportunities):

Word Retrieval Difficulty	Spontaneous Gesture	Gesture With Cue (# of Cues)
1.	+	
2.	+	
3.	–	+ (cues: 2)
4.	–	–
5.	+	

Az:/ This session, the client's scores on Objective 2a (spontaneous gestures) increased from a score of 1 of 5 during last week's session to a score of 3 of 5 (criteria) during today's session. Spontaneous gestures included swinging his arms to represent "home run," a motion to his head to represent "baseball cap," and a thumbs-up letting the group know his dinner last night was good.

Pm:/ Plan to discuss with supervisor how to change procedures for initiating the group's conversation activity, including potentially preselecting the order of activities before the session or assigning who goes first in each activity. This may decrease time spent organizing these aspects of the conversation during the session. The patient's wife asked to speak with the supervising SLP about additional community resources for physical therapy. The SLPA told the wife that she would share this request with her supervising SLP. The SLPA also gave the patient's wife her supervisor's direct phone line.

SOAP NOTE EXAMPLE 2

The client smiled and laughed frequently throughout the session. He indicated he was successful with his homework and felt it helped him recall relaxation techniques, which he indicated he used during his classroom science fair presentation. Stutter-free speech in 2-minute narratives (Goal 4) was targeted during today's session. The client completed 10 of 13 2-minute narratives, with zero (0) disfluencies (76% accuracy). Using narratives about NASCAR (describing features of favorite teams) elicited ample client narration. Plan to review with supervisor current data collection methods for noting number and type of disfluency.

SOAP NOTE EXAMPLE 3

Subjective: Jill was tearful today and reluctant to leave her mom to participate in treatment. Jill's mom attended the first 15 minutes of treatment.

Objective:

Goal 1 (phonologic awareness—syllable identification)
Jill was 100% accurate (20/20) for clapping once per syllable for words read by the SLPA.

Goal 2 (phonologic awareness—identification of initial sound)
Jill was 75% accurate (15/20) for pointing to the initial sound of words read by the SLPA, given a choice of five printed letters.

Goal 3 (phonologic awareness—sound blending)
Jill was 90% accurate (18/20) for blending and producing the correct target word from syllable segments read to her by the SLPA.

Analysis: Jill appeared to enjoy the use of Sponge Bob-related vocabulary during sound blending and initial letter identification tasks. Her scores across all goals have improved from the previous session when accuracy for Goals 1, 2, and 3 were all less than 50%.

Plan: Plan to identify additional topic areas to incorporate into future sessions. Plan to discuss with supervisor the potential use of crayons and drawing during treatment tasks. During the first portion of the session, when Jill experienced difficulty separating from her mom, her om initiated a drawing activity. Jill's mom indicated that Jill enjoys drawing at home and has started writing the letters of her name within drawn images.

CHAPTER 10

Implementing Treatment

To do something, however small, to make others happier and better, is the highest ambition, the most elevating hope, which can inspire a human being.

—John Lubbock

As a speech-language pathology assistant (SLPA), you may be called upon to implement treatment services with individuals who have communicative disorders (American Speech-Language-Hearing Association [ASHA], 2013). This, of course, will be under the direct supervision and instruction of your supervising speech-language pathologist (SLP) (ASHA, 2013). Often, the thought of this is both exciting and intimidating to new SLPAs. When you see an experienced and effective SLP implementing services, it may seem effortless and easy, but in fact it requires very careful planning, specific training, and, in many cases, years of experience.

The term *service delivery model* is used to describe "where, when, and with whom" clinical services in speech-language pathology are provided (Cascella, Purdy, & Dempsey, 2007, p. 259).

In terms of where treatment is provided, this can vary greatly with the population you serve and the setting in which you are employed. Treatment may be provided within the client's environment, such as in his or her classroom, community, home, or work setting. In some settings, this is referred to as a "push-in" (Cirrin et al., 2010) or an "integrated" (Buysse & Bailey, 1993) service delivery model. This contrasts with treatment services provided outside a client's environment, such as in a clinical treatment space. This is often referred to as a "pull-out" (McGinty & Justice, 2006) or a "clinical" (Cascella et al., 2007) service delivery model.

In recent years, *telepractice* has emerged as a new methodology which replaces physical venues for treatment services. For SLPs, telepractice refers to "the application of telecommunications technology to the delivery of speech-language pathology and audiology professional services at a distance by linking clinician to client/patient or clinician to clinician for assessment, intervention, and/or consultation"(ASHA, n.d., Telepractice: Overview, para.1). According to ASHA's scope-of-practice guidelines, if training, supervision, and planning are appropriate, SLPAs may "provide guidance and treatment via telepractice to students, patients, and clients who are selected by the supervising SLP as appropriate for this service delivery model" (ASHA, 2013, Service Delivery, para. 1). If you are asked to provide treatment services via telepractice, many of the concepts discussed in this chapter relative to treatment implementation are applicable to telepractice, but specialized training will also be required (ASHA, n.d.). As an SLPA, you may also be asked to serve as a facilitator for treatment services provided by an SLP via telepractice (ASHA, n.d., Telepractice: Key Issues, Facilitators in Telepractice for Audiology and Speech-Language Services, para. 1). In these instances, you are not the one providing treatment, but rather, you are at the client's location to assist the client while the SLP provides treatment remotely via telecommunication technology. Specialized training is also required to serve as a facilitator for telepractice. A helpful overview for school-based clinicians on this topic is available from Garcia (2013). where, when, and with whom

The *when* of the service delivery model refers to when treatment is provided and addresses the frequency and duration of services, such as the amount of time per session, the number or sessions per week or month, and the total duration of treatment. The *with whom* in service delivery refers to which professional is most appropriate to provide services. In the case of an SLPA, this may mean a decision about whether services are provided solely by an SLP or with the assistance of an SLPA.

Your supervising SLP will determine the optimum delivery model for each client, including where, when, and with whom treatment services are provided. You should familiarize yourself with each of these aspects of your client's service delivery format. *How* treatment is implemented is also highly variable and determined by your supervising SLP. Treatment may be provided to an individual or to a small group of individuals, using a wide array of methods and intervention models (Cascella et al., 2007). How treatment is provided can be described along a spectrum between the two extremes of clinician-directed or client-centered approaches (Roth & Paul, 2007).

Clinician-directed approaches are highly structured and directed by a clinician. The most common forms of clinician-directed approaches are either *drill* or *drill and play* (Roth & Paul, 2007, p. 164). In drill activities, a very specific chain of events occurs. First, the clinician presents a stimulus, such a picture, a written word, a question, or some other method of eliciting a desired response from the client. This is known as the antecedent. The client then produces the required response. This is referred to as the behavior. The clinician responds to this behavior with reinforcement or corrective feedback (also known as the consequence). Generally, this same procedure of *antecedent-behavior-consequence* is then repeated multiple times in a very similar fashion until a required level of accuracy is obtained.

A similar procedure called "drill and play," embeds the *antecedent-behavior-consequence* sequence within some type of motivating activity. For children, this is typically a game or play activity. For example, a game using a small sponge and several bags labelled with a target word can elicit a response from clients (Roth & Paul, 2007). The clinician gives the client the small sponge and asks the client to throw the sponge into one of the bags to select a word to be produced (the antecedent). The client then produces the word labeled on the bag (the behavior). Then the clinician reinforces or provides feedback about the client's production (the consequence).

In client-centered approaches, clinicians give less direction. The emphasis of this approach is on eliciting a desired behavior in a natural context and then responding in a communicative way (Roth & Paul, 2007). The sequence of *antecedent-behavior-consequence* is modified at the levels of the antecedent and consequence. In client-centered approaches, the clinician waits for the client to initiate a behavior spontaneously instead of directly eliciting it. Generally, this is accomplished by structuring the environment to facilitate meaningful and enjoyable communication attempts in a naturally occurring context. For children, this usually means engaging in play activities that are rewarding and motivating and then encouraging communication during play. For adults, this may mean engaging in conversation about topics the client that finds meaningful and interesting. In terms of consequences, rather than providing specific corrective feedback or reinforcements such as *good* or *correct* (as is typical in clinician-directed approaches), the clinician responds to the client's behavior in a communicative manner. For example, if while engaging in a play activity with trains, a client spontaneously uses a targeted behavior, such as saying "my train is going *under* the bridge" (behavior), the clinician would respond in a manner consistent with the communicative context, such as, "I see your train is going under the bridge. My train is traveling *over* the bridge" (the consequence).

In real-world settings, SLPs and SLPAs engage in a blended approach, incorporating elements of both clinician-directed and client-centered approaches, as applicable to the service delivery model, goals of intervention, and the client's needs and preferences. Using either approach requires careful planning and consideration relative to the client, the environment, and your actions as the clinician. The sections that follow highlight some general concepts and things to consider in each aspect.

THINGS TO CONSIDER: THE CLIENT

When it comes to thinking about the client in the scope of successful treatment sessions, there are many avenues to explore, such as things like the client's age, goals, interests, strengths, and weaknesses, and so forth. Many of these details will be discussed in the client's assessment report and treatment plans, compiled by your supervising SLP. In addition to considering the client's individual treatment plan, one of the most important questions is, "Is the client ready to participate in the treatment session?" Although a simple question, it is the most basic and minimal requirement for any successful treatment session.

Cognitive researchers describe two important principles related to client readiness: low road processing and high road processing (Cox, 2007; Meltzer, 2010; Ward, 2009). *Low-road processing* entails attention to basic biologic and physiologic need states, such as hunger, thirst, fatigue, pain, and fear. In contrast, *high-road processing* refers to the set of mental processes that allow people to regulate their thinking and learning. Collectively, high-road processes are referred to as executive control, which includes the ability to pay attention, plan, prioritize, organize, shift between tasks, access working memory, and monitor performance (Cox, 2007; Meltzer, 2010; Ward, 2009). Regardless of the task, these skills are all important to fully participate in treatment sessions and are key components of learning. Of course, the level of complexity demanded of each skill is tailored to the client's abilities, but it is important to understand that if the clients' resources are diverted to low-road processing, they will have limited ability to engage in high-road processing (Ward, 2009). For example, if a client is hungry, in pain, tired, angry, upset, scared, or frustrated, high-road processing becomes challenging and the client's ability to learn is dramatically reduced. As such, a key first step in a successful treatment session is ensuring the clients' basic needs are met so that they can focus on high-road processing.

Developing a strong clinician-client relationship (as discussed below) will address some of the emotional aspects of low-road processing, such as anxiety, frustration, and fear. In terms of biologic needs such as hunger, fatigue, pain, and the need to use the restroom, if these are things you can address in the moment during a session, do so. If not, work with your supervising SLP, the client, the client's family, and related professionals to see how these needs can be met before the client attends the treatment session.

Another important factor related to a client's readiness to participate in treatment is motivation. Motivation plays a key role in successful treatment sessions. Two important elements of motivation are: (1) understanding the purpose of treatment, and (2) seeing a benefit from participation (Moon-Meyer, 2004; Ragan, 2011). As an SLPA, it is outside your scope of practice to discuss the outcomes of treatment overall, but this does not preclude you from explaining the tasks and intended activities of a specific session (ASHA, 2013). Taking time to explain what is planned for an individual session is valuable in helping clients understand what to expect from the session. This, in turn, may carry over to helping the client understand the purpose of treatment and, hopefully, seeing the benefit of participating This will be particularly true if the client can see a connection between the treatment tasks in a specific session and their overall personal goals (Thomas & Storey, 2000).

Another important element in motivation is interest and engagement in the task (Grubbs & Paradise, 2010; Ragan, 2011). Often with young children, this means *make it fun*, and this can apply to adults as well. Beyond knowing why they are there and seeing the benefits of participation, participating in something that is interesting and engaging *to them* will have a positive impact on motivation. Think about the example of physical fitness. Although many of us understand the purpose of exercising on a regular basis and with some effort we may see the benefits of doing so, the motivation to continue participating in physical fitness activities increases if we enjoy them as well. Hence, your job as an SLPA is to get to know your clients and understand what aspects of treatment you can adjust to improve interest, and thereby, motivation in your session.

THINGS TO CONSIDER: THE ENVIRONMENT

Your environment is your stage, and as such, it must be carefully arranged to support the services you provide. If arranged effectively it will aid in the implementation of treatment. If not, it can detract from your effectiveness as a clinician.

All environments where treatment is provided should be clean and safe. Chapter 6 discusses procedures and requirements for disinfecting surfaces and materials. Your employer will have additional specific requirements. Most employers are required to establish minimal environmental safety standards, such as maximum occupancy in a given space, rules about exit accessibility, and procedures for evacuation in case of an emergency. You should familiarize yourself with all the applicable rules. In addition, when arranging the environment for treatment services, you should consider the nature of the sensory environment, the furniture and seating arrangements, and your materials and stimulus presentation methods.

Sensory Environment

Sight and hearing are two important senses to consider when arranging your environment for treatment services. Visually, the environment should be well lit to allow for adequate visual processing of treatment materials. You should also minimize the level of visual distraction in the treatment environment. If there are toys or equipment that will not be used during a particular session, it is generally best to remove them or place them in an area of the room where they will not be a source of distraction for your client. It is also important to provide treatment services in an environment conducive to adequate hearing. This means an environment that is quiet enough for comfortable, conversational levels of speech. You should arrange the environment to eliminate sources of auditory distraction, such as excessive background noise. This may mean closing a door or window to eliminate noise from the outside, or moving to a location that is less noisy overall.

In some instances, you may work with clients with specific vision and/or hearing needs. If so, consult with your supervising SLP, the client and his or her family, or related professionals, such as an audiologist (for hearing issues), to establish an optimum visual and/or hearing environment for that particular client.

Furniture Choice and Seating Arrangement

A big part of the environment is the furniture and seating arrangements. These can enhance or detract from the overall effectiveness of the clinical environment. Ensure that the furniture is suited to the size of your client (Moon-Meyer, 2004). You do not want an adult client seated in a child-sized chair, nor do you want a child client seated in an adult-sized chair. Generally, when tabletop activities are performed, you should select furniture that allows for comfort and free mobility of the arms and hands. The concept of *proximal stability = distal mobility* (Costigan, n.d., slide 27) can ensure that the client is in an optimal position. This means that if the client's trunk is supported and comfortable, he or she will have maximum free use of the upper extremities. An easy way to remember this is "90-90-90" when it comes to seating (Costigan, n.d., slide 40), meaning the hips, knees, and ankles should be in neutral positions at roughly 90-degree angles (Figure 10–1). In some cases it is appropriate to use no furniture at all, as in the case of young children engaged in play activities. In any seating position, if a client has unique motor or physical needs, you should consult with your supervising SLP, the client and their family, and related professionals, such as an occupational therapist, to ensure the client's seating and positioning allow for maximum participation. In terms of seating, maintaining an eye-level position with your clients will optimize communication between you and your client; you do not want to dominate your client by for example, seating yourself in a tall chair while the client is seated on the floor (Moon-Meyer, 2004).

Where you place yourself in relation to the door is also important. It is generally best to position yourself with your back toward the exit (Figure 10–2). This gives the clinician control of the exit if needed, for example, in cases where a client such

Figure 10–1. 90-90-90 seating position.

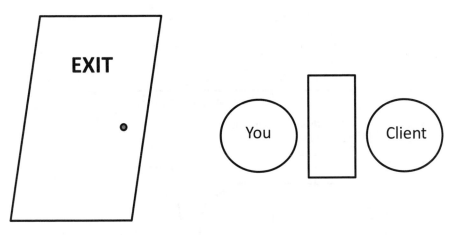

Figure 10–2. Positioning relative to the exit.

as a young child tries to exit the session abruptly (Moon-Meyer, 2004). In addition, there may be situations when the clinician needs to exit the session quickly to obtain assistance. Placing yourself closest to the exit, with your back to the door, ensures you will have a clear path to do so (Moon-Meyer, 2004).

Your position for data collection is also something to consider when arranging furniture and seating. Data collection sheets should be placed to the side of the hand you use to write (Figure 10–3; Moon-Meyer, 2004), regardless of your seating location (e.g., at a table or seated on the floor). This allows you to easily record information and leaves your nondominant hand free for manipulating materials, as needed. In addition, the client and data collection sheet should be positioned so that what you are writing is out of view of the client (Moon-Meyer, 2004). In cases where you are seated at a table and the client is positioned directly across from you, positioning a clipboard at a slight angle may be appropriate to block the client's view of what you are writing. Figure 10–3 depicts a variety of options for

positioning the client in relation to your data sheet, in both individual and group treatment settings. These positions can be adjusted for other seating arrangements, such as on the floor. The key is to arrange your data collection sheet so that it is easily accessible to you but not in view of, or a distraction to, your client.

Materials and Stimulus Presentation Methods

Treatment often involves the use of props, such as pictured items, written material, real objects, and a variety of games or toys (Hegde, 1998). These are often referred to as a stimulus (singular) or stimuli (plural). As discussed in Chapter 7, these items are carefully selected with the guidance of your supervising SLP, based on the unique aspects of your clients and their goals (Hegde, 1998).

Examples of pictured stimuli are things like a picture of a dog to elicit verbal production of the word *dog*, a line drawing of a summer scene to elicit conversation about a recent vacation or

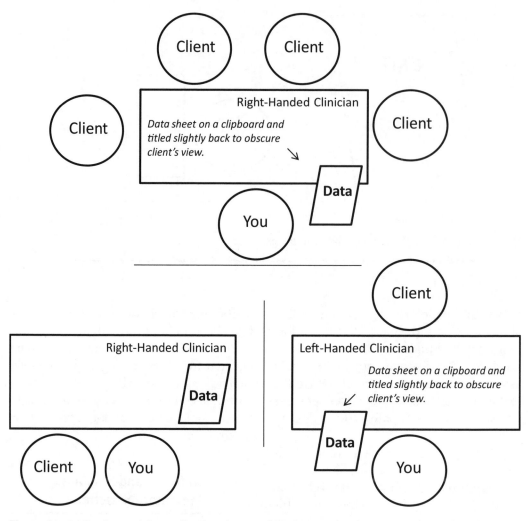

Figure 10–3. Seating and data collection sheet positions.

favored summer activity, or a set of cartoon images the client places in order and then uses to tell a story. Pictured stimuli can also display important concepts, such as a drawing of how to place the tongue when producing a specific sound. Pictured stimuli can be line drawings (black and white or color), color photographs, or a combination of the two. Pictured stimuli can also be combined with written text, as applicable. The images used can be obtained from commercially available sets, magazines, or online sources such as Microsoft Clip Art, Getty Images, or Google Images.

Pictured stimuli should be, "clear, simple, direct, and unambiguous" (Hegde, 1998, p. 154). This means that when clients view stimulus, it should be obvious to them what is intended. Furthermore, pictured stimuli should be attractive and motivating for the client (Hegde, 1998). For example, if a young child is interested in a specific cartoon character, incorporating that character into pictured stimuli may be motivating for that client. Similarly, if a client has a specific interest or hobby, using pictured stimuli with these themes may be particularly rewarding. Whenever possible, using images and pictured stimuli from the client's environment is highly effective. Pictured stimuli should also match the client's age and level of development. Avoid selecting stimuli that are childlike in nature for adults; for young children, select pictured stimuli that are appropriate to their specific developmental level.

In some cases, real-object stimuli may be preferred, such as balls, dolls, toys, or real or simulated daily items, such as kitchen utensils and food items. Chapter 16 discusses ideas for selecting toys and stimuli used for young children engaged in play during treatment activities. Remember too, that objects used by different clients should be cleaned and disinfected between uses, as discussed in Chapter 6.

Written stimuli can also be used. Examples of written stimuli are a textbook from the client's science class to be read by the client to target reading comprehension or to elicit description and conversation; written words, sentences, or paragraphs to be read aloud; or a worksheet with written directions targeting certain grammatical elements. Like pictured stimuli, written stimuli should be direct, effective, and designed to meet their specific intended purpose. They should also match the client's reading abilities and interests. If you are not sure what level of reading material is appropriate for a specific client, speak with your supervising SLP to gain additional details about the client's skills and needs. In addition, ensure the size of any print is appropriate for use with your client. In some cases, cli-

ents have visual impairments that necessitate larger print than would be typical in traditional reading materials. Even for young children who are not literate, presenting pictured or written stimuli in a sequence consistent with their future literacy lays a good foundation for literacy development (Moon-Meyer, 2004). For English speakers, this is a left-to-right, top-to-bottom reading order. Importantly, all stimuli, regardless of form, should be "ethnoculturally appropriate" (Hegde, 1998, p. 154). Chapter 5 provides additional explanation and instruction on this topic. Furthermore, prepare your stimuli in advance of a clinical session and make sure they are presorted in the appropriate order to save time during the session and present a professional and organized impression. For some individuals, you may want to keep the work area clear and have only the stimuli needed for one activity at a time in view. In that case, have the next set of stimuli easily accessible so that you can transition between activities quickly. Lastly, if you are presenting stimuli that require the client to choose a specific target from an array of choices, as in a receptive task where the client points to a specific pictured item named by you, carefully consider the number of choices (Moon-Meyer, 2004). For example, Figure 10–4 displays a scenario in which the client was asked to point to an item described by the clinician. You can see that in the first attempt (#1), the clinician presented four cards (also known as a "field" of four) and then gave the client a command to point to one of them. When the client pointed to one of the cards (e.g., dog), the field of choices became narrowed to the three cards that the client did not select. If the clinician does not replace the card for "dog" for the second trial (#2) before giving the next

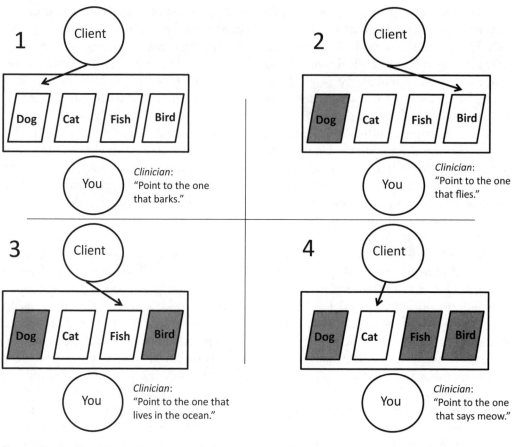

Figure 10–4. Consistency in response choices.

command, the client would then be selecting not from a field of four, as in the first attempt, but from a field of three choices. Similarly, in the third attempt (#3), the choices narrowed even further to only two possibilities, followed by the fourth trial (#4), which was a field of one, because the client had already pointed to all but one item on the table. This decreasing field of choices makes the task easier with each successful attempt. The best method for countering this occurrence is to replace items after each attempt or present a new set of cards for each attempt.

**THINGS TO CONSIDER:
THE CLINICIAN**

Much of responsibility for a positive treatment session outcome rests with the clinicians and her or his behavior. When a session has not gone as anticipated or did not have a positive outcome, the best course of action is to look to your own behaviors and interactions *first* as the primary source of variance. Often, when you do this you will find that there are elements of your performance that negatively affected the outcome. The good news is that if your behaviors can negatively affect the outcome, they can also positively affect. Consider developing a better clinical rapport and a refining your clinical interactions, including things like how you give instructions, model behaviors, and provide hints (also known as prompts). The use of behavioral principles is also a key factor in your interactions during therapy. This is discussed in detail in Chapter 11. Each of these areas will be discussed in the sections that follow.

Clinical Rapport

Developing a positive rapport with clients you serve can have a dramatic impact on treatment services. Rapport is not simply whether your clients "like" you (Pattison & Powell, 1990). Rather, rapport is "the establishment and maintenance of an interactive, harmonious, and communicative relationship" (p. 77). Importantly, rapport can change over time (Pattison & Powell, 1990), meaning that you must work to develop a positive clinician-client rapport initially, and then work to *maintain* the positive relationship over time. Chapter 4 discussed tips for effective communication, which will be very helpful in establishing a strong communicative relationship with your clients.

In addition, an important element of establishing and maintaining a positive rapport is to be sensitive to the client's physical and emotional needs (Pattison & Powell, 1990). The sections above about the environment and the client discussed considerations such as clients' *physical* needs, such as a supportive and comfortable environment, and making sure the clients' basic needs are met. In terms of

emotional needs, keep in mind that clients vary in their feelings and emotions about treatment. Some individuals view it positively and are excited to attend treatment, whereas others feel anxious about treatment activities and communicative tasks (Brumfitt, 2010; Flasher & Fogle, 2004; Holland, 2007). In addition, some individuals may be depressed or have strong emotional reactions to their communicative impairment (Brumfitt, 2010; Flasher & Fogle, 2004; Holland, 2007). The provision of counseling to individuals with communicative disorders is outside the scope of an SLPA (ASHA, 2013). If you are concerned about the psychological well-being of any client you serve, immediately notify your supervising SLP. Two important ways SLPAs can support their client's emotional needs while further establishing a positive rapport are as follows:

1. *Show that you are attentive and focused on your client's needs.* This means limiting discussion about yourself and personal topics. It is appropriate on a limited basis to share personal stories and experiences with your clients, but the focus of treatment sessions should not be on you. In fact, you should limit that total amount of time you spend talking in general (Moon-Meyers, 2004; Pattison & Powell, 1990). You can encourage shy or withdrawn clients to interact with you during a clinical session by (a) allowing for a brief period of small talk at the beginning or end of each session (tailored to their age and abilities), (b) showing a genuine interest in clients' well-being, and (c) communicating slowly, asking open-ended questions, and waiting for and encouraging clients to communicate (Pattison & Powell, 1990).

This is particularly true when you first get to know a client. You should also be conscious of your nonverbal behaviors to ensure that you are welcoming. You do not want to inadvertently convey the wrong messages nonverbally by displaying behaviors such as fidgeting (e.g., tapping your pencil, twirling your hair, shaking your legs) or resting your hands on your chin, because these can make you appear nervous or bored (Moon-Meyer, 2004). In addition, always silence your cell phone and other sources of personal electronic distraction, such as e-mail and text message notifications on electronic devices. It is also professional to place these items out of view of the client since it may give the impression that you are waiting for a call or other contact not related to the client's session. Lastly, starting and ending your clinical sessions on time gives the impression that you are focused on clients' needs and are conscious that their time is valuable.

2. *Structure the session to decrease negative emotions.* Start each session with a brief description of the tasks or activities to be included in each session (Moon-Meyer, 2004). Letting clients know what is planned allows clients who are anxious to prepare for the session's activities. It also reinforces the purpose of the session and helps facilitate shared responsibility for session goals, which in turn helps build positive client-clinician rapport (Roth & Worthington, 2001). Chapter 11 offers suggestions for reinforcement and positive support that can be used to facilitate participation and reduce negative emotions and behaviors associated with treatment. In addi-

tion, consult with your supervising SLP to ensure you are pacing sessions so that activities are not too fast or too slow for each individual client (Roth & Worthington, 2001). This serves to decrease any undue frustration for tasks that are either too easy or boring or tasks that are too difficult. In addition, in general, following a pattern of targeting easier tasks at the beginning and end of the session allows treatment to begin and end on a positive note (Moon-Meyer, 2004; Roth & Worthington, 2001). Lastly, remember to leave time at the end of the session to do the following:

a. Provide a warning shortly before the session ends, especially for clients who may feel frustrated with ending the session or anxious in transitioning to the next activity (Moon-Meyer, 2004).

b. Provide a recap of the client's performance (Roth &Worthington, 2001). This is also an opportunity to highlight any positive accomplishments made that session (Moon-Meyer, 2004).

c. Provide a summary of any home activities or additional outside assignments recommended and assigned by your supervising SLP (Roth &Worthington, 2001).

d. Offer an opportunity for the client to ask questions.

An additional avenue for improving your clinical effectiveness and establishing a positive client-clinician rapport is to give clients an opportunity to provide feedback about the services provided. In allied health fields this is often referred to as customer-oriented care (Reisberg, 1996). One important aspect of customer-oriented care is an opportunity for customers to give both positive and negative feedback about the services provided (Frattali, 1991; Reisberg, 1996). In the case of speech-language pathology, our clients (and their families) are our customers. Feedback from clients can be obtained in a formalized fashion through written or online client satisfaction surveys (Frattali, 1991). Often these measures are developed and administered by your employer (or your supervisor). If your setting uses a client satisfaction survey, familiarize yourself with the questions on the survey.

Informal mechanisms can also be used during individual clinical sessions to obtain client feedback (Frattali, 1991). The use of a rating scale, like those in Figure 10–5 can be helpful for receiving feedback during clinical interaction (Brumfitt,

2010; Wewers & Lowe, 1990). These are examples of visual analog scales (VAS).

A VAS is "a straight line, the end anchors of which are labeled as the extreme boundaries of the sensation, feeling, or response to be measured" (Wewers & Lowe, 1990, p. 13). VAS can be modified and used with any sensation or feeling. VAS have frequently been used as a way for clients to report their pain or mood in clinical settings (Wewers & Lowe, 1990). They have also been used with pictorial representations at the ends of lines to represent applicable extremes (Brumfitt, 2010). Clarifying words, numbers, and or written descriptors can also be added (Wewers & Lowe, 1990). Some advantages of VAS, particularly those with pictorial representations, are that they are less tied

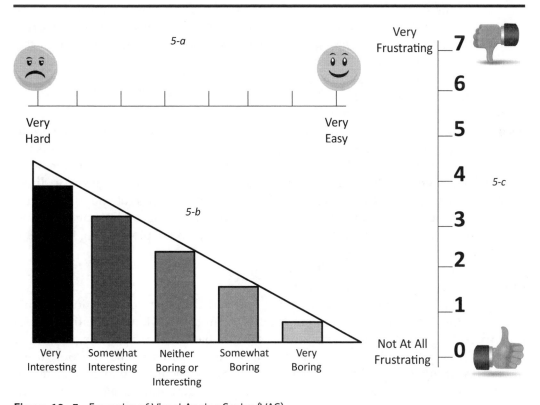

Figure 10–5. Examples of Visual Analog Scales (VAS).

to complex language skills that would be needed, for example, to describe a specific sensation or feeling or to understand a complex verbal or written question about a sensation or feeling (Brumfitt, 2010). This makes them potentially applicable for use with clients with of varying ages and abilities.

Some ways that SLPAs can incorporate VAS into their sessions could be by asking the client to give either general or specific feedback about a treatment task or session. Some things that could be measured with VAS include the following:

- Frustration (frustrated to not frustrated)
- Pain (not painful to painful)
- Difficulty (easy to hard)
- Interest level (boring to interesting)
- Comfort level (comfortable to uncomfortable).

Traditionally, VAS use very specific numeric scales, but for use in speech-language pathology settings, they can simply serve as means of soliciting qualitative (e.g., nonnumeric) and subjective feedback from clients about their experiences, feelings, and attitude about anything related to the clinical session. For example, if the VAS in Figure 10–5a was used and the client pointed close to the "very easy" symbol, you could share that information to share with your supervising SLP, so that she or he could review the task to see if a potential modification is needed for future sessions. Similarly, if you use the scale presented in Figure 10–5c during a treatment task and the client indicated they were "very frustrated" by pointing closest to the 6, you would know that she or he is becoming frustrated with the task and a break may be needed.

As with all clinical procedures, the use of these scales should first be discussed with your supervising SLP to ensure they are appropriate for a specific client. You should obtain guidance in developing an applicable VAS and in establishing how and when to request this type of feedback from the client. Generally, VAS used in this way are most effective when combined with careful instructions (Wewers & Lowe, 1990). Being given a similar VAS more than once allows the client to become comfortable with offering opinions in this fashion. It also provides an opportunity to track the client's opinions over time and across tasks. A VAS is not the only way to elicit client feedback about some aspect of your clinical services. You can also simply ask direct questions (e.g., Are you feeling frustrated? Is this task boring? Am I going too fast?). The key here is to offer an opportunity, appropriate to the client's abilities, for the client to express opinions about the clinical session.

Clinical Interactions

An additional and important aspect to consider when providing treatment is the nature of your clinical interaction with clients, including how you provide directions, the effectiveness of your demonstrations and modeling, and the prompts and scaffolding you deploy during treatment.

Directions

Your verbal and written directions about a treatment task can have a positive or negative impact on if that task is performed accurately and as intended. Your directions to the client should be short and to the point. You should also allow sufficient time for the client to respond before repeating directions (Roth & Worthington, 2001). The form of your directions is important as well and, in general, they should be in declarative form (Roth & Worthington, 2001), such as the following:

Name this picture.

Say the word _____.

Write these words in sentences.

Let's begin.

Tell me what happened this weekend.

Repeat after me.

Place the picture in the box.

Take a card from the stack of cards.

Avoid combining a command and a question, such as, "*Can you* name this picture?" and "*Can you* repeat after me?" In these instances, an appropriate response is for the client to answer yes or no, not for the individual to perform the requested task. Similarly, note that when some commands are converted to questions, such as, "Are you ready to begin?" (instead of "Let's begin."), the question form gives the client an opportunity to say no and not begin the task. In some situations, it is perfectly appropriate and acceptable to request information about a client's readiness to begin, while in others, it may be an opportunity for the client to avoid or escape an undesirable task. In those instances, it is better to avoid asking such a question and stick to a command (Roth & Worthington, 2001).

Demonstration/Modeling

Beyond clinical directions, treatment procedures typically require clinicians to demonstrate and model tasks (Hegde, 1998). The distinction between these two behaviors is that in demonstration, there is no expectation that the client immediately repeats the behavior demonstrated. In modeling, the client is expected to imitate the behavior after it is modeled. Clinicians can provide frequent demonstrations of a desired response to help reinforce a concept or behavior (Roth & Worthington, 2001). For example, the clinician speaking at a slow rate demonstrates slow, controlled speech for an individual who stutters, or a clinician frequently using a specific grammatical form in her conversation offers repeated exposure to this form for an individual with a language impairment.

In the case of modeling, knowing when and how to model is an important skill (Hegde, 1998). Modeling is used when a client can imitate a behavior and when a question, prompt, or physical stimulus is not sufficient to elicit the desired response. Modeling occurs most frequently in the initial stages of developing a behavior (Hegde, 1998; Roth & Worthington, 2001). Box 10–1 has helpful tips for providing effective models.

We rarely use imitation in our daily conversations. As such, when using modeling to elicit a behavior, generally the client's goals will gradually transition to requiring less and less clinician support to elicit a desired response. This is known as *fading* (Hegde, 1998). A related technique is shaping (Hegde, 1998). Shaping occurs when a client is not able to imitate a behavior from a model or when the behavior is complex. Shaping breaks a behavior into small, progressively more complex steps, from easy to difficult, until the final level of performance is obtained (Hegde, 1998).

Box 10–1. Providing an Effective Model

1. *Make sure the stage is set for the client to receive and imitate your model.* Model the behavior only when you have the client's attention and he or she knows that an imitation of the model is to follow. Modeling when clients are not paying attention or when they are not ready to imitate will just require a repetition of the model.

2. *Avoid unnatural models.* Model behaviors as you would like them imitated. For example, this means avoiding overly exaggerating or slowing certain elements to such an extent that they become distorted or inaccurate (Moon-Meyer, 2004).

3. *Avoid ungrammatical utterances in your models* (Moon-Meyer, 2004).

4. *Model language at a level appropriate to the client's abilities* (Moon-Meyer, 2004).

5. *As needed, emphasize target behaviors with communicative changes.* For example, when you model a behavior that is embedded in a sentence or phrase, emphasizing the model using an increased vocal pitch or loudness may be appropriate, as in the sentence, "the boy *is* runn*ing*," when the auxiliary verb + present progressive is the target behavior (Hegde, 1998). Remember Principle 2 (above) and do not overemphasize to the extent that the model becomes unnatural.

Prompts/Scaffolding

A *prompt* is assistance provided by a clinician to facilitate a desired response from a client (Hegde, 1998; Roth & Worthington, 2001). Prompts are generally what we think of as hints. Some clinicians also refer to prompts as *cues*, but generally speaking, we reserve the word *cue* to mean a behavior made by a clinician (verbal or nonverbal) to instruct clients *when* to respond, and use the word *prompt* (visual, auditory, or tactile) to mean facilitating *how* to respond (Roth & Paul, 2007). For example, a clinician tapping the client's hand to signal it is the client's turn to respond would be classified as a cue (as it denotes *when* to respond), whereas a clinician using vocal emphasis to highlight a helpful feature of the required production, such as, "The boy is runn*ing*. What is the girl doing?" would be a prompt (as it offers information about *how* to respond). Box 10–2 lists examples of prompts.

Prompts are used when a stimulus alone is not sufficient to elicit the desired response but when more direct elicitation, such as modeling, is not preferred. The term *scaffolding* is also used to describe the use of prompts (or other assistance) from a listener (or clinician) to enable individuals to communicate a message that would not be possible otherwise (Norris & Hoffman, 1990). As the name denotes, scaf-

Box 10–2. Examples of Visual, Auditory, and Tactile Prompts

Auditory prompts: Prompts *heard* by the client

- Modulating your pitch or loudness to vocally emphasize an important concept ("The *girl* is sad.")
- Verbal questioning to provide details about an important feature (e.g., "Where do you find these?" "The lion is hungry. What does he want to eat?")*
- Verbalizing a cloze sentence (e.g., "You bounce a _____," or "The baby is tired. She wants to go to _____.")*
- Verbalizing the first sound or syllable of a word, the first portion of a sentence, or any part of the required response*

Note. Items highlighted with an *, can also be presented in written form and in that case would be considered visual prompts.

Visual prompts: Prompts *seen* by the client

- Positioning your mouth in the shape of a target phoneme (e.g., placing you lips together to demonstrate /m/)
- A picture of a concept (e.g., a drawing showing the position of the tongue)
- A *written* prompt, reminder, or question (e.g., "Remember to _____," or "This animal lives in the jungle," or "When do we eat these?")
- Gesturing above your head with your hand to indicate a high(er) pitch
- Pantomiming an action related to a targeted response (e.g., yawning when "sleep" is the target response)

Tactile prompts: Prompts *felt* by the client

- Tapping out the syllables of a word on the client's hand
- Placing your hand on the client's throat to indicate voiced production
- Running your finger gently down the client's forearm to represent continuous sound (as in the production of /z/)
- A tactile real object that aids production or comprehension (e.g., a piece of sandpaper and silk to contrast soft versus harsh vocal production)

folding is thought of as a bridge of support provided to clients until they are able to receive similarly complex messages without the support of prompts. The chapters in Part III (Specific Populations and Disorders) provide additional information unique to certain populations, disorders, and activities. In some cases, you may need to provide more than one prompt simultaneously or present successively prompts until a desired response is obtained.

The purposeful, and importantly, documented use of prompts is a vital part of clinical interaction. New clinicians are often not aware of the level of prompting needed by a particular client and in some cases, are not even aware that they are providing prompts to a client. This is problematic since prompts can influence how independently a client performs a task. As discussed in Chapter 8, accurate data collection about clients' performance is critical. If you assist a client in the form of prompts but do not record it in your data it will negatively affect the accuracy of those data. These faulty data may then be used by your supervising SLP to make decisions about client care. In Chapter 7, lesson plans were outlined including columns for "Prompts/Modifications" and "Make It Easier/Make It More Difficult," which are used to describe suggested prompts, modifications, or both that may be recommended for a specific task. Before you implement any treatment, discuss with your supervising SLP the types of appropriate prompts or modifications applicable for a specific client, as well as how these prompts should be recorded in your data. Chapter 8, particularly the section on "Response Independence," offers additional suggestions.

Presenting prompts systematically using some form of hierarchy individualized to the client is equally important. There are two general approaches to hierarchies of prompting: effortful learning and errorless learning (Abel, Schultz, Radermacher, Willmes, & Huber, 2005; Mosall, Choe, Cronin, & Massery, 2012; Sohlberg, Ehlardt, & Kennedy, 2005). In *effortful learning* approaches, prompts are ordered from the least assistance to most assistance, allowing clients to respond with the greatest level of independence first. If clients are not successful, then additional prompts provide greater assistance until the desired response is obtained. For example, in a client-centered approach setting where the clinician plays with a doll and related items with a young client, and is attempting to elicit the word *bottle*, the clinician might say, "Oh the baby is so hungry. What should we give her?" If the client does not respond, two potential prompts, one at each end of the spectrum, are possible. The clinician could say, "The baby needs a bottle. Say bottle." (greatest level of assistance and least level of independence). At the other end of the spectrum, the clinician could give a minimal visual prompt such as simply looking at the bottle (least assistance and greatest level of independence). In the latter example, if the client then responds by saying "a bottle," she or he has done so with minimal assistance and with greater independence than imitating the response "bottle" after it has been modeled by the clinician.

In *errorless learning* approaches, prompts are presented from the greatest assistance to the least assistance. For example, in a clinician-directed approach, such as teaching a client to use a memory device, the clinician might present the steps of accessing the device first by modeling each step and having the client copy the steps (e.g., opening the device, finding the applicable page, identifying information on that page). Next the clinician might provide a model for all but the final step. In that case, the greatest level of assistance (and thereby prompts) was provided first because rather than independently recalling and performing *all* the steps, the client only needed to perform a minimal step (the final one after all previous steps were modeled). Gradually, then, fewer and fewer prompts are provided until the client successfully performs all the steps independently. As an SLPA, you should confirm with your supervising SLP which approach is most applicable to a specific treatment target and to each client's individualized goals.

REFERENCES

Abel, S., Schultz, A., Radermacher, R., Willmes, K., & Huber, W. (2005). Decreasing and increasing cues in naming therapy for aphasia. *Aphasiology, 19*(9), 831–848.

American Speech-Language-Hearing Association. (n.d.). *Telepractice.* Retrieved from http://www.asha.org/Practice-Portal/Professional-Issues/Telepractice/

American Speech-Language-Hearing Association. (2013). *Speech-language pathology assistant scope of practice.* Retrieved from https://www.asha.org/policy/sp2013-00337/#sec1.6.2

Brumfitt, S. (2010). *Psychological well-being and acquired communication impairments.* San Francisco, CA: John Wiley.

Buysse, V., & Bailey, D. B. (1993). Behavioral and developmental outcomes in young children with disabilities in integrated and segregated settings: A review of comparative studies. *Journal of Special Education, 26,* 434–461.

Cascella, R., Purdy, M. H., & Dempsey, J. J. (2007). Clinical service delivery and work settings. In R. Paul & P. Cascella (Eds.), *Introduction to clinical methods in communication disorders* (pp. 259–282). Baltimore, MD: Paul H. Brookes.

Cirrin, F. M., Schooling, T. L., Nelson, N. W., Diehl, S. F., Flynn, P. F., Staskowski, M., . . . Adamczyk, D. F. (2010). Evidence-based systematic review: Effects of different service delivery models on communication outcomes for elementary school-age children. *Language, Speech, and Hearing Services in Schools, 41*(3), 233–264.

Costigan, A. (n.d.). *An introduction to seating and positioning for individuals who use assistive technology.* Retrieved from http://mcn.educ.psu.edu/dbm/S_P_AT _pt1/S_P_AT_HO.pdf

Cox, A. (2007). *No mind left behind: Understanding and fostering executive control—The eight essential brain skills every child needs to thrive.* New York, NY: Penguin.

Flasher, L. V., & Fogle, P. T. (2004). *Counseling skills for speech-language pathologists and audiologists.* Clifton Park, NY: Thomson Delmar Learning.

Frattali, C. (1991, Winter). Measuring client satisfaction. *ASHA Quality Improvement Digest.* Retrieved from http://www.asha.org/SLP/healthcare/Measuring-Client-Satisfaction/

Garcia, C. (2013). *Online manual for the school-based telepractice paraprofessional.* Unpublished manuscript. Retrieved from http://csd.wp.uncg.edu/wp-content/uploads/sites/6/2012/12/OnlineTelepractice-Manual-for-Paraprofessionals.pdf

Grubbs, C., & Paradise, D. (2010). *Making speech therapy fun: Motivating children with autism to speak.* Retrieved from file:///C:/Users/000666547/Downloads/1446-Grubbs-Christine.pdf

Hegde, M. N. (1998). *Treatment procedures in communicative disorders* (3rd ed.). Austin, TX: Pro-Ed.

Holland, A. (2007). *Counseling in communication disorders: A wellness perspective.* San Diego, CA: Plural.

McGinty, A. S., & Justice, L. M. (2006). Classroom-based versus pull-out interventions: A review of the experimental evidence. *EBP Briefs, 1*(1), 1–25.

Meltzer, L. (2010). *Promoting executive function in the classroom.* New York, NY: Guilford.

Moon-Meyer, S. (2004). *Survival guide for the beginning speech-language clinician.* Austin, TX: Pro-Ed.

Mosall, A., Choe, Y., Cronin, M., & Massery, M. (2012). *Effortful vs. errorless learning in computer-mediated home practice* [Presentation]. Retrieved from file:///C:/Users/000666547/Downloads/5082%20Effortful%20vs%20Errorless%20Learning%20in%20Computer%20Mediated%20Home%20Treatment.pdf

Norris, J. A., & Hoffman, P. R. (1990). Language intervention within naturalistic environments. *Language, Speech, and Hearing Services in Schools, 21,* 72–84.

Pattison, G. A., & Powell, T. W. (1990). Establishing rapport with young children during speech and language diagnostic evaluations. *National Student Speech Language and Hearing Association Journal, 17,* 77–80.

Ragan, T. (2011). 10 ways to motivate the unmotivated student [Web blog]. Retrieved from https://blog.asha.org/2011/04/05/10-ways-to-motivate-the-unmotivated-student/

Reisberg, M. (1996). Customer satisfaction in health care. *Perspectives on Administration and Supervision, 6*(2), 12–15.

Roth, F., & Paul, R. (2007).Communication intervention. In R. Paul & P. Cascella (Eds.), *Introduction to clinical methods in communication disorders* (2nd ed.) (pp. 157–178). Baltimore, MD: Paul H. Brookes.

Roth, F. R., & Worthington, C. K. (2001). *Treatment resource manual for speech-language pathology.* Albany, NY: Delmar.

Sohlberg, M. M., Ehlardt, L., & Kennedy, M. (2005). Instructional techniques in cognitive rehabilitation: A preliminary report. *Seminars in Speech and Language, 26,* 268–279.

Thomas, B., & Storey, E. (2000, April). Motivating the elderly client in long-term care. *Advance for Physical Therapy and Rehab Medicine.* Retrieved from http://physical-therapy.advanceweb.com/

Ward, S. (2009). *Executive function skills for the SLP* [Presentation]. Retrieved from http://www.asha.org/Events/convention/handouts/2009/1718_Ward_Sarah_2/

Wewers, M. E., & Lowe, N. K. (1990). A critical review of visual analogue scales in the measurement of clinical phenomena. *Residential Nursing Health, 13*(4), 227–236.

CHAPTER 11

Using Behavioral Principles

Human behavior flows from three main sources: desire, emotion, and knowledge.

—Plato (Greek philosopher)

The topic of this chapter is behaviorism and its application in the field of speech-language pathology. Behaviorism is broadly defined as a systematic approach to understanding human behavior from the perspective of the environment and its control or influence. Without further discussion, it may not be immediately obvious to the novice clinician why an entire chapter in a handbook for speech-language pathology assistants (SLPAs) is devoted to this topic. There are several reasons why this topic has relevance for

SLPAs, including the following (Maul, Findley, & Nicolson- Adams, 2016, p. 3):

a. "there is a well-established evidence base for the efficacy of methods based on behaviorism,

b. many clients on speech-language pathologists' (SLPs) caseloads are likely to exhibit challenging behaviors,

c. there is an increasing need for SLPs to collaborate with board-certified behavior analysts (BCBAs) in providing assessment and intervention for children with behavior disorders, and

d. the principles of behaviorism are broadly applicable across types and levels of severity of communicative disorders."

This chapter reviews basic principles of behaviorism, including operant conditioning and the important concept of positive behavioral interventions and support. The information in the chapter ties back to Chapter 10 in many ways. Along with each of the recommendations discussed under the heading Things to Consider in Chapter 10, the use of behavioral principles has relevance to what SLPAs take into consideration about the clinical environment, the client, and their own behavior. This is true for any client seen by an SLPA, but behaviorism and positive behavioral supports are particularly relevant in understanding and changing behaviors that interfere with successful participation in meaningful and productive activities, including behaviors that interfere with the services provided by SLPs and thereby SLPAs.

OPERANT CONDITIONING

How an SLPA responds to a client's communication, whether elicited or produced spontaneously, plays an important role in the treatment process. At a very basic level, the job of the SLP is to design treatment that creates, increases, and in some cases decreases specific behaviors (Hegde, 1998). Behaviors targeted are typically those of communication (Roth & Worthington, 2001), although in recent years the scope of an SLP has extended to behaviors outside of communication, such as swallowing (ASHA, 2007). Operant condition-

ing is a theory used to explain how human behaviors can be influenced (either positively or negatively) by the consequences that follow a behavior (Mowrer, 1982). Clinician-directed treatments rely heavily on this theory and the principles of *reinforcement* and *punishment* (Roth & Paul, 2007), but these concepts are also applicable to client-centered treatment approaches. As discussed in Chapter 10, a framework of antecedent-behavior-consequence is used in both types of approaches. The principles of reinforcement and punishment explain how the consequence of a behavior will affect its occurrence and frequency.

Reinforcement

Reinforcement increases the frequency of a behavior (Hegde, 1998). There are two types of reinforcement: positive reinforcement and negative reinforcement. A positive reinforcer is a rewarding item, event, or action that is presented in response to a desired behavior, and a negative reinforcer is an unpleasant item, event, or action that is removed in response to a desired behavior. Although both positive and negative reinforcement increase the frequency of a desired behavior, negative reinforcement is not commonly used in clinical settings in the field of speech-language pathology (Roth & Worthington, 2001).

Positive reinforcement (and thereby positive reinforcers) are common in the field of speech-language pathology and are classified as primary or secondary. Primary reinforcement is physiologically or biologically driven. Food is one of the most common examples of a primary reinforcer (Roth & Worthington, 2001). The use of food as reinforcement, however, should be done with caution (Hegde, 1998) and only under the direction of your supervising SLP. Given the potential for food allergies and sensitivities, specific parental preferences, and religious or cultural considerations, parental consent is typically sought for the use of food as a reinforcement during treatment sessions.

Secondary reinforcers are items, events, or actions that a client learns are rewarding. Secondary reinforcers are commonly used in the field of speech-language pathology and include social rewards, tokens, and performance feedback (Box 11–1).

Box 11–1. Examples of Secondary Reinforcers

Social Rewards

A social reward is an action such as smiling, eye contact, or verbal praise, given in response to a desired behavior (Roth & Worthington, 2001). Social rewards give clients immediate positive feedback about the accuracy of a desired response. Social rewards of a communicative nature (such as those that would naturally occur with a successful communication exchange) are commonly used in client-centered treatment approaches.

Tokens

A token is an item given in response to a desired behavior. The item itself is not particularly rewarding, but tokens can be accrued and exchanged for a specific reward. Examples of tokens commonly used in the field of speech-language pathology are points, check marks, stickers, and chips. The use of token systems is more common in clinician-directed than client-centered approaches to treatment and is frequently utilized, particularly in settings with children, to reward both communicative behaviors targeted in treatment and behaviors related to participation in treatment, such as attention and participation (Hegde, 1998).

Performance Feedback

Performance feedback is information provided to the client about a desired behavior(s). This type of feedback is also called *informative feedback* because it provides information about the client's performance (Hegde, 1998). It can presented verbally or in written form and includes information such as percent correct, frequency of occurrence, biofeedback, or numerical ratings of the client's performance. It is not necessarily intended to be praise but can be combined with either tokens or social rewards. Responding with the phrase, "Excellent work, you kept your rate slow that time," is an example of social reward ("excellent work") + performance feedback ("you kept your rate slow that time"). Combinations of this nature can be highly effective (Moon-Meyer, 2004).

Punishment

In contrast to reinforcement, punishment decreases the frequency of a behavior. Punishment is generally categorized as either Type I or Type II (Roth & Worthington, 2001). Type I punishment involves an adverse consequence to an undesired

behavior. In the field of speech-language pathology, a common form of Type I punishment is corrective feedback, including verbal, nonverbal, and mechanical corrective feedback (Hegde, 1998; Box 11–2). As with reinforcement, punishment may be used in response to the communicative behaviors targeted in treatment or behav-

---

Box 11–2. Examples of Corrective Feedback

Verbal Corrective Feedback

Verbal corrective feedback is typically a minimally adverse verbal response, such as "no," "try again," and "incorrect," to a behavior that the clinician judges to be inadequate or inaccurate for some reason (Hegde, 1998). It gives the client immediate feedback about the inaccuracy or inappropriateness of a specific response. As with combining social reward and performance feedback (reinforcement), verbal corrective feedback can also provide the client with specific information about the inaccuracy of a response, such as "no, remember to place your tongue between your teeth."

Nonverbal Corrective Feedback

Nonverbal corrective feedback is similar to verbal corrective feedback but delivered in a gesture, such as a hand single to denote the need to slow speech rate for an individual who stutters, or some other nonverbal signal (Hegde, 1998). Generally, nonverbal feedback is best used in combination with verbal feedback, such as saying "slow down" (verbal feedback) while providing a hand motion to represent a slowed rate (Hegde, 1998).

Mechanical Corrective Feedback

Mechanical corrective feedback includes visual or auditory signals given by an external device, such as a computer, in response to an inaccurate, inadequate, or inappropriate response (Hegde, 1998). Increasingly, computer programs are used to give this type of feedback in response to a variety of related behaviors. Commonly, the programs combine mechanical corrective feedback with reinforcement (Hegde, 1998), such as a low pitch tone or flashing signal to indicate an inaccurate response and the word *correct* combined with a visual image of a happy face to indicate accurate production, both during the same task.

iors that interfere with treatment, such as aggressive or uncooperative behaviors (Hegde, 1998).

Type II punishment consists of removing a pleasant condition in response to an undesired behavior (Roth & Worthington, 2001). The two most common types of Type II punishment used in the field of speech-language pathology are time-out and response costs (Hegde, 1998; Roth & Worthington, 2001; Box 11–3).

New clinicians may be reluctant to provide punishment, given the negative connotation associated with the word *punishment* (Hegde, 1998). It is correct to be cautious about the use of punishment. However, as you can see from the examples provided, some forms of punishment, such as corrective feedback, can be minimally aversive and still serve the important purpose of providing feedback about an inaccurate response. Generally though, only very minimally aversive forms of punishment should be used. Punishment (particularly Type II punishment) should be used only with the guidance of your supervising SLP and only after reinforcement of a desired behavior has been inef-

fective (Bopp, Brown, & Mirenda, 2004). Working closely with your supervising SLP to ensure you have adequate knowledge and skills in the use of reinforcement and punishment is critical.

Effective Use of Operant Principles

The key to using both reinforcement or punishment is to do so specifically and with an understanding of its purpose and impact. The use of these techniques first requires an understanding of what will serve as an effective reinforcement (increase a desired behavior) or punishment (decrease an undesired behavior), and whether something serves as a reinforcement" versus a punishment depends in part on the individual. A classic example of this with regard to punishment is when a novice clinician inaccurately believes that a timeout from participating in treatment will be a form of punishment for an undesired behavior (e.g., a loud aggressive comment), only to find that in fact the incidence of that behavior increases. In that case, the brief and temporary removal

---

Box 11–3. Time-out and Response Cost

Time-out

Time-out involves "temporary isolation or removal of a client to an environment with limited opportunity to receive positive reinforcement" (Roth & Worthington, 2001, p. 15). An example of this with a young client might be turning his or her chair to a blank wall in the treatment room for a brief period.

Response Cost

Response cost involves removing a previously earned positive reinforcer (Hegde, 1998; Roth & Worthington, 2001). This is commonly done with the use of tokens, by removing a token earned in response to an undesired behavior.

from the treatment session was actually a reward for the client. Similar effects can also be seen, for example, when a clinician gives attention to an undesired behavior and finds that the behavior increases. In that case, the clinicians' attention was reinforcing for the client, resulting in an increase in the frequency of the undesired behavior in an attempt to get additional clinician attention.

Identifying what reinforcement is most applicable for a given client and in which context is key to using operant principles effectively. Reinforcement assessment checklists like those in Appendix 11–A and 11–B identify several types of reinforcement (auditory, visual, tactile) that might apply to a specific individual. Training and practical application is also imperative to ensure you implement these techniques effectively. Specific instruction from your supervising SLP, as well as having her or him evaluate your effectiveness in deploying these techniques, is a top pri-

ority. Several additional tips in deploying effective operant principles are as follows:

1. *Emphasize the positive.* Use positive reinforcement first and most readily. Positive praise, particularly descriptive praise, is very powerful in shaping behaviors and also in building self-esteem.
2. *Use descriptive praise for reinforcement and avoid evaluative praise* (Soclof, 2010). Descriptive praise tells clients specifically why they earned praise or reinforcement (e.g., "Great focus. That time you kept your tongue tip up," or "Good, you corrected all the spelling errors in this sentence"), whereas evaluative praise provides only a generic comment about performance, not linked to the behavior itself (e.g., "good girl," "nice work"; Soclof, 2010). Table 11–1 contains several examples of descriptive and evaluative praise.

Table 11–1. Examples of Evaluative Versus Descriptive Praise

Evaluative Praise	Descriptive Praise
"Good job."	"You worked hard on this reading comprehension sheet. You were able to determine the main point and the conclusion."
"You are so strong."	"You pushed that finger right into the playdoh, you made a pancake—that is using those fingers muscles and making them strong."
"Good girl."	"You said the 's' sound clearly, you put your tongue right behind your teeth and that 's' sound came right out."
"You are so smart."	"You got a match! They are the same—two horses!" or "You got two pegs into the pegboard—two more to go."
"You are a great artist."	"I like the way you used the black border around the pink. It really makes the pink color pop out."
"You are the best at coloring."	"I love to look at this picture. All the rainbow colors make me smile."
"You are so nice."	"You picked up Mark's scarf after it fell on the floor. That is a kind thing to do."
"I am so proud of you, you got all A's."	"This report card shows a lot of effort and hard work, you should be proud of yourself."

Source: Reprinted with permission from Soclof, A. (2010). *The absolute best way to motivate your clients.* Retrieved from http://www.SpeechPathology.com

3. *Establish a behavior code.* A behavior code consists of the rules of participation in treatment. These will vary but may be things like waiting for the clinician to explain a task before the client begins, staying seated in the chair during the treatment session, and not interrupting someone when they are speaking. For some clients, this code may need to be written, visually displayed, or both and explained each session. Behavior codes in group treatment (discussed in Chapter 12) can be highly valuable since they establish a uniform code of conduct and expectations across all group members.

4. *Combine corrective feedback with descriptive praise.* Corrective feedback (and in particular verbal corrective feedback) can shape the nature of production and offer suggestions for improvement (e.g., correct feedback + descriptive praise; Soclof, 2010). However, corrective feedback that is generic in nature can be perceived as criticism, which is associated with negative emotions (Soclof, 2010). Table 11–2 offers suggestions for shaping feedback from criticism to corrective feedback and combining it with descriptive praise.

5. *Avoid the OK syndrome* (Moon-Meyer, 2004). The "OK" syndrome is when a clinician frequently says "OK," for things such as a conversational filler (e.g., "OK, let's begin"), tagging questions (e.g., "Read this paragraph, OK?"), and in response to a client's behavior (e.g., "OK." or "OK, not quite, let's try again"; Moon-Meyer, 2004). As you can see in each of these examples, removing the "OK" actually adds clarity and specificity to the clinician's verbal statements. In particular, using "OK" in response to clients' behavior is problematic because it is a vague comment that does not assist clients in understanding whether their response was accurate or inaccurate, desired or undesired, and so on.

Table 11–2. Criticism Versus Corrective Feedback + Descriptive Praise

Criticism	Corrective Feedback + Descriptive Praise
"This is a sloppy paper!"	"This word here and this letter here are on the line. Here is a good amount of space between the words. Can you try that with the rest of the line?"
"Stop saying you can't do this, you can if you try!"	"You are halfway through the maze, only a little more to go."
"It is not enough times!"	"You said the 'r' sound five times correctly, five more to go!"
"Stop fidgeting, sit down, and finish."	"You knew baby and mommy, now show me the dog."
"Stop running and yelling."	"You walked all the way from your class to the steps using a quiet voice—only a few more steps to go using a quiet voice and steady feet."
"You won't be able to play any of the games you like if you don't hurry up and finish your work."	"You did a whole worksheet. One more to go before we play 'Operation.'"

Source: Reprinted with permission from Soclof, A. (2010). *The absolute best way to motivate your clients.* Retrieved from http://www.SpeechPathology.com

6. *Place your emphasis on the target behavior, not the activity.* Often, in treatment with young children, games are used as a vehicle for eliciting target behaviors. This may create the mirage that the game is the emphasis of treatment and not the target behaviors (Moon-Meyer, 2004, p. 313). To avoid this, clinicians must tie reinforcement to treatment targets. For example you could use some aspect of game performance as a reinforcer, but only provide the reinforcer when a target behavior meets a criterion (e.g., saying /r/ five times correctly and moving five spaces, using the past-tense verb to collect a certain score or move a given number of spaces).

POSITIVE BEHAVIORAL INTERVENTIONS AND SUPPORTS

Beyond the use of behaviorism (and operant conditioning) to help shape treatment targets, SLPs participate in an approach known as positive behavioral interventions and supports (PBIS). PBIS is designed for understanding and changing behaviors that interfere with successful participation in meaningful and productive activities, including the presence of a wide variety of challenging behaviors such as withdrawal, screaming, repetitive behaviors, aggression, tantrums, and self-injury (Bopp et al., 2004; Dunlap, 2005). PBIS is an " . . . approach for assisting school personnel in adopting and organizing evidence-based behavioral interventions into an integrated continuum that enhances academic and social behavior outcomes for all students" (Office of Special Education and Programs, n.d.-a,

What is PBIS). PBIS has been widely studied for use with individuals with severe developmental disabilities, particularly individuals with autism spectrum disorder (ASD), but it has also been applied to children and adults with other types of disabilities and individuals without disabilities (Bopp et al., 2004; Dunlap, 2005). When used school-wide, it is also referred to as School-Wide Positive Behavior Supports (Office of Special Education and Programs, n.d.-a.).

PBIS is a person-centered approach (Carr et al., 2002) that focuses on:

1. Modifying specific aspects of the environment to prevent problem behaviors from occurring (antecedent)
2. Teaching new skills to replace problem behaviors (behavior)
3. Using functional consequences to encourage positive behavior (consequence).

PBIS addresses all three aspects of the antecedent-behavior-consequence chain, but with the important underlying assumption that challenging behaviors are "not just a response that should be reduced or eliminated; rather, they represent an individual's best attempt to transmit a message or meet a need" (Bopp et al., 2004, p. 5). For example, perhaps an individual who is screaming or acting aggressively toward a classmate is attempting to say, "I want X," "I don't want X," or "I need X" (p. 5). PBIS addresses such challenging behavior through the lens of its function. Box 11–4 contains a description and examples of several common functions of challenging behavior. Other authors have parsed these behaviors into even finer categories of function, such as the following (Otten & Tuttle, 2010, pp. 19–20):

Box 11–4. Common Functions of Challenging Behavior

Escape or Avoidance

The behavior is an attempt to get out of doing something the individual does not want to do.

> Example: During a social group, Scott does not want to take a turn so he pinches another student to get out of his turn.

Attention Seeking

The behavior gets the attention of a parent, teacher, sibling, peer, or other person in the individual's environment.

> Example: When Amy notices her teaching giving attention to another student, she screams to regain her teacher's attention.

Seeking Access to Materials

The behavior gets access to a preferred item or participation in a preferred activity.

> Example: While sitting with her peers at story time, Susan see a musical toy she loves on the table next to her, grabs it, and begins to play music on it.

Sensory Stimulation (Also Known as Automatic Reinforcement)

The behavior feels good to the individual.

> Example: During speech-therapy, instead of engaging in a shared reading activity, Bill repeatedly flips through the pages of the book because he likes the way it looks, feels or both.

---

1. Getting attention or a reaction
2. Obtaining a sense of power or control
3. Meeting a sensory need
4. Communicating a feeling
5. Expressing a lack of understanding
6. Escaping or avoiding something

PBIS is commonly described with three tiers (Figure 11–1). Tier 1, also known as universal or primary, targets developing a high-quality learning environment for all students. This tier focuses on school-wide efforts, such as establishing school-wide classroom standards and routines that encourage expected behaviors and discourage problem behaviors (Office of Special Education and Programs, n.d.-b). Two common examples of supports at this level are school-wide behavior codes (Figure 11–2) and acknowledgment reward systems (Figure 11–3; Dunlap, Goodman, McEvoy Wayne, & Paris, 2010).

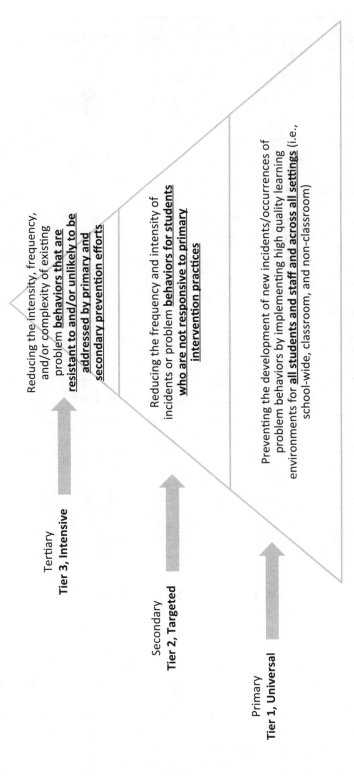

Figure 11–1. PBIS tiers of intervention and support. Adapted from Office of Special Education and Programs (n.d.–b, What is Tier 3 of PBIS).

Tertiary
Tier 3, Intensive

Reducing the intensity, frequency, and/or complexity of existing problem <u>**behaviors that are resistant to and/or unlikely to be addressed by primary and secondary prevention efforts**</u>

Secondary
Tier 2, Targeted

Reducing the frequency and intensity of incidents or problem <u>**behaviors for students who are not responsive to primary intervention practices**</u>

Primary
Tier 1, Universal

Preventing the development of new incidents/occurrences of problem behaviors by implementing high quality learning environments for <u>**all students and staff and across all settings**</u> (i.e., school-wide, classroom, and non-classroom)

SHORE ELEMENTARY SCHOOL
SHARKS
SOAR AT SHORE!

CLASSROOM EXPECTATIONS

BE RESPECTFUL
Listen to all directions
Use quiet voices
Raise your hand and wait your turn to speak
Be friendly and polite to everyone

BE RESPONSIBLE
Be prepared by bringing all supplies
Follow directions the first time they are given
Complete all assigned tasks
Keep cubbies, desks, and classrooms clean

BE SAFE
Keep your hands, feet, and objects to yourself
Stay in assigned seat
Walk at all times

Figure 11–2. School-wide behavior code.

FINS UP!

_____
was being FINtastic!

Issued by: _____ Date: _____

SHORE ELEMENTARY SCHOOL

Figure 11–3. School-Wide acknowledgment system.

Tier 2, also known as secondary or targeted, is focused on behaviors that interventions and supports have been unsuccessful at addressing in Tier 1. Tier 2 interventions and supports could be instruction in self-regulation and social skills, increased adult supervision, more opportunities for positive reinforcement, and increased access to academic support. Simple behavioral contacts might also be deployed in Tier 2 (Figures 11–4, 11–5, and 11–6).

Tier 3, also known as tertiary or intensive, is the most intensive and focuses on an individual student and behavior for which both Tier 1 and Tier 2 interventions and supports have been unsuccessful. Any successful techniques from Tier 1 and Tier 2 would continue, but Tier 3 typically includes a formal and individualized functional behavioral analysis (FBA, discussed below) for a student-specific challenging behavior. FBA is followed by individualized and often intensive guidance and instruction in using new skills as a replacement for the problem behavior and/or rearrangement of the antecedent environment so that problems can be prevented and desirable behaviors can be encouraged.

Given its person-centered foundations, PBIS is established with an understanding of the "needs, goals, strengths, and preferences of the individual" (Buschbacher & Fox, 2003, p. 218). The concepts of choice, self determination, and lifestyle enhancement are embedded within all levels of PBIS (p. 218). The essential steps of PBIS, and particularly Tier 3 interventions and supports, are presented in Figure 11–7.

As the first step in PBIS illustrates, PBIS is a team effort across all levels of

---

POSITIVE BEHAVIOR CONTRACT

The following is an agreement between _____ and _____.

The student will _____ and the teacher will _____.

The following conditions apply:

1. _____

2. _____

3. _____

This contract is void if the student fails to achieve the goal.

The contract will be reviewed on _____.

Student Signature/Date: _____

Teacher Signature/Date: _____

Figure 11–4. Positive behavior contract (student).

★★★★★★★★★★★★ MY CONTRACT ★★★★★★★★★★★★

Name: _____

Date: _____

These are my goals:

1. _____

2. _____

3. _____

These are my consequences if I don't meet my goals:

_____

_____

_____

These are my rewards/positive consequences if I meet my goals:

_____

_____

_____

My contract will be reviewed on: _____

Signatures:

_____

_____

_____

SOAR LIKE AN EAGLE
HUBBARD MIDDLE SCHOOL

Figure 11–5. Positive behavior contract (student).

the approach. Studies have shown more positive outcomes for PBIS intervention when team decision making is employed (Goh & Bambara, 2012). PBIS teams in Tier 3 are individually formed to meet the unique needs of a specific student. Members of the team include first and foremost the individual and his or her family members, as well as individuals who know the student well and who will be implementing interventions and supports (Office of Special Education and

HOME/SCHOOL BEHAVIOR PLAN

The school and parent(s) agree to support each other, work together, and create consistent expectations for _____ (student's name).

The reason we are developing this plan is because _____ has been having a problem with _____ (behavior in school).

Positive behaviors to be increased:

Behaviors to be decreased:

The school agrees to:

Parent(s) agree to:

When will this plan be explained to the student?

Next meeting date to review progress:

School Staff Signature: _____

Parent(s)/Guardian(s) Signatures: _____

Figure 11–6. Positive behavior contract (home/parent).

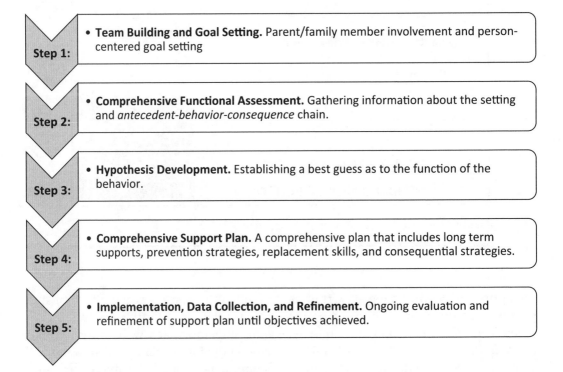

Step 1:
• **Team Building and Goal Setting.** Parent/family member involvement and person-centered goal setting

Step 2:
• **Comprehensive Functional Assessment.** Gathering information about the setting and *antecedent-behavior-consequence* chain.

Step 3:
• **Hypothesis Development.** Establishing a best guess as to the function of the behavior.

Step 4:
• **Comprehensive Support Plan.** A comprehensive plan that includes long term supports, prevention strategies, replacement skills, and consequential strategies.

Step 5:
• **Implementation, Data Collection, and Refinement.** Ongoing evaluation and refinement of support plan until objectives achieved.

Figure 11–7. Five essential steps of PBIS. Adapted from Buschbacher and Fox (2003, p. 219).

Programs, n.d.-c). Other examples of team members include school administrators, teachers, social workers, school psychologists, applied behavioral analysis (ABA) therapists, speech-language pathologists, and support personnel such as aides and SLPAs. An ABA therapist is a team member whose role may not be familiar to an SLPA. Box 11–5 contains a description of ABA therapy and the therapists who provide this service. As an SLPA you might be called upon to collaborate with members of a PBIS team and assist with implementing interventions and supports.

Functional Behavioral Analysis

Before we review a few key PBIS treatment approaches, it is important to discuss the concept of FBA. FBA is an individualized strategy to identify the purpose or function of a challenging behavior so that team members can develop a plan to modify the variable(s) that maintain the behavior and/or teach appropriate replacement behaviors using positive interventions. Essentially, FBA is used to better understand the pattern, purpose, and function of a specific behavior by identifying events that precede (antecedents) and follow (consequences) a challenging behavior. It is an integral part of PBIS, especially Tier 3 interventions and supports. It is typically accomplished through (ASHA, n.d.-b.; Neidert, Rooker, Bayles & Miller, 2013)

1. Describing the behavior;
2. Interviewing those who know the individual to identify the events, times, and situations that give rise to the behavior(s) and the consequences that seem to maintain the behavior(s);

3. Developing a hypothesis or hypotheses to explain these situations and the reinforcers that maintain them;
4. Collecting data through direct observation to systematically test and support or refute the hypothesis or hypotheses.

As noted in Box 11–5, BCBAs and BCBA-Ds have specialized training in this area, but FBA, similar to PBIS, is a team effort. The outcome of an FBA is commonly a behavioral intervention plan (BIP). This chapter's appendices contain samples of informal (Appendix 11–C) and more formal (Appendix 11–D) BIPs. It is important to note, however, that the scope and form of BIPs vary greatly, according to the setting and recommendations of the PBIS team. Some essential elements common to any BIP include (Otten & Tuttle, 2010, pp. 204–205):

1. A description of an acceptable or desired replacement behavior(s) which serves a similar function as the challenging behavior
2. A plan for directly teaching that behavior(s)
3. Prevention strategies to remove or modify the antecedent triggers on the challenging behavior
4. A planned system for reinforcement when a desired behavior occurs
5. Logical undesired consequences if the undesired or challenging behavior occurs

As with other aspects of PBIS, you may be asked to participate in specific aspects of a BIP. In doing so, it is critical that you work with your supervising SLP to ensure you have a good foundation in basic behavioral principles and you fully

Box 11–5. ABA Therapy and ABA Therapists

What is ABA?

According to ASHA, ABA is a " . . . systematic application and evaluation of principles of behavior analysis for the improvement of specific behaviors" (American Speech and Hearing Association, n.d.-a., para 1), including the use of behavior management principles such as learning, stimuli, responses, consequences, positive reinforcement, negative reinforcement, punishment, and extinction. Common treatment techniques used in ABA therapy include prompting, cueing, modeling, chaining, differential reinforcement, and fading.

What is an ABA Therapist?

An ABA therapist is a general term used to denote an individual who provides ABA therapy. Levels of training and professional certification of those who do so vary, as noted below (Psychology Today, n.d.):

- **Registered Behavior Technician**
  A registered behavior technician is an individual, with a minimum of a high school diploma and 40 hours of specialized training, who is registered by the Behavior Analyst Certification Board (BACB) to work under the direct supervision of a BCBA or BCaBA (see below for definitions).

- **BCaBA**
  A board-certified assistant behavior analyst (BCaBA) is an individual who holds an undergraduate degree and specialized training in ABA, who is certified by the BACB to serve in a supportive role in the provision of ABA services. A BCaBA cannot provide services alone, but can work in therapeutic settings when supervised by someone who is certified at a higher level.

- **BCBA or BCBA-D**
  A board-certified behavior analyst (BCBA) is an individual with a master level degree. A BCBA-D is an individual with a doctoral degree. Both have specialized training and education in the area of ABA. BCBAs and BCBA-Ds are approved by the BACB to independently perform a wide array of ABA services, including FBA, ABA treatment and intervention, and supervise registered behavioral technicians and BCaBAs.

understand the tenants of PBIS in your specific setting and for the individual exhibiting challenging behaviors.

Key Approaches of PBIS

Related treatment approaches used within PBIS include functional communication training (FCT) and visual supports. Given the customized nature of materials needed for these approaches, SLPAs can play a key role in the creation of materials for their supervising SLPs and PBIS team. As an SLPA, you may also be asked to assist in implementation of these techniques.

Functional Communication Training

FCT is a form of PBIS, "designed to reduce problem behaviors by replacing them with meaningful or functional communication—whether verbal or gestural (Texas Statewide Leadership for Autism, 2009, p. 1). FCT is designed to "teach socially acceptable communication alternatives to problem behavior" (Bopp et al., 2004, p. 6). The first step in this process is a careful assessment of the meaning or "message(s)" conveyed by a problem behavior and antecedents in the environment related to that behavior (Beukelman & Mirenda, 2013). This is achieved through a detailed and comprehensive assessment, much like FBA, described above, undertaken collaboratively with the client, his or her family, individuals in the client's environment, and related professionals such as the SLP, psychologist, and teacher (Bopp et al., 2004).

Once the message (or meaning of a behavior) is deciphered, the next step is to establish a new and more effective means of conveying that information. This new method must be equivalent in meaning and one that can be conveyed by the client effectively and efficiently in his or her environment. Often, FCT is used with individuals with severely limited or no expressive communication abilities, and thus, augmentative and alternative communication (AAC) is employed to convey messages through words or short phrases, manual signs, gestures, pictured symbols, or written words. Chapter 18 discusses the use of AAC in greater detail, including elements of AAC systems that may be applicable within FCT.

Once a suitable alternative to a problem behavior is identified, an intervention plan is established. This plan addresses instruction in the use of the new behavior, as well as training and collaboration with individuals in the client's environment to ensure socially meaningful and appropriate consequences are in place to generalize the new behavior to the client's environment. Typically, the intervention plan is systematic in nature and embedded within a BIP and PBIS (although it can also exist as a stand-alone goal and approach). Generally it employs several of the behavioral principles described above, such as modeling, shaping, prompts, and the principles of operant conditioning.

Visual Supports

Visual support approaches to facilitate PBIS include both visual schedules and visual modeling. The central premise behind both approaches is to offer instruction, context, and visual information that can assist individuals in modifying and participating effectively in a behavioral chain (antecedent-behavior-consequence) that is challenging for them. Visual supports are customized to the unique needs of an individual and can assist in navigating any number activities such as social communication, activities of daily living, or school-related (academic) activities. Box 11–6 lists a few examples of applicable targets for these approaches, but as these examples show, the possibilities are infinite.

Visual Schedules. Visual schedules are displays of activities, steps, or rules applicable to a specific individual's routine(s) (Beukelman & Mirenda, 2013; Bopp et al., 2004). Visual schedules can display routines across days, weeks, or hours, and at a high level of detail for a very specific routine (e.g., using the bathroom, doing the laundry, baking a cake). The purpose of a visual schedule is to "provide the individual with a way to predict or understand upcoming events in order to reduce problem behaviors and increase independence" (Bopp et al., 2004, p. 14). The use of visual schedules is based on the knowledge that many individuals of all ages, particularly individuals with developmental disabilities, benefit from highly structured environments (Beukelman & Mirenda, 2013; Bopp et al., 2004). Visual schedules are often augmented with verbal input provided to the individual. Figures 11–8, 11–9, and 11–10 show examples of visual schedules. As is evident in Figure 11–9, some visual schedules have a

---

Box 11–6. Examples of Social Communication, Activities of Daily Living, and School–Related (Academic) Scenarios Applicable to Visual Supports

Social Communication

- Requesting items
- Giving compliments
- Interacting with peers
- Expressing affection or dislike

Activities of Daily Living (ADLs)

- Ordering a drink at Starbucks
- Going to the dentist
- Tying shoes
- Doing laundry
- Brushing teeth
- Attending a movie

Academic (School–Related)

- Participating in storytime
- Checking a book out from the library
- Requesting assistance in class
- Attending a school-wide assembly or other school event
- Lining up on the playground after recess

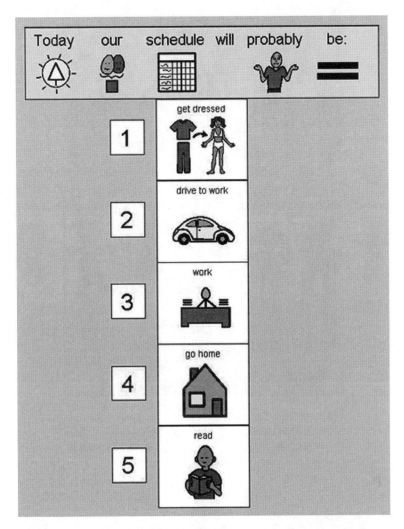

Figure 11–8. Sample visual schedule: Daily schedule, using line drawings. Copyright 2018 Boardmaker. All rights reserved. Used with permission. Boardmaker is a trademark of Tobii Dynavox.

place to denote that a specific step in the routine has been completed (e.g., moving a symbol to the "done" column, crossing off the task after completion, assigning a token such as a happy face). Visual schedules commonly also included aided symbols, such as real objects, photographs, line drawings, or written words, which can be used during the task to facilitate communication.

For use with young children, a variant of the visual schedules above has rules and scripts displayed within a storybook format (Buschbacher, 2018). Social stories designed to convey information about appropriate social behavior, and in particular the commercially available product Social Stories™, have been shown to be effective in reducing problem behavior in individuals with ASD (Pane, Sidener,

Figure 11–9. Sample visual schedule: Daily schedule, using written words, with space to note task completion. Copyright 2013 Indiana University: Indiana Resource Center for Autism. Used with permission.

Figure 11–10. Sample visual schedule: Daily schedule, using real color photographs.

Vladescu, & Nirgudkar, 2015). Similar techniques have been applied to individuals with other types of disabilities and for non-social scripts and routines. The central premise behind using a storybook format is to capitalize on the facilitative aspects of children's literature to help young children navigate a specific routine and behavioral chain (Buschbacher, 2018). The stories are designed to include patterns common to children's literature, including the use of rhyme; repetition of words, phrases, sentences, and refrains; and other patterns that facilitate prediction and processing by young children. Box 11–7 lists several patterns found in children's literature which can be used to create individualized stories of this

---

Box 11–7. Patterns in Predictable Children's Books (Yaworski, n.d.)

Chain or Circular Story

- Plot is interlinked so that the ending leads back to the beginning.

Cumulative Story

- Each time a new event occurs, all previous events in the story are repeated.

Familiar Story

- The story is organized by a recognizable theme, such as days of week or numbers.

Pattern Stories

- Scenes are repeated with some variation.

Question and Answer

- The same or similar questions are repeated throughout the story.

Repetition of Phrase

- Word order in a phrase or sentence is repeated.

Rhyme

- Rhyming words, refrains, or patterns are used throughout the story.

Songbooks

- Familiar songs with predictable elements, such as repetitive phrase are incorporated in the story.

nature. Similar to FCT, the use of visual schedules in any format is preceded by a careful assessment and formulation of a systematic intervention plan for implementation in the client's environment.

Video Modeling

Video modeling is a variant of the visual schedules discussed above, but facilitated by technology that uses video recording and display equipment to provide a visual model of a targeted behavioral chain or routine (Franzone & Collet-Klingenberg, 2008). Video models can be used for a specific individual to target a specific challenging behavior or for schoolwide PBIS, such as videos that "teach and raise awareness of school-wide PBIS

expectations (e.g., be safe), routines (e.g., walk in the hallway), school engagement (e.g., launch PBIS initiatives), special topics (e.g., cyberbullying), and staff responsibilities (e.g., active supervision on the playground)" (Robin, Hirsch, MacSuga-Gage, & Kennedy, 2017, p. 1).

There are several forms of video modeling, including basic video modeling, video self-modeling, point-of-view video modeling, and video prompting, and Box 11–8 describes each. Voice-overs can be included to increase comprehension of the video, either as narration (e.g., "I insert 3 quarters into the machine. I select M&Ms by pressing the large button below them") or to describe the target behavior or rule (e.g., "Students in line at the cafeteria keep their hands to

---

Box 11–8. Types of Video Modeling
(Franzone & Collet-Klingenberg, 2008)

Basic Video Modeling

- Video displays someone besides the learner engaging in the target behavior or skill.

Video Self-Modeling

- The video displays the learner engaging in the target behavior or skill.

Point-of-View Video Modeling

- The video displays the target behavior or skill recorded from the perspective of the learner (i.e., as if being viewed through the learner's eyes).

Video Prompting

- The video displays the target behavior or skill broken down into steps, using any of the formats above, but a pause is inserted after each step for the client to attempt the step just viewed (before viewing the subsequent steps in the sequence).

themselves and do not touch or pinch other students") (Sigafoos, O'Reilly, & de la Cruz, 2007). A variety of prompts can be used before, during, or after the video is viewed, as can a series of fading techniques once the student begins to develop the target behaviors (Sigafoos, O'Reilly, & de la Cruz, 2007). Each of these decisions (and the type of video to utilize) would be determined by your supervising SLP, the PBIS team, or both. In cases of Tier 3 intervention, the behavioral chain targeted within a video model is established via an FBA. The BIP also includes needed details about data collection and monitoring methods for use alongside video modeling (LaCava, 2008). All of these factors are critical to the success of video modeling for reducing challenging behaviors (Sigafoos, O'Reilly, & de la Cruz, 2007).

REFERENCES

American Speech-Language-Hearing Association. (n.d.-a.). *Applied behavior analysis and communication services.* Retrieved from https://www.asha.org/NJC/Applied-Behavior-Analysis-and-Communication-Services/

American Speech-Language-Hearing Association. (n.d.-b.). *Challenging behavior as communication.* Retrieved from: https://www.asha.org/NJC/Challenging-Behavior-as-Communication/

American Speech-Language-Hearing Association. (2007). *Scope of practice in speech-language pathology.* Retrieved from https://www.asha.org/policy/sp2016-00343/

Beukelman, D., & Mirenda, P. (2013). *Augmentative and alternative communication: Supporting children and adults with complex communication needs* (4th ed.). Baltimore, MD: Brookes.

Bopp, K. D., Brown, K. E., & Mirenda, P. (2004). Speech-language pathologists' roles in the delivery of positive behavior supports for individuals with developmental disabilities. *American Journal of Speech-Language Pathology, 13,* 5–19.

Buschbacher, P. (2018). *Routine scripts and rule books for young children: Evidence-based PBS strategies* [Presentation]. Retrieved from http://www.speechpathology.com/

Buschbacher, P., & Fox, L. (2003). Understanding and intervening with the challenging behavior of young children with autism spectrum disorders. *Language, Speech, and Hearing Services in Schools, 34*(3), 217–227. doi:10.1044/0161-1461(2003/018)

Carr, E. G., Dunlap, G., Horner, R. H., Koegel, R. L., Turnbull, A. P., Sailor, W., . . . Fox, L. (2002). Positive behavior support: Evolution of an applied science. *Journal of Positive Behavior Intervention, 4,* 4–16.

Dunlap, G. (2005). Positive behavior supports: An overview. *Perspectives on Language Learning and Education, 12,* 3–6. doi:10.1044/lle12.1.3

Dunlap, K., Goodman, S., McEvoy Wayne, C., & Paris, F. (2010). *School-Wide Behavioral Supports and Intervention: Implementation Guide.* Retrieved from http://www.ccresa.org/Files/Uploads/348/Positive_Behavior_Support_Impl.pdf

Ennis, R. P., Hirsch, S. E., MacSuga-Gage, A. S., & Kennedy M. J. (2017): Positive behavioral interventions and supports in pictures: Using videos to support schoolwide implementation, *Preventing School Failure: Alternative Education for Children and Youth. 62*(1) 1–12. doi: 10.1080/1045988X.2017.1287048

Franzone, E., & Collet-Klingenberg, L. (2008). *Overview of video modeling.* Madison, WI: The National Professional Development Center on Autism Spectrum Disorders, Waisman Center, University of Wisconsin.

Goh, A. E., & Bambara, L. M. (2012). Individualized positive behavior support in school settings: A meta-analysis. *Remedial and Special Education 33*(5) 271–286.

Hegde, M. N. (1998). *Treatment procedures in communicative disorders* (3rd ed.). Austin, TX: Pro-Ed.

LaCava, P. (2008). *Video modeling: An online training module.* (Kansas City: University of Kansas, Special Education Department). In Ohio Center for Autism and Low Incidence (OCALI), Autism Internet Modules (http://www.autisminternetmodules.org). Columbus, OH: OCALI.

Maul, C. A., Findley, B. R., & Nicolson-Adams, A. (2016). *Behavioral principles in communicative disorders: Applications to assessment and treatment.* San Diego, CA: Plural.

Moon-Meyer, S. (2004). *Survival guide for the beginning speech-language clinician*. Austin, TX: Pro-Ed.

Mowrer, D. E. (1982). *Methods of modifying speech behaviors: Learning theory in speech pathology*. Prospect Heights, IL: Waveland.

Neidert, P. L., Rooker, G. W., Bayles, M. W., & Miller, J. R. (2013). Functional analysis of problem behavior. In D. D. Reed, F. D. D. Reed, & J. K. Luiselli (Eds.), *Handbook of crisis intervention and developmental disabilities: Issues in clinical child psychology* (pp. 147–167). New York, NY: Springer.

Office of Special Education and Programs. (n.d.-a.). *PBIS frequently asked questions*. Retrieved from https://www.pbis.org/school/swpbis-for-beginners/pbis-faqs

Office of Special Education and Programs. (n.d.-b.). *What is Tier 3 of PBIS?* Retrieved from https://www.pbis.org/school/tier-3-supports/what-is-tier-3-pbis

Office of Special Education and Programs. (n.d.-c.). *What are Student-Level Tier 3 Systems?* Retrieved from https://www.pbis.org/school/tier-3-supports/what-are-student-level-tier-3-systems

Otten, K. L., & Tuttle, J. L. (2010). *How to reach and teach children with challenging behavior (K-8): Practical, ready-to-use interventions that work*. San Francisco, CA: Jossey-Bass.

Pane, H. M., Sidener, T. M., Vladescu, J. C., & Nirgudkar, A. (2015). Evaluating function based Social Stories™ with children with autism. *Behavior Modification, 39*(6), 912–931.

Psychology Today. (n.d.). *Applied behavioral analysis*. Retrieved from https://www.psychologytoday.com/us/therapy-types/applied-behavior-analysis

Roth, F., & Paul, R. (2007).Communication intervention. In R. Paul & P. Cascella (Eds.), *Introduction to clinical methods in communication disorders* (pp. 157–178). Baltimore, MD: Brookes.

Roth, F. R., & Worthington, C. K. (2001). *Treatment resource manual for speech-language pathology*. Albany, NY: Delmar.

Sigafoos, J., O'Reilly, M., & de la Cruz, B. (2007). *How to use video modeling and video prompting*. Austin, TX: Pro-Ed.

Soclof, A. (2010). *The absolute best way to motivate your clients*. Retrieved from http://www.SpeechPathology.com

Texas Statewide Leadership for Autism. (2009). *Texas guide for effective teaching: Functional communication training*. Retrieved from https://www.gvsu.edu/cms4/asset/64CB422AED08-43F0-F795CA9DE364B6BE/functional communication.pdf

Yaworski, J. (n.d.) *Kinds of predictable books*. Retrieved from http://courses.wcupa.edu/jyaworsk/Courses/EDR510/PredictableBooks.htm

REINFORCER ASSESSMENT

Name_____ Date_____

(Favorites) Completed by: Student Parent Teacher

Toys _____   Friend/person _____

_____   Place _____

_____   Game _____

Snacks _____   Outdoor activity _____

_____   Sport _____

_____   Color _____

Foods _____   Movie _____

_____   T. V. Show _____

_____   Song _____

Drinks _____   Character _____

_____

For students with sensory needs   (Sensory Preferences)
Include likes & dislikes

Auditory _____   Tactile _____

Visual _____   Kinesthetic _____

Olfactory _____   Gustatory _____

© 2015 Traci Bender

APPENDIX 11–B
Reinforcement Assessment (Possible Reinforcer)

POSSIBLE REINFORCERS

SOCIAL

Free time	Eat outside
Listen to music	Tutor
Recess	Note home
Extra recess	Special job
Teacher helper	Class party
Custodian helper	Teach lesson
Dancing	Hugs
Tickles	Massage
Squeezes	Pressure
Line leader	Take a walk
Singing	
Library helper	
Praise	
Pat on the back	
High five	
Run errands	
Board game	
Eat with a friend	
Principal helper	
Sit anywhere	
Cafeteria helper	
Phone call home	
No homework	
Work outside	
Smiles/gestures	
Hear a story	

TANGIBLE

Computer	Sidewalk chalk
iPad	Yo-yo
Favorite snack	Marbles
Favorite toy	Make-up
Stickers	Balls
Write on board	Bubbles
Color	Dressing up
Paint	Ice cream
Clay	Legos
Playdough	Smiley face
Movie	Slinky
Puzzles	Flashlight
Use a pen	Microphone
No shoes	Whistle
Hand stamp	Kite
Nail polish	Use sharpies
Comic book	Sensory bin
video	Lava lamp
Read a book	Shaving cream
Use a camera	koosh balls
Cutting/pasting	Flipbook
Certificate/award	Treasure box
Sit in teacher chair	
Hold stuffed animal	
Ticket to dance/party	
Textured items	

© 2015 Traci Bender

Source: Bender, T. (2015). *Creating a behavior intervention plan* [Blog post]. Retrieved from http://www.thebenderbunch.com/2016/05/creating-behavior-intervention-planbip.html. Copyright 2015 Traci Bender. All rights reserved. Used with permission.

Sample Behavioral Intervention Plan (BIP)—Informal

Behavior Intervention Plan

Name Liz Schoolhouse   Start Date   10/5/15

Behavior	Liz is always blurting out in class.
Function	The function of Liz's behavior is to seek attention. She gets little attention from her classmates and has few friends.
Desired Behavior	Liz will raise her hand for permission to speak and wait for the teacher to call on her.
Proactive Plan	Liz will use a cool points chart that will allow her to self-monitor her blurting out. The chart will be checked each hour and reinforcement will be awarded contingent upon points earned. Give verbal praise each time Liz does not blurt out.
Reactive Plan	If Liz begins to blurt out, behavior will be ignored the first 2 times. After that, the teacher will correct Liz by reminding her of the appropriate behavior.
Reinforcers	A reinforcer, iPad B reinforcer, dolls C reinforcer, M&Ms
Data Collection	Cool point charts will be used as data for number of blurt outs and graphed on a frequency chart. If no progress after 2 weeks, plan will be modified.
Notes	

©2015 Traci Bender

Source: Bender, T. (2015). *Creating a behavior intervention plan* [Blog post]. Retrieved from http://www
.thebenderbunch.com/2016/05/creating-behavior-intervention-planbip.html. Copyright 2015 Traci
Bender. All rights reserved. Used with permission.

Sample Behavioral Intervention Plan (BIP)—Formal

Behavior Intervention Plan

1. Description of targeted behavior

*Describe the behavior. What does the behavior look like?
*Identify frequency (how often it occurs), intensity (how severe is it), and/or the duration (how long the behavior lasts).

Sample

John's targeted behaviors include yelling out, screaming, making loud disruptive noises, hiding in the corner and/or running out of the classroom and around the campus.

Data taken 3/03/15 - 03/13/15
Frequency - John displayed non-compliant behaviors 7/10 days. According to frequency data collected daily for 10 days, the percentage of non-compliant behaviors displayed ranged from 40% to 100% of John's school day.

Intensity - All behaviors range from mild to moderate, with no severe incidences.

2. Functional Behavior Assessment Data

Setting:
*Where does the behavior occur? Is it a particular class, time of day, recess, bus, when child is tired?

Sample

The behaviors occur during instruction and written assignments in the self-contained classroom and during lunch.

Antecedents:
*What happens just before the behavior occurs? What triggers the behavior?

Sample

Behaviors occur when students is not allowed to change the rules or make up his own assignments, when asked to follow directions, when he does not like the lunch choices.

Function:
*What is the student trying to achieve? What are they getting or avoiding?

Sample

John exhibits these behaviors to seek control and get what he wants.

© 2015 Traci Bender

3. Replacement Behaviors (Task Analysis)

*Identify the positive behavior that will be taught to replace the negative behavior. This must be related to the function.

Sample

John will be taught to follow directions by the special education teacher through direct instruction, modeling, non-verbal cues, and practicing for at least 15 minutes, 3 times a week. He will be taught the following steps:

1. Wait patiently for the directions before beginning an activity.
2. Listen carefully to the directions given.
3. Follow the directions given, while staying calm.

4. Proactive Strategies (Individualized Positive Behavior Change Strategies)

*What positive supports will be used to encourage the replacement behavior?
*What accommodations/modifications will be made to support the student? (examples)

Sample

Use a token board reward system with John each time one of the replacement behaviors occurs.
Allow John opportunities to make up his own directions contingent upon earning his tokens.
Provide immediate positive feedback.
Provide positive teacher attention when John is following directions.
Do not focus on work completion, but reinforce following directions. Ex. Do not say,
"Good job, you finished your work." Say, "Good job, thank you for following directions" or "John, I like the way you handled that situation."

5. Positive Strategies to Modify the Environment

*What environmental supports will be used to promote the replacement behavior (seating, calm down area, room arrangement, signs)?

Sample

Display rules and expectations for following directions and review them daily.
Tape a visual reminder of the replacement behaviors on the corner of John's desk.
Provide John with a designated calm down area and a calm down kit for when he is having a difficult time following directions.

6. Reactive Strategies

*What strategies will be used when behaviors occur (prompting, loss of points, de-escalating strategies)?

Ignore minimally disruptive behaviors (planned ignoring)
Give John two choices - the first should be following directions and a reminder of the reinforcement, the second should be the inappropriate behavior and a reminder of the consequence. Give choices calmly and walk away.
Remind John of calming strategies and calm down area
If behaviors become too disruptive to other students, TA 1 will take the students to Mrs. Wright's room while the teacher and TA 2 remain in the classroom with John.

7. Progress Monitoring

*How will progress be monitored and data collected to ensure effectiveness of the behavior plan?
*Who will collect the data?
*How often will it be collected?
*How and when will the data be reviewed (informal meeting, telephone, IEP meeting)?

The special education teacher or staff will collect data randomly throughout the week during 10 different directives, charting compliance or non-compliance.
Data will be analyzed and reviewed every two weeks by the special education teacher.
Continue with each "following directions" step in the task analysis until all steps are mastered.
The special education teacher and John's mother can make mutually agreed minor adjustments to the behavior plan via phone as needed.

8. Intervention Outcome Process

*Identify start and review dates
*Note data here

The behavior plan will begin on _____ and the special education teacher and John's parent will review the plan on _____.

CHAPTER 12

Group Therapy

Jennifer A. Ostergren and Sarah Guzzino-Herrick

*Unity is strength . . . when there is teamwork and
collaboration, wonderful things can be achieved.*

—Mattie Stepanek (nationally recognized poet and peace advocate.
Mattie died at age 13 of complications related to dysautonomic
mitochondrial myopathy, a rare form of muscular dystrophy.)

As has been mentioned, you may be asked to provide treatment services under the supervision and guidance of your supervising speech-language pathologist (SLP) (American Speech-Language-Hearing Association [ASHA], 2013). These services may be delivered to a single individual or to a small group of individuals (Cas-

cella, Purdy, & Dempsey, 2007). Provision of treatment services to small groups of individuals is common in a variety of settings, including school settings for children (Mire, 2007) and medical and community settings for adults (Elman, 2007). Chapter 10 shares ideas for implementing treatment services that are applicable to both individual and group treatment models. The sections that follow focus on the unique aspects of group models of treatment that warrant additional consideration.

The purpose of group treatment varies (Roth & Worthington, 2001) but can include the following:

1. Teaching participants a new communication skill at an introductory level
2. Providing participants with practice in skills established in an individual session
3. Providing participants with socialization, self-help, and/or counseling

Not all groups are appropriate for a speech-language pathology assistant (SLPA) to lead. For example, groups in which counseling and adjustment is the primary (or secondary) purpose would not be appropriate for implementation by an SLPA. Group intervention can occur concurrently with individual sessions or as the sole source of intervention (Roth & Worthington, 2001). It may be provided early, late, or throughout the client's course of treatment. In some cases, group sessions will comprise individuals with similar skills, abilities, and intervention goals, whereas in other instances, group members will be individuals with diverse skills, abilities, and intervention goals (Elman, 2007; Luterman, 2008; Moon-Meyer, 2004). Groups can range in size from as small as two individuals to as large as an entire classroom, as may be the case in community-based groups or in the case of a self-contained classroom in a school setting (Cascella et al., 2007; Elman, 2007). A self-contained classroom is common for students with special needs. Self-contained classrooms place a small

group of pupils with special needs with generally one instructor (often assisted by paraprofessionals) for most of the day (Mattinson, 2011; Schubert & Baxter, 1982; Walker, 2009).

The role of the clinician during group treatment can be directive or nondirective (Roth & Worthington, 2001), based on the purpose of the group. In the case of a directive model, the clinician "sets the agenda, chooses the materials and activities, provides specific instruction, and gives corrective feedback" (Roth & Worthington, 2001, p. 25). In a nondirective role, the group members participate in these activities and the clinician serves as a facilitator in helping group members to accomplish the group's goal(s). An example of a nondirective group model is that of peer-mediated groups. According to Carter and Kennedy (2006), peer-mediated support interventions involve equipping one or more peers, without disabilities, to provide ongoing social and/or academic support to special needs peers of a similar age, under the guidance of educators, paraprofessionals, or other school staff. This intervention is thought to promote independence, due to the students involved becoming more acquainted with working together and leading their own progress. This support arrangement consists of the following: identifying students with a disability and their peers who would benefit from involvement, equipping peers to provide support, arranging opportunities for students to interact and support one another, and monitoring and offering guidance when needed (McCauley & Prelock, 2013).

In any form, clinicians working with groups maintain responsibility for ensuring that group dynamics and communication among group members support apositive learning and social environment for all members. Similar to individual sessions, group treatment activities should be driven by a specific set of goals, applicable to either individual group members or a collective group goal, shared by all members.

Table 12–1 contains a list of several advantages and disadvantages of group treatment. As with any aspect of treatment, your supervising SLP will weigh the advantages and disadvantages of group treatment in deciding when and if it is applicable to a client's needs (ASHA, 2013). She or he will also be responsible for establishing the size, composition, and purpose of group intervention, as well as recommending group activities to target treatment goals.

Moon-Meyer (2004) coined an important term: "therapy in a group" (p. 262). This warrants additional consideration, in contrast with group therapy. According to Moon-Meyer, therapy in a group is not the same as group therapy. Rather, therapy in a group employs the same tenets of an individual session but with multiple clients present. As an example, consider a small group of third graders in a school setting with the following treatment goals:

- John has a treatment goal targeting /r/ sounds in the final position of words.
- Sue has a treatment goal targeting the reduction of disfluencies in conversational speech.
- Bill has a social interaction and pragmatic treatment goal.

Using a *therapy in a group* model, time is split between each individual in targeting treatment goals. When John is practicing /r/ sounds in words, the clinician

Table 12–1. Advantages and Disadvantages of Group Therapy

Advantages of Group Therapy	Disadvantages of Group Therapy
• Group participants may motivate each other or offer insight and assistance that a clinician cannot readily provide.	• Individual participants may receive less direct attention from the clinician.
• More opportunities exist for natural speaking situations, socialization, and peer interactions. This may enhance carryover and generalization of a target behavior.	• Some participants may be reluctant to participate fully in group interactions, particularly those who are shy or self-conscious.
• Participants have an opportunity to observe group members and may recognize that others have problems similar to their own.	• Some participants may monopolize group interactions.
• Group interactions, especially when the clinician takes a nondirective role, may decrease dependence of the clinician and thereby increase client independence.	• Generally there are fewer opportunities per participant per increment of time to engage in a specific behavior (compared with individual sessions). This may mean fewer opportunities to address specific weaknesses and less direct practice of a specific skill.
	• The pace of the group (or the rate of progress) may not be exactly matched with each participant.

Source: Roth and Worthington, 2007, p. 26.

interacts with him, providing feedback and correction to shape accurate production of target words. While this occurs, Sue and Bill wait for their turn. Next, Sue receives the clinician's attention, practicing fluent speech in short narratives. Again, the clinician focuses her attention on Sue, while John and Bill now wait. Finally, it is Bill's turn, and the clinician turns her efforts to discussing sample scenarios of appropriate and inappropriate personal space diagrams, while group members John and Sue now wait. As you can see from this interaction, there is very little interaction *between* the group members themselves, as well as a reduction in the total amount of interaction each group member has with the clinician. This is problematic, particularly when you consider the amount of treatment received per the amount of participation. If this were, for example, a 30-minute session, each participant would have received roughly 10 minutes of *treatment* and 20 minutes of *waiting*. This is not group therapy. None of the advantages of group therapy (described above) could be realized with this model (e.g., group participants motivated by each other, group participants engaging in natural speaking situations), but all of the disadvantages are magnified (e.g., less direct attention from the clinician, fewer opportunities to practice). In this instance, a group member's time is better spent engaging in other activities and attending only an individual session with the clinician for 10 minutes.

As this example shows, the main distinguishing feature of group therapy and that of therapy in a group is interaction, both between the clients and with the clinician. In terms of client interactions, Moon-Meyer (2004) outlines two types of interaction that should be considered:

non-goal-related interaction and goal-related interaction. With non-goal-related interaction, as the name suggests, the interaction between clients does not target the treatment goal, as in the case of waiting their turn or performing tasks not related to their treatment goal. In contrast, goal-directed interactions target each of the client's treatment goals. Maximizing the amount of goal-directed interaction should always be your primary goal during group sessions. This, of course, is easiest when individuals share a similar goal, but with careful planning, group therapy and maximum goal-directed interaction can also be achieved when individuals do not share similar goals.

CHARACTERISTICS OF EFFECTIVE GROUP DYNAMICS

The term *effectiveness* refers to "the extent to which a specific intervention, regimen, or service, when deployed in routine practice, does what it is intended to do" (Baum, 1998, p. 237, cited in Last, 1983). Travis (1957) outlined five characteristics that aid in effective group dynamics, including creating a positive atmosphere, facilitating observation, making tools available, providing opportunities for repeated experiences, and helping to reduce barriers. Each is a factor to consider in designing and/or modifying the dynamics of a group treatment session.

In *creating a positive atmosphere*, as an SLPA, you must demonstrate acceptance, respect, and belonging for each individual. This process may be implemented through your behaviors of speech, facial expressions, postures, and so forth, which should all communicate a positive and welcoming attitude toward group members. This will set the foundation for group interaction. In addition, you must be conscious of the fact that the world is viewed differently by others. Therefore, not projecting your own attitudes on the group will benefit the group atmosphere. Furthermore, allowing group members to participate in selecting and planning activities will influence this as well and create a sense of belonging within that group.

By exhibiting these behaviors and attitudes, you also promote the next characteristic of an effective group dynamic: *facilitating observation*. This means that you assume that group members will be influenced by the behavior(s) they observe, both your behavior and those of the other group members. One issue in this area is placing undue pressure on a group member to respond. You can be mindful of how you introduce group activities and what will be required of group members. You want to ensure the group dynamic is such that group members can participate with ease and pleasure. In addition, as much as possible, use naturally occurring, intrinsic rewards over artificial rewards (such as tokens or "good work"). In educational settings, it is common for students to become influenced by their group members, especially if those members seem to be doing better than them (Travis, 1957). For example, when a student struggles to produce a target utterance, this may create anxiety within the student, especially when she observes overt and artificial praise given to other students. This may decrease future participation in group activities.

The third characteristic of effective group therapy dynamics is *making tools available*. Use of the proper tools to complement the group and individual goal(s) is critical. You can plan in advance of group sessions by listing the materials needed to implement group treatment. This information can be listed on the lesson plan for that session (see Chapter 7). You should make sure all materials are modified to meet each group member's abilities and that there are ample materials, accessible to all members. You will want to ensure, however, that emphasis is on the interactions of group members and the goals of the group session. Chapter 10 discusses the concept of the "game mirage" (Moon-Meyer, 2004). This applies to groups as well. You can avoid the game mirage and reinforce goals of group treatment by providing an introduction to the session, stating the goals to be targeted, elaborating on them during the session, and then concluding with a summary of the group session (Vinson, 2009, p. 310).

Opportunities for repeated experience is also a characteristic of effective group dynamics. This does not mean learning will take place solely through repetition of an activity, as discussed in Chapter 10 relative to clinician-directed treatment that employs drill activities. It does mean, though, that group dynamics and learning are enhanced through opportunities to practice skills with diverse peers who may differ in gender, age, and status (e.g., authority figure vs. peer).

Reducing barriers is the final factor to consider in ensuring a positive group dynamic. This can vary greatly but would include the group leader analyzing factors that impeded the effectiveness of the group, the group dynamics, or group learning. In the field of augmentative and alternative communication (AAC), researchers describe barriers that may impede the use of AAC. These principles can also be applied to group dynamics as well and include opportunity barriers and access barriers (Beukelman & Mirenda, 2005). Opportunity barriers are factors outside the individual that may affect the individual or group dynamics. Three opportunity barriers that may be particularly relevant to your work as an SLPA in group sessions are skills, attitude, and knowledge barriers. These pertain to having the skills and knowledge needed to be effective in a group situation and your attitude toward group situations. If any of these are areas of concern, you can work with your supervising SLP to ensure you have the adequate skills, abilities, and attitudes to successfully run a group session. Access barriers relate to "the capacities, attitudes, and resources" of the individual, including "a lack of ability or difficulty with manipulation and management of objects, problems with cognitive function and decision making, literacy problems, and/or sensory-perceptual impairments (i.e., vision or hearing impairments)" (Roth & Worthington, 2001, p. 116). Here, too, you can work with your supervising SLP to identify any barriers in these areas applicable to group members and their participation in group treatment.

SAMPLE GROUP ACTIVITIES

The activities used in group sessions are a vehicle for obtaining specific goals and can vary greatly, per the group's purpose. As discussed in Chapter 7, lesson plans serve the purpose of directing specific elements of a given session, such as the goals to be targeted, materials to be used, potential prompts or assistance, and data collection methods. Carefully prepared and detailed lesson plans for group treatment sessions will serve a similar purpose.

Although an extensive review of all applicable activities used within group treatment sessions, across the multitude of settings and clients an SLPA may serve, is beyond the scope of this chapter, Table 12–2 contains a sampling of activities for children. Box 12–1 contains a list of suggested activities for adults.

In addition, Chapters 13 and 16 also contain additional examples of treatment activities that can be adapted to group dynamics. Ideas for activities can also be found in resources devoted to group approaches for specific age groups or disorders. For example, *Group Treatment of Neurogenic Communication Disorders: The Expert Clinician's Approach* (Elman, 2007) provides a comprehensive review of group treatment approaches for individuals with neurogenic disorders, such as aphasia, traumatic brain injury, and dementia. Similarly, *Group Treatment for Asperger Syndrome: A Social Skills Curriculum* (Adams, 2006) provides a valuable resource in the area of group treatment for Asperger syndrome. A sample of activities suggested by Adams (2006) for social skills is listed in Appendix 12–A.

Table 12–2. Sample Group Activities for Children

Activity	Suggested Target Area(s)
Shared book reading, card games such as Go Fish, board games, and Tic-Tac-Toe (Figure 12–1) using target sounds	Articulation
Shared reading activities, story retelling rope (Figure 12–2), and comic strips (Figure 12–3)	Language comprehension, verbal expression, writing, WH-questions
Venn diagrams (Figure 12–4) and visual aids, comparing and contrasting topics like sports, foods, presidents, and holidays	Curriculum-based information, language comprehension, language expression, vocabulary, same/different, narrative writing
Theme-based art and creative endeavors, such as coloring, crafts, and building projects	Following directions, sequencing, vocabulary, and verbal expression
Obstacle course and building activities	Prepositions
Hangman	Spelling
Treasure or scavenger hunts, conversational ladder (Figure 12–5), conversational starter cards (e.g., If you could have any superhero powers, what would they be? What would you buy if you won a million dollars? If you could invent a video game, what would it be like?), off-campus outings, and role-play (e.g., student becomes the teacher)	Verbal expression, stuttering and disfluency, and social skills

Tic-Tac-Toe

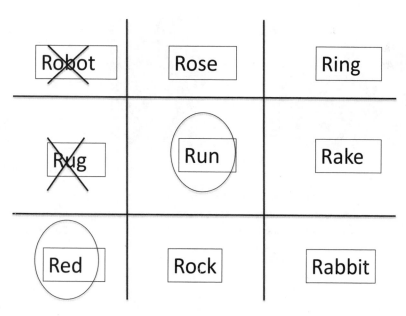

Figure 12–1. Sample group activity: Tic-Tac-Toe with target words.

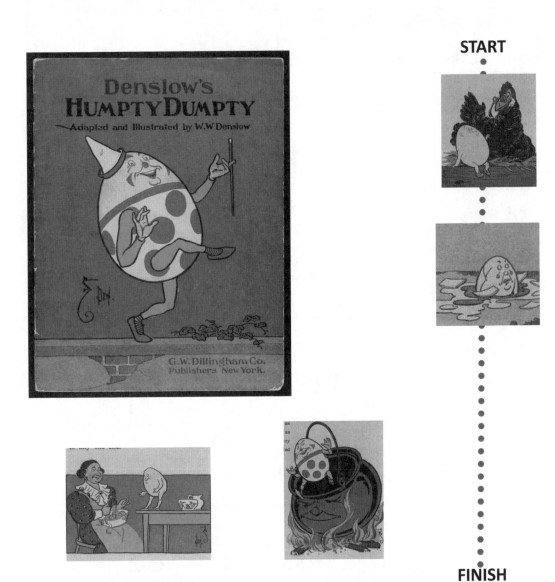

START

FINISH

Figure 12–2. Sample group activity: Story retelling rope, using Denslow's *Humpty Dumpty*. *Note.* Group members engage in a shared book reading and then retell the story, placing images from the book along a rope to guide retelling. Images in the public domain. Courtesy of U.S. Library of Congress Rare Book and Special Collections Division.

Comic strip

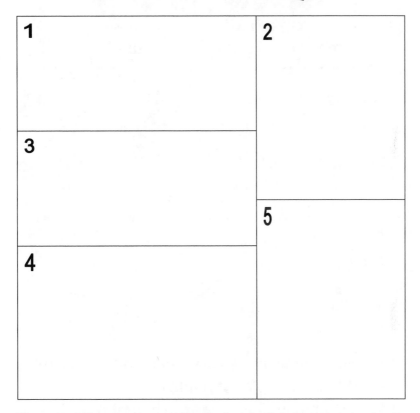

Figure 12–3. Sample group activity: Comic strip. *Note.* Group members create and tell a story by drawing images in the comic strip boxes or using the provided images, arranged and placed in the boxes.

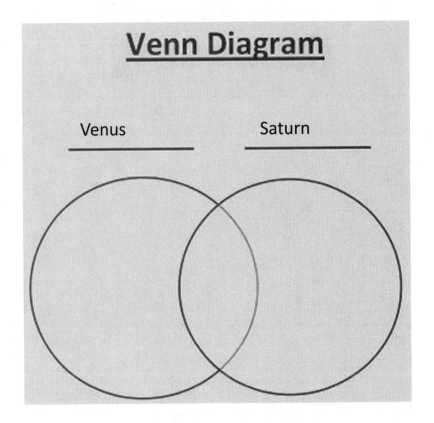

Venn Diagram

Venus   Saturn
_____   _____

1. How many moons does each planet have?
2. What is the planet made of?
3. How many rings does the planet have?

Figure 12–4. Sample group activity: Venn diagram. *Note.* Group members discuss attributes of related/unrelated items.

Figure 12–5. Sample group activity: Conversation ladder. *Note.* Group members rank and discuss contrasting concepts (e.g., easiest/most difficult speaking situations, most/least favored activity in school, etc.).

Box 12–1. Suggested Activities for Adult Groups

- Role-play real-life activities, using communication strategies, conflict resolution, self-advocacy techniques, and so forth.
- Charades-based activities using gestures, drawing, writing, and description
- Facilitated discussion centered on favorite activities/hobbies, recent events, strategy use, problem solving, and so forth.
- Performance, either impromptu (e.g., group script reading) or group activities centered on a specific performance (e.g., putting on a play for family, friends, community members)
- Poem reading, either impromptu or planned
- Community outings to practice daily living skills (e.g., money use, conversations with strangers, map reading, effective medical visits)
- Team activities, such as scavenger hunts, building activities, board or card games, cooking activities, and so forth
- A movie club centered on having facilitated discussion about selected movies watched by group members
- A book club centered on reading a book and facilitated discussion about its content

APPLYING CLASSROOM MANAGEMENT PRINCIPLES TO GROUP TREATMENT

In the field of education, teachers commonly work with groups of students, using techniques known as classroom management techniques. These are a set of principles that involve the actions of the teacher "to create a learning environment that encourages positive social interaction, active engagement in learning, and self-motivation" (Burden, 2006, p. 4). Many of these principles are also applicable to the services SLPs and SLPAs provide during group treatment. Research in this area suggests that several key factors underlie effective teaching and positively functioning classroom environments (Parsonson, 2012, p. 17), as follows:

1. Clear, simple rules and expectations that are consistently and fairly applied.
As an SLPA, it will be important for you to establish the rules of the group session. An example of applicable rules for children may be the following (Adams, 2006, p. 9):

- Raise your hands before you talk.
- Keep good eye contact.
- Listen when others are talking.
- Take turns talking about topics of interest.
- Use your inside voice.

These can be modified for adults as well. It is important to inform members of the rules at a level appropriate to the age, abilities, and purpose of the group. For young children, this may mean posting something in the group environment, similar to Figure 12–6, and then reviewing this information at the beginning of each session and as needed, given any potential rule violations.

2. Predictable events and routines, including cues and signals about upcoming activities.
Chapter 10 discusses similar concepts in the area of visual schedules. The samples of visual schedules provided in Chapter 10 can be adapted to represent the agenda of activities planned for a group session. For adult, literate clients, this can be accomplished by providing a written agenda for group sessions, similar to those used in business meetings. You can also maintain consistency in the design of group sessions by starting each session with a consistent opening activity, such as greetings and updates, followed by a core activity (that changes on a regular basis) and then a consistent closing activity. After a few sessions, as applicable, clients can begin to actively participate (or even lead) these opening and closing activities.

3. Frequent use of specific and descriptive praise, including verbal and nonverbal praise.
Chapter 10 provides a thorough discussion of operant conditioning and positive behavioral supports, both of which are applicable to the use of reinforcement and praise. The section on the effective use of operant principles provides several helpful examples of descriptive versus evaluative praise and effective reinforcement techniques. In the area of classroom management, Bradley, Pauley, and Pauley (2006) also suggest that teachers *know their students* and their personalities, motives, and desires as an important factor in the use of praise and reinforcement. This is good advice for SLPAs as well.

Relative to disruptive behaviors, researchers in the area of classroom management specifically warn against the use

Looking Eyes	
Listening Ears	
Quiet Voices	
Helping Hands	

Figure 12–6. Visual rules for posting in group environments with children. Images courtesy of Microsoft Corporation © 2013.

of any of the teacher behaviors listed in Box 12–2 in response to disruptive student behavior. Instead, when student behaviors become disruptive, a Three-Step Response Plan is recommended in classroom settings (Burden, 2006; Figure 12–7). This plan employs the principles of least intervention, which states that "when dealing with routine classroom behavior, misbehavior should be corrected with the simplest, least intrusive intervention that will work" (Slavin, 2006, as cited in Burden, 2006, p. 215). Each of these suggestions can also be used by SLPAs during group sessions to restore order when disruptive behavior is present.

4. Matching tasks to the skills and abilities of the learners.

In the field of education, this is known as *differentiated instruction* and is achieved when the teacher accommodates student

---

Box 12–2. Behaviors to Avoid in Response to Disruptive Behavior (Burden, 2006)

1. Harsh and humiliating reprimands
2. Threats
3. Nagging
4. Forced apologies
5. Sarcastic remarks
6. Group punishment
7. Assigning extra work
8. Reducing grades
9. Writing as punishment
10. Physical labor or exercise
11. Corporal punishment

STEP 1	STEP 2	STEP 3
SITUATIONAL ASSISTANCE	**MILD RESPONSE**	**MODERATE RESPONSE**
Help the student cope with the situation and keep the student on task.	*Use non-punishing actions to help the student return to the task.*	*Remove desired stimulus to decrease unwanted behavior.*
Sample Teacher Actions: •Remove distracting objects •Reinforce desired behavior •Boost interest •Provide assistance •Redirect behavior •Modify environment	Sample Teacher Actions: •Ignore the behavior •Use nonverbal cues (e.g., eye gaze, facial expression, etc.) •Call on the student to respond/answer a question •Give reminder of class rules or verbal reprimand •Ask, "What should you be doing?"	Sample Teacher Actions: •Withdraw privileges •Change seating •Place student in time-out •Contact parents •Have student visit the principle

Figure 12–7. Illustration of a Three-Step Response for addressing disruptive behavior in group settings. Adapted from Burden (2006, p. 220).

differences in "readiness levels, interests, and learning profiles," thereby achieving an optimum learning environment for all learners (Subban, 2006, p. 940). Matching tasks to group members' skills and abilities also reduces frustration and/or boredom, which is often associated with disruptive behavior (Parsonson, 2012).

SLPs are generally very good at achieving differentiated instruction given an individual treatment session. The key is to maintain this same level of differentiation during group sessions. This requires careful planning. Just as teachers plan for their classroom activities, SLPAs must also plan carefully and work with the supervising SLP to ensure an effective lesson plan is in place for each group session. In fact, as discussed in Chapter 7, the idea of lesson planning is borrowed from the field of education and the research surrounding classroom management. Remember that one element of an effective lesson plan includes ways to modify tasks, if needed. To do this in a timely fashion requires that you carefully observe group member behavior and implement modification, as needed, *during* group sessions. Using effective data collection is also important as this information can then be used by your supervising SLP to make additional modifications prior

to the next session. Chapter 10 (particularly the sections on "Things to Consider: The Client" and "Things to Consider: The Environment") offers additional suggestions in potential modifications to ensure the environment is supportive and the client is ready and able to participate fully in treatment activities.

DATA COLLECTION DURING GROUP SESSIONS

All the techniques discussed in Chapter 8 also apply to recording the performance of group members during group sessions. The importance of doing so accurately and consistently is equally important in both group and individual sessions. Collecting data during group sessions may be even more challenging, however, given the nature of the session and the need to attend to the needs of multiple members simultaneously. Appendix 12–B and the companion website of this textbook contain a sample data collection sheet for use during a group session. Many of the sample data sheets provided in Chapter 8 can also be easily modified for group sessions. Box 12–3 contains some additional tips for collecting data during group treatment.

Box 12–3. Tips for Collecting Data in Group Sessions

■ Discuss with your supervising SLP employing different techniques, such as the following:

  ■ *Timed Data Collection:* Collecting data on one group member the first 5 minutes, the next group member the following 5 minutes, and so forth.

  ■ *Rotating Data Collection:* Collecting data on one goal, per client, per session and then rotating to a different goal, per client the next session, and so forth, until you have collected data on all goals for all clients, then start the rotating process all over again.

■ Make sure to prepare your data sheets in advance, completing as much as possible prior to the session, including prerecording group member names, goals, codes for scoring, and so forth.

■ Think creatively about where you will keep your data collection sheets within a group dynamic to ensure they are accessible to you but not readily in view of group members.

■ Be aware of the prompts you provide, both for data collection purposes (as recommended in Chapter 8) and also *across* group members. It may be that the prompts provided to one group member affect (either positively or negatively) the performance of another group member. For example, a student prompted using a tactile cue for the /s/ phoneme (e.g., sliding the pointer finger on the table) may influence her group mate to use the same technique for practicing her /g/ words, which would result in an error in the production of /g/. Having a way to note the relationship of all prompts is helpful if you or your supervising SLP suspect this may be the case.

REFERENCES

Adams, L. (2006). *Group treatment for Asperger syndrome: A social skills curriculum.* San Diego, CA: Plural.

American Speech-Language-Hearing Association (ASHA). (2013). *Speech-language pathology assistant scope of practice.* Retrieved from http://www.asha.org/policy

Beukelman, D. R., & Mirenda, P. (2005). *Augmentative and alternative communication: Supporting children and adults with complex communication needs.* Baltimore, MD: Brookes.

Bradley, D. F., Pauley, J. A., & Pauley, J. F. (2006). *Effective classroom management: Six keys to success.* Lanham, MD: Rowman & Littlefield Education.

Burden, P. (2006). *Classroom management: Creating a successful K–12 learning community.* Hoboken, NJ: Wiley.

Carter, E. W., & Kennedy, C. H. (2006). Promoting access to the general curriculum using peer support strategies. *Research and Practice for Persons With Severe Disabilities, 31,* 284–292.

Cascella, R., Purdy, M. H., & Dempsey, J. J. (2007). Clinical service delivery and work settings.

In R. Paul & P. Cascella (Eds.), *Introduction to clinical methods in communication disorders* (pp. 259–282). Baltimore, MD: Brookes.

Elman, R. J. (2007). *Group treatment of neurogenic communication disorders: The expert clinician's approach* (2nd ed.). San Diego, CA: Plural.

Last, J. M. (1983). *A dictionary of epidemiology.* New York, NY: Oxford University Press.

Luterman, D. (2008). *Counseling persons with communication disorders and their families.* Austin, TX: Pro-Ed.

Mattinson, R. E. (2011). Comparison of students classified ED in self-contained classrooms and a self-contained school. *Education and Treatment of Children, 34*(1), 15–33.

McCauley, R., & Prelock, P. (Eds.). (2013). *Treatment of autism spectrum disorders: Evidence-based intervention strategies for communication and social interactions.* Baltimore, MD: Brookes.

Mire, S. (2007). Workload analysis: IEP and the group size factors in calculating workload. *School Based Issues,* 18–20.

Moon-Meyer, S. (2004). *Survival guide for the beginning speech-language clinician.* Austin, TX: Pro-Ed.

Parsonson, B. S. (2012). Evidence-based classroom behavior management strategies. *Kairanranga, 13*(1), 16–23.

Roth, F. R., & Worthington, C. K. (2001). *Treatment resource manual for speech-language pathology.* Albany, NY: Delmar.

Schubert, N. A., & Baxter, M. B. (1982). The self-contained open classroom as a viable learning environment. *Education, 102,* 411–415.

Subban, P. (2006). Differentiated instruction: A Research Basis. *International Education Journal, 7*(7), 935–947.

Travis, L. E. (1957). *Handbook of speech pathology.* New York, NY: Appleton-Century-Crofts.

Vinson, B. P. (2009). *Workplace skills and professional issues in speech-language pathology.* San Diego, CA: Plural.

Walker, K. (2009). Self-contained classrooms: Research brief. *Education Partnerships,* 1–3.

APPENDIX 11–A

Social Skills Group Activities (Adams, 2006)

Activity	Ages	Objective	Materials	Procedure
Dice Talk	3–5 years old	Child will use eye contact in communication.	▪ A small sized box ▪ Plain paper to cover box ▪ Marker ▪ Tape	Find a small box that can be covered with paper and used as a dice for this communication game. Use a size that is easy and fun for little hands to toss. Wrap the box in plain paper. On the faces of the dice, write questions or statements to elicit answers from the children. For example, on the six faces of the dice, you could write: ▪ Name an animal that lives in the zoo. ▪ Tell me a food you like to eat ▪ What animal lives on a farm? ▪ What is something you like to drink? ▪ Tell me an animal that lives on a farm. ▪ Name a toy you like to play with. Explain to the children that they each will get a turn to toss the dice, and they get to answer the question that lands on top. Tell them that they will answer to you, and they must look in your eyes as they talk to you. Explain that looking at people as they talk to them is a good thing we all need to practice.
Bowling	3–5 years old	Child will learn turn-taking in a group activity.	▪ Plastic bowling pins and ball ▪ Masking tape	Set up the pins, placing a piece of tape on the floor to mark where the children should stand when throwing the ball. Arrange the children in a line behind the masking tape. Explain that each child will get a turn when he or she steps up to the line.

Activity	Ages	Objective	Materials	Procedure
Bowling *continued*				Show the children how to go to the back of the line after their turn. If there are so many children that the wait in line is quite long, have two bowling sets to increase the children's turn taking and lessen the demand on their patience.
Pumpkin Decorating	6–9 years old	Child will use turn-taking in group activity.	■ One large pumpkin ■ Pretty fall leaves of various shapes and colors ■ Yarn ■ Markers ■ Construction paper ■ Scissors ■ Tape ■ Slips of numbered paper and a hat to draw them out to determine turn-taking order	Tell the group they get to decorate a pumpkin, giving it a face, hair, and ears. Instruct the children that they are free to use any of the materials, but they must take turns adding decorations to the pumpkin. Allow them a brief time to discuss possible decorating ideas; if necessary, prompt their creativity with suggestions such as, "Leaves for hair? A mouth out of yarn? Draw ears with a marker?" Draw numbers out of a hat to determine the order they go in, informing them everyone may each have as many turns as necessary to fully decorate the pumpkin.
Big Muscles!	6–9 years old	Child will participate in role-play with the group.	■ Heavy objects and light objects *Heavy/Light* cans of soup/feathers detergent jug/foam cups hammer/crayon dictionary/leaf rock/cotton balls	Talk about things that are heavy and light and ask the children for the meaning of each word. Children can pretend to be weightlifters and take turns lifting the objects. Each child can win a medal for his or her big muscles.

continues

Appendix 11–A. *continued*

Activity	Ages	Objective	Materials	Procedure
I'll Be Your Server	10–12 years old	Child will use eye contact when speaking and listening.	▪ Refreshments (one item for each student to distribute to group) ▪ Server's apron (optional)	Inform students that they will each have a turn being a waiter, passing out refreshments to the rest of the group. Instruct students that good communication, including eye contact, is important to being a waiter as well as being a consumer. Have students choose the refreshment items they will distribute. Let them take turns passing out the items, using eye contact as they ask each group member, "Would you like some____?" Remind group members also to make eye contact as they are waited on.
Student Teacher	10–12 years old	Child will use eye contact, topic maintenance, and appropriate length of communication	▪ None	Explain to the group that, for this activity, the teacher will be the student, and the students will give feedback to the teacher regarding topic maintenance. Instruct the students to think of topics for the teacher to present. Examples may include: what I did over the weekend, how to make a peanut butter and jelly sandwich, the reasons I became a teacher, my favorite foods, games I played when I was a child, and so on. Show the students a signal (such as raising a hand or pointing a finger at you) they may use if they hear the presentation go off topic. Be sure to wander off topic as you present and respond to students' signals to get back on topic.

Source: Adams, L. (2006). *Group treatment for Asperger syndrome: A social skills curriculum.* © Copyright 2006 Plural Publishing, Inc. All rights reserved. Reprinted with permission.

APPENDIX 11–B
Group Data Collection Sheet

Group Time: _____ Location: _____ Date: _____ (Length of Session: _____)

Members Present: _____

Group Activity: _____

NOTES FOR SESSION: _____

Member Name: _____

Objective(s)	Data Tally	Data Summary	Comments

NOTES FOR SESSION: _____

Member Name: _____

Objective(s)	Data Tally	Data Summary	Comments

NOTES FOR SESSION: _____

Member Name: _____

Objective(s)	Data Tally	Data Summary	Comments

NOTES FOR SESSION: _____

Member Name: _____

Objective(s)	Data Tally	Data Summary	Comments

PART III

Treatment for Specific Populations and Disorders

CHAPTER 13

Speech Sound Remediation for Children

Lei Sun

Words mean more than what is set down on paper. It takes the human voice to infuse them with deeper meaning.

—Maya Angelou (American author, poet, and recipient of the National Medal of the Arts and the President's Medal of Freedom)

The caseload of speech-language pathologists (SLPs) commonly includes individuals with speech sound disorders (SSD), especially for SLPs working in school settings, with preschoolers and young school-age children (ages 3–9 years). According to the American Speech-Language-Hearing Association's (ASHA's) 2012 schools survey, students with articulation and phonological disorders were the most commonly reported individuals on the caseload of school-based SLPs (ASHA, 2012). As such, speech-language pathology assistants (SLPAs) working in school settings must be knowledgeable about this topic. This chapter provides an overview of SSD, including speech sound development and classification and general and specific guidelines for treating SSD. This chapter is not meant to be a substitute for more in-depth reading and resources; rather, it can serve as a complement to your introductory coursework on the topic.

Before we discuss sound remediation, it is important to review some key concepts. A *phoneme* is a family of very similar sounds. For example, we produce the /t/ in *tea, tool,* and *take* slightly different, but we all perceive the first sound as /t/. A phoneme is the smallest linguistic unit of sound that can signal a difference in meaning. As an example, if we change the first sound of *tea* to /k/, then it will be a different word, *key,* which has a totally different meaning from *tea.* The concept of signaling a difference in meaning through a change of sound is very important for speech intervention. Usually, we use *virgules* such as /t/ for the ideal description of the sound (i.e., the way the sound should be produced) and *brackets* [t] for the actual sound produced by an individual. The International Phonetic Alphabet (IPA) is commonly used to represent the sounds of oral language. Appendix 4–B in Chapter 4 contains a list of core IPA symbols.

Speech intelligibility is a measure of how much a listener can understand someone else's speech. It can be targeted directly or indirectly, depending on the goals and objectives set by an SLP. The priority of treatment goals may vary across children in speech and language therapy. In some instances, speech sounds are not necessarily targeted if, for example, a child has limited verbal output or if language intervention is the priority. A lack

of speech intelligibility is often addressed in younger children because of the significant negative impact it can have on social interaction and future academic performance (e.g., literacy). Usually, a child can be easily understood by age 5 years, although some sounds develop later such as /s, z, ʃ, θ, ð/ (which is appropriate for a 5-year-old; Peña-Brooks & Hegde, 2007). Children diagnosed with intellectual disabilities, early speech or language delay, autism, and other speech-language-related impairments may require more time to develop speech sounds (Bernthal, Bankson, & Flipsen, 2013). In some instances, inconsistent speech sound production and persistent use of age-inappropriate phonological processes, such as error patterns known as liquid gliding (using /w/ to replace /r/), final consonant deletion (deleting sounds in the final position) are observed beyond age 9 years. For children with speech-language disorders, speech can be targeted directly or indirectly, depending on overall speech intelligibility and the extent to which speech errors negatively affect the child's daily life, social interaction, and academic performance.

To consider individual differences in acquiring speech sounds, it is important to become familiar with speech acquisition norms and realize that there is no cutoff age for the development of a single sound. For example, /s/ starts to emerge around age 3 years and may not be mastered until the age 8 years. It usually takes longer to develop later developing sounds compared with early developing sounds, such as /h, m, w, p/. As a foundation for a discussion of speech sound remediation, the following section provides an overview about speech sound classification, speech sound acquisition, and common phonological processes.

SPEECH SOUND CLASSIFICATION

Classifications of sounds, based on their place (where along the vocal tract the consonant is formed), voicing (whether the vocal folds are vibrating during the production), and manner (how the sound is formed; Peña-Brooks & Hegde, 2007,), is an important foundation for understanding how to elicit target sounds. Figure 13–1 contains a place-voice-manner (PVM) chart, denoting place of articulation, whether the consonant shown is voiced or voiceless, and manner of articulation for different sounds (Bowen, 2011; http://speech-language-therapy.com/images/pvmchart.png).

Familiarity with this classification system is helpful for understanding the similarity and differences across sounds. For example, if a child's target sound is /s/ and the child is able to produce /t/ consistently, clinicians can take advantage of place similarity and use /t/ to elicit /s/. Similarly, clinicians can use voice on and off to train the voiced sounds by helping the child feel the vibration of the voice box by, for example, having the child touch his or her own neck when the child produces voiced sounds. A vowel chart is also provided for review, as vowels can be used to elicit some consonant production (Figure 13–2).

SPEECH SOUND DEVELOPMENT

Consonants

SLPs frequently use speech sound developmental norms and sequences to determine eligibility for treatment of SSD,

	MANNER		VOICING	PLACE						
				Bilabial	Labiodental	Interdental	Alveolar	Palatal	Velar	Glottal
OBSTRUENTS	Stop		Voiceless	p			t		k	ʔ
			Voiced	b			d		g	
	Fricative		Voiceless		f		s	ʃ		h
			Voiced		v	ð	z	ʒ		
	Affricate		Voiceless					tʃ		
			Voiced					dʒ		
SONORANTS	Nasal		Voiced	m			n			
	LIQUID	Lateral	Voiced				l			
		Rhotic	Voiced					r		
	Glide		Voiced	w					j	w

Figure 13–1. Place-Voice-Manner (PVM) Chart. Reprinted with permission from Bowen, C. (2011). *Communication disorders glossary*. Retrieved August 10, 2013, from http://www.speech-language-therapy.com/index.php?option=com_content&view=article&id=14&Itemid=123.

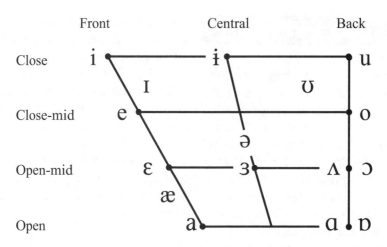

Figure 13–2. English vowels, classified based on position of the tongue. Image courtesy of Wikimedia Commons.

such as Sander (1972), Templin (1957), and Smit, Hand, Freilinger, Bernthal, and Bird (1990; Gordon-Brannan & Weiss, 2007). Due to different methodologies and criteria used when researchers developed speech norms, different sequences of speech sound acquisition have been reported. Despite these minor differences, the order of acquisition of sounds and sound classes is very similar across norms. For example, in general, stops, nasals, and glides develop early, and liquids, fricatives, and affricates develop later. Clinicians must keep in mind though, that the position of the sound (e.g., whether the sound appears in the initial, medial, or final position of a word) can also affect how long it takes children to acquire a sound. As an example, /t/ in initial position (*tea, toy, tale*) may be mastered around age three years, but /t/ in final position (*cat, feet*) may not be mastered until around age four years. Generally speaking, if the sound emerges in one position, sound production in other positions should be expected soon. Medial sounds usually (but not always) take slightly longer to acquire, compared with sounds in initial and final positions.

A helpful classification of sound development was that developed by Shriberg (1993), which divided the 24 English speech sounds into three categories: early eight, middle eight, and late eight. Lof (2017) used this classification to compare common speech acquisition norms and found that children master the early eight sounds around age three years, the middle eight sounds between ages 3 and 7 years (with /t, k, g, ŋ, f/ often acquired by age 4 and /v, tʃ, dʒ/ developing between ages 5 and 7), and the late eight sounds usually between 6 and 8 years of age (Table 13–1).

Consonant Clusters/Blends

Consonant clusters, or blends (e.g., combination of consonants), usually develop after the child's oral motor control and coordination are more mature. Box 13–1 contains a list of common consonant clusters.

Table 13–1. Shriberg's Three Categories of Speech Sound Developmental Sequence

Early eight	/m, b, j, n, w, d, p, h/
Middle eight	/t, k, g, ŋ, f, v, tʃ, dʒ/
Late eight	/ s, z, l, r, ʃ, ʒ, θ, ð/

Source: Shriberg, 1993.

Box 13–1. Common Consonant Clusters

■ L blends: pl-, kl-, fl-
■ S blends: sp-, sm-, sn-, st-, sk-
■ R blends: gr-, br-, dr-, kr-

Consonant clusters can be in the initial position or final position (-pt, -ks, -ft, -sk, etc.) and can be a combination of two consonants or three consonants (spr-, spl-, thr-, -kst). Like consonant acquisition, consonant clusters follow a general acquisition sequence, which varies based on the position of the cluster. Usually, consonant clusters begin to develop between 3:6 and 4:0 years, when children have developed a good amount of consonants and is ready to combine them. Therefore, it is unrealistic to work on consonant clusters when a child has only a limited number of consonants in her or his phonetic inventory (i.e., sounds that the child is able to produce consistently), has not yet developed the sounds included in the clusters, or when the child is too young. It is always good to practice single consonants (e.g., /s/) until their sound production stabilizes and then introduce associated consonant clusters (e.g., sm-, sn-, sp-, st-, etc.).

Keep in mind that consonant clusters take longer to develop, and some may be mastered after age 8 years for some children (e.g., thr-, skw-, str-, spr-, etc.; Peña-Brooks & Hegde, 2007). In addition, clinicians generally consider consonant acquisition when working on clusters. As an example, it is appropriate for a 5-year-old to say *fwog* instead of *frog*, as /r/ is still developing. In general, it is more important to help the child be aware of a cluster that has two or three sounds in it, rather than the perfect production of each individual phoneme in the cluster. For example, it is more critical to produce /f/ and /r/ in *frog* even though it sounds like *fwog* than only producing one sound in the cluster as in *fog*, because *fog* is a different word and carries a very different meaning from *frog*. In contrast, *fwog* still carries the meaning of *frog* even though it does not sound the way it should.

Vowels

Most children have no difficulty acquiring vowels. Vowels usually develop early, except /ɚ, ɝ/, which are usually mastered before age 5 years because tongue retraction is required to produce these two r-colored vowels. If a child shows difficulty producing vowels, more serious speech issues or structural issues may be indicated. When a child has difficulty producing vowels, sounds that carry real meanings can be used to elicit the vowels. For example, "haha," "uhoh," "ouch," and "owie." C (consonant), V (vowel), and VC (vowel-consonant) words that represent different daily utterances should also be included to facilitate both vowels and early developing consonants to expand the child's sound inventory. For example, up, hi, bye, no, boo, my, nana, mama, dada. If a child cannot differentiate between two vowels, minimal contrasts or pairs (which will be reviewed under the phonemic, linguistically-based, and phonology treatment approaches) are often used in treatment to target perception and production training.

COMMON PHONOLOGICAL PROCESSES

During the time when children learn to talk like adults, they simplify adults' speech by using predictable "error" patterns called phonological processes. The use of phonological processes is related to speech sound acquisition. For example, a child uses /t/ to replace /k/ (velar fronting) when the child is still in the process of developing the /k/ sound. All children use phonological processes when developing their speech sounds. However, children with speech delays or SSD use phonological processes beyond an appropriate age range, which makes the speech errors age inappropriate. Keep in mind

that some children who have impairments in other areas, such as cognition and language, may use the processes for a much longer period of time. Some phonological processes may be eliminated early, such as initial and final consonant deletion and velar fronting, but some phonological processes may take longer to be suppressed, such as liquid gliding and stopping of voiced and voiceless "th (/θ/)." As such, sometimes goals may target specific patterns or phonological processes instead of particular sounds, such as "XX will improve speech intelligibility by reducing final consonant deletion." As an SLPA, it is important to have a basic concept of some common phonological processes (Table 13–2).

GENERAL TREATMENT PRINCIPLES

In general, treatment can be viewed as "a continuum of activities comprising three stages: establishment, facilitation of gen-

Table 13–2. Common Phonological Processes

Phonological Process	Description	Examples
Final consonant deletion	A final consonant is omitted/deleted from a word	ca for cat, cu for cup
Initial consonant deletion	An initial consonant is omitted/deleted from a word	at for fat, ake for lake
Syllable deletion	A syllable (especially a weak/unstressed syllable) is omitted/deleted from a word	puter for computer, nana for banana
Cluster reduction	One phoneme of the cluster is deleted from the cluster	fag for flag, fog for frog
Stopping of fricatives	Stops replace fricatives and affricates	top for sop, poo for zoo
Velar fronting	Alveolar stops (/t, d/) replace velar sounds (/k, g, ŋ/)	tea for key, do for go
Liquid gliding	Glides (/w, j/) replace liquids (/l, r/)	wake for lake, yeg for leg
Devoicing	Voiceless consonants replace voiced consonants	nos for nose, pik for pig
Assimilation	One sound becomes more like a neighboring sound. It could be due to place or manner.	lellow for yellow, take for cake

Source: Peña-Brooks and Hegde, 2007.

eralization, and maintenance" (Bernthal et al., 2013, p. 270). Figure 13–3 presents this continuum. Treatment starts with eliciting the target sound, gradually moves to stabilizing the speech sound production in all positions and increasing linguistic levels (from words to conversation), and then maintaining consistent speech sound production in different settings, contexts, and with different communication partners, through self-monitoring.

The first step in the treatment process is to establish appropriate treatment goals and objectives. This is the job of your supervising SLP (ASHA, 2013). As an SLPA, it is critical that for each treatment objective, you are able to accurately identify target sounds, production level (i.e., syllable, word, phrase or sentence, spontaneous speech), accuracy level (e.g., 70%, 7 of 10 trials), prompt level (e.g., minimal, maximal prompting), and setting (usually in speech therapy). Chapter 7 offers general suggestions in this regard. Remember that an objective may be written in various ways, but it should always contain those elements. An example of a common speech sound remediation objective is, "L.B. will produce /s/ and /s/ blends at word level with 80% accuracy with

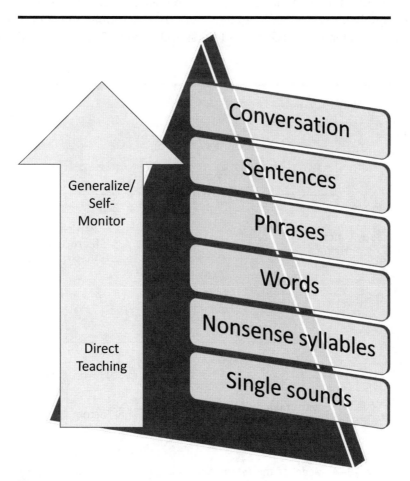

Figure 13–3. Hierarchy of speech sound remediation.

minimal prompting in three consecutive speech therapy sessions." Using this objective as an example, can you identify the elements listed above?

Intervention remediating SSD is generally divided into two major treatment approaches: phonetic/motor-based/articulation treatment approaches; and phonemic/linguistically-based/phonologic treatment approaches. Although the two treatment approaches stems from distinctive theories and clinical observations, it is impossible to separate the function (linguistic/phonemic) from the form (motor-based/phonetic) as they are two sides of the same coin. As you implement treatment, it is important to keep this in mind. Phonology is only one aspect of language and intervention to remediate SSDs should always be considered in the larger scope of language and its purpose. The ultimate goal is to improve a child's overall speech intelligibility, in order to convey meaning efficiently and effectively, and to assist the child to function better in her or his daily life. The World Health Organization's *International Classification of Functioning, Disability and Health* (World Health Organization, 2001) highlights this relationship, which should be the cornerstone of speech sound remediation (Figure 13–4). Effective and functional intervention targets both form (body structures and functions) and function (meaningful use of speech sounds, along with language rules, to function well in daily activities).

A traditional view of remediating speech errors uses discrete skills (e.g., not

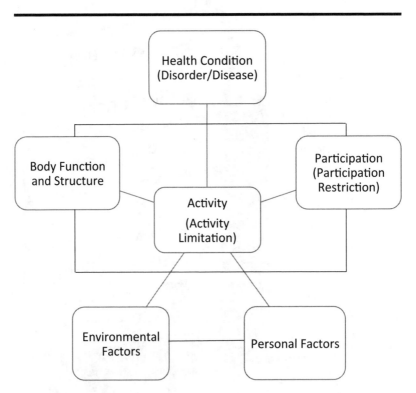

Figure 13–4. Model of the *International Classification of Functioning, Disability, and Health.*

viewing phonology as part of language) and a "drill-and-kill" method. Although maximizing accurate production is key to improving speech intelligibility, it may be that with this method, students overgeneralize speech sound production (e.g., use the target sound in words that do not contain the target sound). This further compromises effective communication. Students may also respond poorly to drill activities. The gold standard in speech sound remediation should always be effective, efficient, and functional treatment activities. Box 13–2 depicts an example of this approach within a treatment session.

PRIMARY TREATMENT APPROACHES

Although we divide treatment approaches into two main categories (phonetic/motor-based/articulation; phonemic/linguistically-based/phonologic), it is impossible to work on form and function separately. The difference across different treatment approaches is in how

each approach organizes and sequences treatment targets, which is determined according to the child's severity of SSD. For example, clinicians use phonetic treatment approaches, such as using a variety of cues (e.g., visual, tactile, verbal) or external tools (e.g., tongue depressor), to elicit a target sound. Once the sound is stimulable and produced consistently, phonemic treatment approaches should be used to facilitate target discrimination and sound production. Therefore, a combination of the phonetic and phonemic approaches is recommended, depending on the child's needs and strengths. Table 13–3 briefly summarizes the general differences between the phonetic and phonemic treatment approaches.

Phonetic/Motor–Based/Articulation Treatment Approach

A traditional approach to phonetic training has been commonly used since the 1970s (Van Riper & Erickson, 1996). Using this approach, the child gradually moves along the continuum of treatment from

---

Box 13–2. Sample Speech Sound Remediation Session

1. Start the treatment session by having the child practice target sounds at the appropriate linguistic level (e.g., word, phrase, sentence) for a short amount of time.
2. Have the child use target words in naturalistic activities. For younger children, play-based activities are an excellent option. Language-based activities, such as shared book reading, are especially good for children with language impairments (LI) and SSD. Literacy-based treatment activities, incorporating phonological awareness activities for preschoolers, and conventional reading and writing for older children, are also highly valuable. Chapter 16 offers additional suggestions.
3. End the session by reviewing target sounds and speech homework.

Table 13–3. Core Differences: Phonetic Versus Phonemic Approaches

Phonetic Approach	Phonemic Approach
Focus on teaching correct production of individual sounds	Focus on learning correct production through contrasting sounds
Use of nonsense/made up syllables/words is allowed	Only use meaningful real words
Appropriate for limited speech errors	Appropriate for identified erred patterns
Good for nonstimulable sounds	Good for stimulable sounds
Start with phonemes or nonsense syllables	Start with words

Sources: Bernthal, Bankson, and Flipsen, 2013; Peña-Brooks and Hegde, 2007.

perceptual/ear training, sound establishment, sound stabilization, transfer/carryover, and then maintenance. Some elements of the traditional approach can be separately incorporated into treatment as needed, without implementing the entire method.

Perceptual Training/Ear Training

Perceptual training is used at the beginning of a traditional approach if the child has difficulty discriminating between the desired sound (i.e., the target speech sound) and the undesired sound (i.e., the sound that the child produces instead). If the child does not have auditory discrimination problems, treatment moves forward to the sound establishment phase. Before perceptual training, training words should be selected based on the child's present level. However, it may not be an appropriate activity if the child has difficulty understanding what you expect him or her to do. Your modeling is always necessary to ensure each child's understanding of the task in order to successfully implement the activity. During perceptual training, the child's correct responses and errors should be carefully monitored. It is important to keep in mind that per-

ceptual training does not automatically lead to correct sound production and improved speech intelligibility. However, perceptual training can increase awareness of the target phoneme and can be added before or during production training. The use of perceptual training may or may not be evident in a child's treatment objectives. An example of an objective including perceptual training may be, "XX will independently distinguish _____ sound (desired sound) from _____ sound (undesired sound) with minimal prompting when presented with picture cards, with 80% accuracy in two consecutive sessions." Table 13–4 summarizes different methods for ear training.

Sound Establishment/Sound Elicitation

Sound elicitation often starts with a phoneme (e.g., fricatives), syllable (e.g., target phoneme + schwa, especially stops/pə/ and liquids /lə/), or word (e.g., meaningful and functional CVC (consonant-vowel-consonant words). Your supervising SLP will determine which level facilitates production more easily for each child and the child's ultimate goal in communication. A common treatment objective at this level of training may be,

Table 13–4. Perceptual Ear Training Methods

Traditional Approach	Identification	Clinician directs the child's attention to how the speech sound feels in the mouth. Clinician uses objects to describe the characteristics of the speech sound (e.g., /t/ is a ticking sound, /f/ is an angry cat sound). A common task may be for the child to ring a bell or raise his or her hand when hearing a target sound.
	Isolation	Child is asked to identify the target sound in increasing linguistic levels (syllables, words, phrases, sentences).
	Stimulation	Similar to auditory bombardment (see below), clinician provides child with maximal auditory stimuli of the target sound, through varying loudness, stress (e.g., add stress to syllable containing the target sound), and duration of the sound (prolong the target sound).
	Discrimination	Clinician produces sounds and the child is asked to make judgments of correct and incorrect productions.
Auditory Bombardment		Tasks blend the target sound into all activities and emphasize it through shared book reading, language/literacy games, play, conversation, and so forth. For example, if the target sound is /s/, the clinician may read a book about superheros (Superman, Spiderman, Sandman, etc.), highlighting /s/ while reading the book. Similarly, the clinician may emphasize /s/ in conversation ("it'S Super Silly, iSn't it?" "That'S hiS not yourS").
Minimal Pair		Clinician uses pairs of words containing undesirable sound (e.g., [t]replaces /s/, [t] is the undesirable sound) and desirable sound (/s/ is the desirable sound) along with written words and corresponding pictures. For example, the child is asked to hand pictures named to the clinician (sea-tea, sue-two).

Source: Bernthal, Bankson, and Flipsen, 2013.

"XX will produce _____ sound in _____ position (initial or final) at word (or syllable-CV, VC; [consonant-vowel or vowel-consonant) level with minimal prompting with 70% accuracy in two consecutive sessions." Table 13–5 summarizes several techniques used to elicit target sounds. Keep in mind though, that more than one technique may be needed. The combination of techniques depends on the child's needs and how the child responds to each technique. All the techniques listed are used to elicit speech sounds in isolation. Conversational speech is dynamic and variable; it considers the influence from neighboring sounds (i.e., the consonant or vowel that comes before and after the sound) and suprasegmental features (e.g., stress, intonation), rather than the combination of isolated speech sounds. Therefore, additional attention is generally given to transferring learned, isolated speech sounds to more connected running speech, and then to generalization to different settings and with varied communication partners. As an additional reference, consult *Articulatory and Phonological Impairments: A Clinical Focus* by Jacqueline Bauman-Waengler (2012) and *Eliciting Sounds: Techniques and Strategies for Clinicians* by Secord, Boyce, Donohue, Fox, and Shine (2007).

Sound Stabilization

Once the target sound is successfully elicited, phonetic treatment then focuses on stabilizing sound production in all

Table 13–5. Common Techniques for Eliciting Speech Sounds

Sound-Evoking Technique	Procedures
Imitation	Ask the child to watch, listen, and repeat the target sound. A mirror can be used (e.g., watch me, listen, and make the sound just like I do-/s/).
Phonetic Placement	Clinician uses visual and tactile cues and describes where to place the articulators in order to produce the target sound. A mouth puppet and mirror can be used with younger children. Oral structure graphs can be used with older children (first grade and up). External tools such as a tongue depressor should be used as the last resort.
Contextual Cues/ Co-Articulation	Clinician identifies key words (words in which the child can produce the target sound correctly) and word contexts (the neighboring sounds that can facilitate the correct production of the target sound without additional training). Clinician uses this advantage to help the child feel and hear the target sound and attempt to transfer the correct target production to other words. Usually the information can be gathered from contextual testing done by the SLP. For example, /s/ may be produced easily in clusters/blends (st, sp, sn, etc.) rather than singletons (sun, sit, etc.;Williams, 1991). For example, /s/ may be produced easily after /t/ due to similar placement (bright-sun, hot-soup, etc.). Velar sounds may be easily produced after high-back vowels (/u, ʊ/).
Sound Modification/ Shaping	Clinician uses a sound that is already in the child's phonetic inventory (the child can produce the sound correctly and independently) and shapes it to the target sound. For example, if the child can produce /l/, /l/ is shaped into /r/ by asking the child to slide the tongue tip slowly back along the roof of the mouth.
Tactile-Kinesthetic	Clinician manipulates the child's articulators externally on the face and neck to guide speech sound production.

Sources: Bernthal, Bankson, and Flipsen, 2013; Bauman-Waengler, 2012; Gordon-Brannan and Weiss, 2007.

positions of words and at varied levels of complexity. Generally, objectives start with the lowest level (i.e., when the child requires great assistance from the clinician) and progresses to higher levels (i.e., when the clinician starts to fade prompting, in order to achieve correct *independent* speech sound production). For example, if the child successfully produces /s/ in final position (*kiss, face*), treatment then moves forward to initial (*sun, see*) and then medial position (*seesaw, castle*), which automatically incorporates two-syllable words. Once the child finishes the sound production in one position or one level (syllable, word), the clinician incorporates a review to ensure sound stabilization while moving forward to the next level. An example of a common treatment objective at this level would be, "XX will produce _____ sound in _____ position (initial, medial or final) at word level with minimal prompting with 70% accuracy in two consecutive sessions" or "XX will produce _____ sound in all positions at sentence level with minimal prompting with 70% accuracy in two consecutive sessions." Table 13–6 provides treatment suggestions for this type of objective.

Speech Homework

To improve speech intelligibility, clients must practice correct speech sound production. Because 30 minutes or an hour a week of treatment does not provide

Table 13–6. Sound Stabilization Sample Activities

Level	Treatment Suggestions
Word	Target sound can first be elicited in final or initial position and then gradually moved to medial position. The purpose of treatment is to stabilize the sound production in all word positions. *Potential Activities:* 1. Incorporate target words into board games or any type of game. For example, using target words to play Go Fish, the child must produce the word correctly to receive the correct card. 2. Use games as reinforcement to elicit maximal correct sound production. For example, the child must produce the word correctly three times before moving the pawn. *Suggested games:* Go Fish, chess, fishing game, memory game, bowling, safari, Hangman (good for children with a large vocabulary size)
Phrase/sentence	Incorporate phrases that contain the target sound. Carrier phrases start with the same phrase and only fill in different words that contain the target sound to complete the sentence. *Potential Activities:* 1. Set a scene that facilitates the use of carrier phrases. e.g., I see a _____ (target sound /l/: lake, lamp, line, etc). 2. To increase the difficulty, two target words can be included in one phrase. e.g., I "like" the _____ (target sound /l/: lake, lamp, line, etc).
Sentence	Start with simple and short sentences containing one target word and then gradually increase the complexity of the sentence and the number of target words. *Potential Activities:* 1. If the child is able to read, use ready-made materials and ask the child to read sentences. 2. If the child has higher language abilities, ask the child to make up a sentence using the practiced target word. For example, I like to go to beach and pick up "seashells" out of the "sand."
Conversation	The purpose of the conversation level is to help the child be more aware of his or her own speech errors and develop effective self-monitoring strategies. It requires a certain level of metalinguistic skill and may be more appropriate for older children and children with good language skills. *Potential Activities:* 1. Use audio recording: record part of the session, play it back to the child, identify and discuss the speech errors. We must be cautious about the child's emotional and psychological changes when using this method. Do not make the child feel that he or she is the center of the attention (put the child on the spot). 2. Ask the child to fill out the speech rating chart to evaluate his or her own speech for each session using letter grades (A, B, C). A speech diary can be created to use at home to continue the self-monitoring process. 3. Discuss developing effective strategies with the child, tailored specifically for him or her. For example, use of the secret visual code shared between the classroom teacher, the child, and the clinician as a reminder when needed.

Source: Bernthal, Bankson, and Flipsen, 2013.

sufficient practice, speech homework is necessary. Creating a speech file for the child and sending home a list of practice words after each session is recommended. As an SLPA, you may be asked to assist your supervising SLP in creating these materials (ASHA, 2013). The practice words should be words that were practiced in treatment sessions for which correct sound production has been established. Usually 10 to 15 minutes of practice a day is sufficient to maintain and stabilize correct sound production. A note for the parent or caregiver regarding how to use the speech homework and a signature and/or initial line for the parent or caregiver to confirm the completion of the speech homework is recommended. Appendix 13–A contains a sample speech homework sheet.

Phonemic/Linguistically–Based/ Phonologic Treatment Approach

The focus of phonemic/linguistically-based/phonology treatment is to replace erred patterns and to establish sound contrasts (Bernthal et al., 2013). This treatment approach is more appropriate for children whose speech errors can be identified by patterns and phonological processes, such as final consonant deletion, velar fronting, liquid gliding, and cluster reduction. Because the child uses patterns, his or her speech intelligibility is usually much lower than the child who has articulation disorders with fewer speech errors. Children with phonological disorders usually have difficulty distinguishing targets sound from error sounds. For example, a child who uses liquid gliding may have difficulty distinguishing the difference between *lake* and *wake* that results in incorrect production. In contrast, a child

with an articulation disorder may be able to differentiate between /w/ and /r/ but struggle to produce /r/. Therefore, which treatment approach (phonetic or phonemic) is most effective and beneficial depends on the child's ability to contrast the sounds and produce the target with minimal assistance (i.e., the sound is stimulable). If a child understands the difference between the sounds, the clinician can facilitate sound production using the sound-evoking techniques reviewed earlier. If the child struggles with differentiating the error sound and the target sound, training on perception of contrasts and then production of contrasts will be the focus. Your supervising SLP will determine the most appropriate approach for each client (ASHA, 2013).

Providing the treatment that meets the child's needs to improve the child's overall speech intelligibility is the ultimate goal. An indication of using phonologically-based treatment activities may not always be evident in an objective. An objective using this approach may look like the examples presented in the sound stabilization section, such as "XX will produce _____ sound in _____ position (initial, medial, or final) at word level with minimal prompting with 80% accuracy in two consecutive sessions." The use of treatment approaches depends on the child's deficits and severity of SSD. The sections that follow provide an overview of three evidence- and phonologically-based treatment approaches.

Minimal Oppositions/Minimal Pairs

Word pairs are used in a minimal opposition/minimal pair contrast approach. A phoneme already in the child's inventory is used to contrast with the target sound/desired sound (Barlow & Gierut, 2002). For example, if the child uses /w/ to replace /r/, it shows that the child is able to produce /w/ (in the child's inventory) but may not understand the contrast between /w/ and /r/. Treatment then focuses on the use of /w/ in the child's inventory to contrast with the target sound /r/. The goal of this treatment is to help the child understand that different sounds represent different words and meanings and that correct sound production is important for successful communication. Therefore, a change of one sound will change the word and intended meaning, which may cause communica-

tion breakdowns. As an example, if the child asks for a picture of *tea* instead of *key* when she really wants *key,* receiving the wrong picture card of *tea* will be the consequence of incorrect sound production. The procedure of minimal pair training is presented in Figure 13–5.

Maximal Oppositions Contrast

Maximal oppositions contrast uses the same procedure as minimal oppositions contrast (above). The only difference is in the selection of word pairs (Gierut, 1989). The word pair *tea-key* is different only in

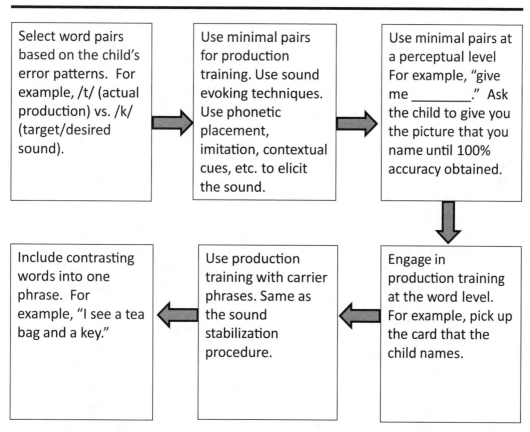

Figure 13–5. Minimal opposition/minimal pairs approach flowchart. Based on Bernthal, Bankson, and Flipsen (2013).

one feature: that of place. If "k-m" pairs are used, greater phonological change in the phonology system can be made, because /k/ and /m/ differ on place, manner, and nasality of production. Therefore, in maximal opposition training, /m/ would be used if it was already in the child's inventory, to contrast with/k/ (the target sound). The purpose of this approach is to promote better generalization to other sounds and greater overall change of the child's phonological system through maximal contrast. The same flowchart for minimal oppositions contrast (see Figure 13–5) can be used for maximal oppositions contrast, with the only change being the selection of a sound already in the child's repertoire that maximally contrasts with the target sound.

Multiple Oppositions Therapy

The multiple oppositions approach is based on minimal oppositions (as above). The aim of this approach is to achieve maximum phonological reorganization in a systematic way. Instead of targeting one contrast at a time, this approach targets several contrasts simultaneously (Williams, 1993, 2000). This approach is good for children who have multiple sound errors and tend to use one sound to replace several. For example, if the child uses /t/ to replace /s, f, k/, it is most efficient and effective to target all three substitutions at once. In this instance, three different pairs of contrasts are used, including t-s (*cheat-cheese*), t-f (*cheat-chief*), and t-k (*cheat-cheek*), with 10 words in each pair. The therapy procedure is similar to minimal oppositions (see Figure 13–5). First, the clinician names words and the child sorts them into different piles for perception training (one pile for each of three target sounds: /s, f, k/). When the child is able to successfully differentiate these sound contrasts, treatment focuses on production training. Clinicians can also ask the child to sort the named words into different piles to work on perception and production simultaneously.

Speech and Language Ability

Tying speech therapy to daily life and functional communication is the goal when working with children who have limited language ability. Being able to communicate needs and wants is a priority. Therefore, targeting functional words and phrases and high-frequency words is highly recommended. Treatment begins with CVC words that are highly functional and frequently used in daily life such as *hi, bye, no, help, want, go, me, mom, dad*. How intelligible the word and phrase should be depends on the child's current speech and language functioning and other related health issues. Sometimes, approximation (i.e., close production of the target word) is acceptable if the child is not able to produce clear speech sounds, but approximation of the sound or word serves the communication purpose.

Working With School–Age Children With SSD

Children who start to develop phonics and phonological awareness may benefit from using phonological awareness activities to indirectly improve speech sound production. Phonological awareness is the individual's awareness of the sound structure of spoken words (Justice, Gillon, McNeill, & Schuele, 2013). Development of phonological awareness is important for learning to read. As phonological awareness brings the child's attention to the sound and syllable (e.g., alliteration of the sound at the beginning or at the end, syllable segmenting and blending), it is beneficial to incorporate these tasks into treatment to facilitate speech sound production and phonological awareness simultaneously. If the child uses syllable deletion, writing down the words and clapping out the syllables may increase the child's awareness of the syllable boundary and syllable structure. An example of this would be for the word *computer*. This is a three-syllable word. If the child tends to say *puter*, clinicians can show the child a picture along with the written word and clap out or highlight the syllables. Some children can quickly "fix" their speech errors through auditory and visual prompting. For alliteration, clinicians can ask the child to sort the cards into different piles based on the position of the sound and then use these target words to practice sound production. If the child enjoys spelling, spelling can also be used as a building block to facilitate awareness of speech sounds and speech errors.

Targeting Grammatical Morphemes at the Same Time

Final consonant deletion (FCD) is a one of the common phonological processes that may persist beyond appropriate age. What makes FCD important as a treatment target is its negative impact on grammatical morphemes. Grammatical morphemes carry additional meaning, like plural-s (indicates number) and tense markers (indicate time). If a child tends to delete all final sounds, it will not only significantly affect the child's speech intelligibility but also prevent the child from delivering meaningful messages. For example, when the child is explaining what happened last night to her friend, deletion of final consonants has a negative impact, as in "I see two ca__ cha__ a mou__" versus "I see two cats chase a mouse." Without the final consonants, the intended message is confusing. Another example is the deletion of plurals. If the child says, "my dog like to fight with each other" for "my dogs like to fight with each other," without the producing /s/ at the end of *dogs*, the listener may be puzzled about how many dogs the child has. Thus, /t, d, ŋ, s, z/ in the final position are very important because they carry additional grammatical meaning for present progressive tense (wash*ing*), regular past tense (walk*ed*) and plurals (dog*s*). According to Tyler, Lewis, Haskill, and Tolbert (2002), working on morphosyntax (morphology and syntax) can lead to cross-domain change in phonology. Therefore, instead of working on FCD in general, clinicians can target those specific final sounds that carry additional grammatical meaning to also facilitate positive changes in phonology and other language components (morphosyntax and pragmatics).

The Use of Nonspeech Oral Motor Exercises and Activities (NSOME)

Nonspeech oral motor exercises (NSOME) are activities, such as blowing bubbles, sucking straws, chewing tube, tongue wagging, and kissing, used to improve speech intelligibility. NSOME are frequently questioned by researchers regarding the direct relationship between

NSOME and improving speech intelligibility (Forrest, 2002; Lof, 2003). The rationales behind not using NSOME for children with SSD are as follows (Forrest, 2002):

1. Speech needs more than the strength of articulators. One purpose of NSOME is to strengthen oral muscles to improve speech intelligibility.
2. Breaking speech production down into individual and isolated motor components is not sufficient to learn an overall skill. Speech production requires very sophisticated fine motor control and coordination in a timely fashion. Therefore, exercising each articulator separately does not improve overall skills required for speech.
3. Even though the structures used in speech and nonspeech activities may be the same, the structures are used differently in these two types of activities.

The best way to improve speech intelligibility is to actually work on speech sounds and practice the sounds in a meaningful context (e.g., words, phrases) daily, because speech movement is different from other gross motor and fine motor movements. Effective ways of treating speech errors include the following:

1. Provide ear training, if necessary.
2. Work on speech sound production intensively using meaningful words at different levels (i.e., word, phrase, sentence, conversation).
3. Incorporate curriculum-based and literacy-related activities to promote generalization of correct sound production.
4. Provide speech homework for daily practice under the parent's or caregiver's supervision.

5. Help the child develop and implement self-monitoring strategies to self-correct error sounds in daily life.

Selecting Treatment Materials

A wide selection of articulation cards is available. However, as an SLPA, you will be required to select appropriate training words for the child, either in support of your supervising SLP's session or before you implement treatment with a client (ASHA, 2013). Box 13–3 contains a list of important elements to consider in selecting these materials.

When selecting stimuli, the target word should be easily identified. Real objects or pictures of real objects and actions that contain the target sound may be more effective and functional for younger children. Line drawing pictures, word lists, or reading passages may be more suitable for older children who are reading or are beginning to read. Ready-made articulation cards are convenient and can save time on preparation. However, keep in mind that selection of these materials must be done before each session to maximize learning outcomes. Appropriate training words should be selected to best facilitate target sound production. Functional target sounds used frequently in the child's daily life and words, selected from the child's curriculum should be used to facilitate generalization and maximize treatment gains.

Individualized training materials are highly recommended and they should always be meaningful to the child. Therefore, selection of words based on the child's language level is important in facilitating both speech and language development. Using pictures with written words printed on the above or below

> ## Box 13–3. Things to Consider When Selecting Treatment Materials
>
> ■ **Syllable shape:** Syllable shape is the number of syllables in the word. Fewer syllables make it easier for the child to produce the target sound.
> ■ **Neighboring sounds:** Neighboring sounds are the sounds that come before and after the target sound, which may influence the target sound. For example, /uk/ will be easier than /ek/ when eliciting /k/ in VC syllable production because the tongue position of /u/ is closer to the tongue position of /k/ (high-back vowel /u/ vs. mid-front vowel /e/).
> ■ **Stress:** Stress can be used to highlight the target sound. If the target sound is stressed, it may be easier for the child to pick up the sound.
> ■ **Cluster or singleton:** The use of singletons or blends depends on how easy it is to facilitate production of the target sound. For example, /s/ may be produced more easily in consonant clusters (st-, sn-) than singleton (Williams, 1991).
> ■ **Frequency:** High-frequency words are more functional and common in daily life. However, error production from old habits may be more difficult to correct. In that case, consider staying away from the high-frequency words that are consistently produced incorrectly until the target sound can be produced consistently.

may increase print awareness and sight word learning while working on the target sound. Choosing target words meaningful for the child and appropriate for the child's language level will facilitate generalization of sound production and increase the child's vocabulary repertoire. Starting with early developing words, such as concrete objects and visible action words, especially for younger children, may be helpful. If the child does not know the target word (e.g., *seesaw*), clinicians can talk about the word (e.g., "you can find it in the playground, one end goes up and one end goes down,") and link it to the child's personal experience.

Speech therapy should never be only drill and sound practice. When a child makes the link between the word, the letter, the sound, and the concept, the word will be stored in long-term memory more easily and become part of the child's vocabulary repertoire.

Most children who have SSD may have comorbid language delays or disorders, which may make addressing distorted speech sound(s) through language- and literacy-based treatment activities more effective. Language- and literacy-based treatment can even facilitate and support language development and learning for children who have SSD without other developmental or language learning issues. The focus of language- and literacy-based treatment goes beyond correct speech production. For example, through shared book reading, clinicians can highlight target sound(s) and emphasize and elaborate on related word and content knowledge. These types of activities can be blended into the treatment session to facilitate speech and language development simultaneously. Box 13–4 has suggestions for creating language- and literacy-based treatment activities. Chapter 16 (particularly its sections on books as play) provide additional suggestions.

Making Speech Sessions Fun and Motivating

Treatment sessions should never be drill-and-kill, but maximal training opportunities and practice must be provided to stabilize the target sound production. As maximum repetition is inevitable, clinicians must keep the speech session interesting and motivational. If the child is also working on language, fun activities can be blended into the session to make the session feel less like work. As stated earlier, language- and literacy-based activities should always be part of the treatment to facilitate both speech and language production. How to divide the session and how much time to spend on speech sound production and language learning depends on the priorities for the child and how the child responds to the treatment. You can work with your supervising SLP in discussing a good balance for each child. No matter the types of activities, keeping them fun and motivational is critical. Use short games and language- and literacy-based activities creatively to keep the speech session fun and provide maximal opportunity for practice. Table 13–7 provides sample activities that can be easily modified and expanded.

Box 13–4. Suggestions of Language- and Literacy-Based Treatment Activities

1. *Select a book that is appropriate for the child's language and reading level.* The book can be chosen from the pool of reading materials used in the classroom or home. That way, the teacher or parent can carry over the learning to different settings to promote generalization. Collaboration with other professionals and the parent to select appropriate and motivating treatment materials is crucial.
2. *Pre-read the book and highlight the words containing the target sound.*
3. *While you read the book with the child, emphasize the target sound and talk about the target words* (e.g., offer definition, synonym, antonym, homonym).
4. *After reading the book, help the child retell the story using target words and pictures from the book.*
5. *Incorporate arts and crafts after the reading activities to make retelling the story fun and easy.*

Table 13–7. Sample Games and Treatment Activities

Sample Activity	Materials	General Procedure
Fishing	Fish-shape magnets Fishing poles Training words	Attach target words to the back of fish-shape magnets. Child uses fishing pole to catch the fish and says the target words.
Bowling	Bowling ball and pins Training words	Attach target words to the bowling pins. Child knocks down bowling pins and says the word on the pin(s).
Safari	Flashlight(s) Training words	Place target words around the room. Give the child a flashlight. Turn off the light. Ask the child to find all target words using the flashlight.
Arts & Crafts	Scissors, glue, varied materials, Training words	Procedure varies depending on the art project. Use target words as part of the materials to complete the project.
Board Game	Candyland, Chutes & Ladders, Bingo, etc.	Procedure varies depending on the board game. Child has to say the target word(s) before moving the game piece.
Card Game	Memory games, Go Fish, etc.	Procedure varies depending on the card game. Use target words as game cards to compete with each other. Minimal pairs can be used as cards for Go Fish game.
Toys/Games	Train set, Genga, etc.	Procedure varies depending on the game. Various toys and games can be used. Child has to produce the target words before receiving or moving a game piece.

The purpose of these activities is to use simple and easy games and activities without creating additional cognitive and linguistic demands and to focus on maximizing opportunities for target sound production.

Treatment is a dynamic process. As such, clinicians need to have an open mind regarding the trial-and-error process. Keeping the speech session fun and effective is the goal; thus, finding an effective approach to facilitate target sound production through a short and quick experimental trial may be required. It is also critical to keep in mind that every child must be treated individually, even though she or he may have the same goal or work on the same sound(s) as others. It is very common to see that children respond to the same treatment approach or treatment activity differently. Therefore, creating individualized treatment activities is necessary.

In a school setting, group treatment can be used instead of individual sessions. Many of the activities discussed in Table 13–7 can be adapted for groups of children. Chapter 12 also offers suggestions for how to adapt activities. How to group children to address each child's speech and language goal(s) can be very challenging, but effective group sessions have the advantage of facilitating speech and language development through peer modeling. Using peers to model correct production and transferring practice into fun and competitive games may make training more enjoyable and motivational.

Lastly, iPads or other high-technology devices can be attractive and fun for children. Several apps designed for speech sound remediation can be used along with ready-made articulation cards. However, some children may be distracted by these devices, which may result in difficulty managing the session. Therefore, consider how to best use these devices without creating a negative impact on speech and language learning.

Monitoring Progress and Tracking Clinical Data

To ensure the effectiveness of interventions, clinicians must consistently track the frequency of correct production of the target sound in relation to the child's progress toward speech goal(s). Creating a general clinical data sheet that can be quickly modified for each child is highly recommended. Clinical data must be collected during each session. Audio recording each session to ensure the accuracy of the data is also necessary. Appendix 13–B is a sample data sheet. All data sheets should include quantitative data (e.g., numbers, such as percentages, number of prompts) and qualitative data (e.g., clinical observations that cannot be quantified easily by numbers). Chapter 8 offers additional suggestions for data collection. The appendices of Chapter 8 contain generic data sheets that can be modified for SSD treatment. Data sheets with the following components are very helpful:

1. Target sound: the sound(s) the child was working on in the session
2. Position: initial (I), medial (M), or final (F) position
3. Accuracy of production
4. Type of prompt provided

5. Qualitative clinical observation. Clinical observation should be brief but informative. Information should include the client's level of participation (e.g., attention, behavior), the training materials used, and any noted client strengths and weaknesses evident while implementing treatment.

If language is also addressed during the session, progress regarding language learning should be documented separately. Use a separate data sheet for each goal addressed in the child's treatment plan. As stated earlier, the purpose of data collection is to ensure the effectiveness of the intervention. Therefore, if a child does not progress at a desired and reasonable pace, treatment activities need to be modified by your supervising SLP. Thus, data need to be effectively conveyed to your supervising SLP. Chapter 9 has additional suggestions on how to summarize this information in a modified subjective, objective, assessment, and plan (SOAP) note format.

REFERENCES

American Speech-Language-Hearing Association. (2012). *2012 Schools survey report: SLP caseload characteristics.* Retrieved from http://www.asha.org/research/memberdata/schoolssurvey/

American Speech-Language-Hearing Association. (2013). *Speech-language pathology assistant scope of practice.* Retrieved from https://www.asha.org/policy/sp2013-00337/#sec1.6.2

Barlow, J., & Gierut, J. (2002). Minimal pair approaches to phonological remediation. *Seminars in Speech and Language, 23*(1), 57–67. doi:10.1055/s-2002-24969

Bauman-Waengler, J. (2012). *Articulatory and phonological impairments: A clinical focus* (4th ed.). Boston, MA: Pearson.

Bernthal, J., Bankson, N., & Flipsen, P. (2013). *Articulation and phonological disorders: Speech sound disorders in children* (7th ed.). Upper Saddle River, NJ: Pearson.

Bowen, C. (2011). *Communication disorders glossary.* Retrieved from http://www.speech-language-therapy.com/index.php?option=com_content&view=article&id=14&Itemid=123

Forrest, K. (2002). Are oral-motor exercises useful in the treatment of phonological/articulatory disorders? *Seminars in Speech and Language, 23,* 15–25. doi:10.1055/s-2002-23508

Gierut, J. (1989). Maximal oppositions approach to phonological treatment. *Journal of Speech and Hearing Research, 54,* 9–19. doi:10.1044/jshd.5401.09

Gordon-Brannan, M. E., & Weiss, C. E. (2007). *Clinical management of articulation and phonologic disorders* (3rd ed.). Baltimore, MD: Lippincott, Williams & Wilkins.

Justice, L., Gillon, G., McNeill, B., & Schuele, C. M. (2013). Phonological awareness: Description, assessment, and intervention. In J. E. Bernthal, N. W. Bankson, & P. Flipsen (Eds.), *Articulation and phonological disorders: Speech sound disorders in children* (7th ed., pp. 355–382). Upper Saddle River, NJ: Pearson.

Lof, G. (2003). Oral motor exercises and treatment outcomes. *Perspectives on Language, Learning, and Education, 10*(1), 7–12.

Lof, G. (2017, March). *What works for speech sound disorders: Using evidence to guide practice* [PowerPoint slides]. Presentation at the Mississippi Speech-Language-Hearing Association Annual Conference, Natchez, MS. Retrieved from https://www.z2systems.com/neon/resource/msha/files/Handouts/2017/Lof%20handout.pdf

Peña-Brooks, A., & Hegde, M. N. (2007). *Assessment and treatment of articulation and phonological disorders in children: A dual-level text* (2nd ed.). Austin, TX: Pro-Ed.

Sander, E. (1972). Do we know when speech sounds are learned? *Journal of Speech and Hearing Disorders, 37,* 55–63.

Secord, W. A., Boyce, S. E., Donohue, J. S., Fox, R. A., & Shine, R. E. (2007). *Eliciting sounds: Techniques and strategies for clinicians* (2nd ed.). Clifton Park, NY: Delmar Cengage Learning.

Shriberg, L. (1993). Four new speech and prosody-voice measures for genetics research and other studies in developmental phonological disorders. *Journal of Speech and Hearing Research, 36,* 105–140.

Smit, A., Hand, L., Freilinger, J., Bernthal, J., & Bird, A. (1990). The Iowa articulation norms project and its Nebraska replication. *Journal of Speech and Hearing Disorders, 55,* 779–798.

Templin, M. (1957). *Certain language skills in children.* Minneapolis, MN: University of Minnesota Press.

Tyler, A., Lewis, K., Haskill, A., & Tolbert, L. (2002). Efficacy and cross-domain effects of a morphosyntax and a phonology intervention. *Language, Speech and Hearing Services in Schools, 33,* 52–66. doi:10.1044/0161-1461(2002/005)

Van Riper, C., & Erickson, R. (1996). *Speech correction: An introduction to speech pathology and audiology* (7th ed.). Englewood Cliffs, NJ: Prentice-Hall.

Williams, A. L. (1991). Generalization patterns associated with training least phonological knowledge. *Journal of Speech and Hearing Research, 34,* 722–733.

Williams, A. L. (1993). Phonological reorganization: A qualitative measure of phonological improvement. *American Journal of Speech-Language Pathology, 2,* 44–51.

Williams, A. L. (2000). Multiple oppositions: Case studies of variables in phonological intervention. *American Journal of Speech-Language Pathology, 9,* 289–299.

World Health Organization. (2001). *International Classification of Functioning, Disability and Health (ICF).* Geneva, Switzerland: Author.

APPENDIX 13–A
Sample SSD Homework Sheet

Please give this speech homework sheet to your parent. Say each word correctly *10 times* a day with your parent. Pay attention to the sound you make. Remember to show your parent what you have learned in your speech session. Please ask your parent to put *a check mark for each word* after you say the word correctly 10 times. After you finish saying all the words correctly, please ask your parent to *initial at the bottom for each day you practice*. Please remember to bring your speech folder with you next time when you come to the speech room.

Keep up the good work!!   _____/Speech teacher

Target words—/s/ in initial position	Day 1	Day 2	Day 3	Day 4	Day 5	Day 6	Day 7
Sun							
Sea							
Say							
Saw							
Parent's Initials							

APPENDIX 13–B
Sample SSD Treatment Data Collection Form

Target Sound	Position (I/M/F)	Speech sound production (+ correct production, – incorrect production) **Prompt system** (**1.** Physical [placement] **2.** Visual **3.** Verbal **4.** No prompt/independent)
/k/	I (initial)	–/3 (explanation: incorrect with physical prompt provided), –/2, –/2+3 (incorrect with visual and verbal combined), +/3 (correct with physical prompt provided), +/3, +/3 . . . _____ *correct production* /_____ *total number of production in one session (correct + incorrect)* = _____*% accuracy*

Clinical Observation (qualitative)

Fully participated. Word level: one- and two-syllable words used. Responds best to physical prompt (articulation placement with tongue depressor). Starting to positively react to visual prompt. Mirror used throughout.

CHAPTER 14

Early Intervention

Margaret Vento-Wilson

INTRODUCTION

Watch and listen to a young child talk! You may be amused, impressed, puzzled, or curious, and you are bound to learn something. You will learn that when young children talk, they interact with and influence other persons; they talk about what they are doing, or are about to do, or want someone else to do; they say sounds or words, or phrases. And having noticed these things, you will have learned something about language. (Lahey, 1988, p. 1)

So opens Margaret Lahey's textbook on language development. This quote is on

the first page of the first chapter because of the primacy of the message, which serves to remind all practitioners that as much theoretical knowledge we may have about language, and as much as we have been taught by university professors about this remarkable phenomenon, children themselves are our best and truest teachers, and should always inform and drive our intervention.

When I was in graduate school, I used every opportunity to interact with two of my young nieces to test out what I had recently learned. I remember one encounter with Kate, my then three-year-old niece, who told me a complicated story about playing at the park with her best friend the day before. In the midst of the telling, she remarked with great emotion, "And then she felled me down!" Although I understood her perfectly, her sentence violated the semantic and syntactic rules of English. Upon first glance, the rule violations did not look complicated, but when I got home that evening, I analyzed what she had done in that sentence, and here is what I discovered (Goldberg & Jackendoff, 2004; Nadathur, 2017; Pinker, 1999; Smith, 1970; Wright, 2002):

1. She correctly selected a *move and change* verb to describe the event, which implies action or a change of state.
2. She further specified by using a resultative verb, which implies a completed action.
3. She maintained faithfulness to verb class, in that both the verbs *to fall* and *to push* involve a causative action with a resulting event.
4. She maintained faithfulness to the past tense form of *fall* and generated the word *fell*.
5. She applied the morphological rules for marking a weak verb by adding *–ed* to a strong verb, which typically involves a vowel change—from *f<u>a</u>ll* to *f<u>e</u>ll*.
6. She incorrectly chose the verb *to fall*, rather than *to push*, and in an attempt to reconcile the morphological requirements for regular past tense markedness, she applied the *–ed*. All of which resulted in a redundancy of markedness.
7. In selecting the verb *to fall*, she inadvertently changed the source of agency: The verb *to fall* is involuntary, which does not require an agent, and the verb *to push* is volitional, and requires an agent.
8. She merged internal and external causation.
9. She altered the transitivity of the verb: The verb *to fall* is an intransitive verb, which means that the action does not transfer to an object, and the verb *to push* is transitive, which means that it requires an object to receive the action.

Unbelievably, my three-year-old niece accomplished all this in a split second, and all before she was able to tie her own shoes!

If you had any doubts about the complexity of language before you began this chapter, I suspect that those doubts have now been erased. But I enjoin you not to let this complexity chase you away. As complex as it is, in the end, language is simply the way we as humans use symbols to interact with others. You are a fluent speaker of your native language, and you have been manipulating linguistic symbols your whole life. And now as a speech-language pathologist assistant (SLPA), you will have the opportunity to help others use language this same way, but with a bird's eye view of the construct of language.

Playing a part in the acquisition and early development of a child's language is wonderfully fun and I cannot recommend it highly enough. I cannot think of a single day in my work with children that has not made me smile, and I can think of only a few that have not made me laugh out loud. However, I must caution you that successful outcomes never *just happen*. Rather, they are the result of an SLPA's strong theoretical base, well-conducted intervention, and ongoing self-reflection to support continued improvement. This chapter has been written to support your work as an SLPA in early intervention, and the information presented here addresses the first two components of successful outcomes, but only you can address the third component (Figure 14–1).

THE WORK OF CHILDREN

Upon birth, children are tasked with an immense job that seems almost impossible when described in detail. In their first few years, typically developing children make the transformation from a nonverbal state to a verbal state and learn to comprehend, manipulate, construct, and produce their native language fluently (Bates & Goodman, 1997; Brown, 1973; Pinker, 1996). This remarkable transformation involves many stages and hierarchies, several which are described below.

Table 14–1 presents some of the milestones of language development as described by Bates (2003) in her extensive

Figure 14–1. Children ready for early intervention. Courtesy of Bing Images, free to share and use commercially.

Table 14–1. Developmental Model of Language Acquisition

Age Range	Milestone	Definition
0 to 3 months	Initial state of the system	The infant prefers to listen to sounds in the native language, as opposed to non-native languages.
		The infant can hear all phonetic contrasts used in the languages of the world.
3 to 6 months	Perception and production of vowels	The infant coos and imitates vowels only.
		Vowel perception is organized along language-specific lines.
6 to 8 months	Babbling in consonant-vowel segments (e.g., Ba, Baba)	
8 to 10 months	Word comprehension	The infant starts to lose sensitivity to consonants outside its native language.
12 to 13 months	Word production	The infant begins to name objects and people.
16 to 20 months	Word combinations	Vocabulary acceleration occurs.
		Relational words begin to appear (verbs and adjectives).
24 to 36 months	Grammaticization	Function words begin to appear (prepositions, articles).
		Inflectional morphology emerges (verb tense).
		Sentence complexity increases.
3 year to adulthood	Late Developments	Vocabulary growth continues.
		The child demonstrates increased comprehension and use of rare and complex forms.
		Sentence-level grammar is reorganized for the purpose of discourse.

Source: Bates, 2003, p. 15.

work on language acquisition. Dramatic growth occurs in receptive and expressive vocabulary in the first 30 months of life (Bates, 2003).

In this same approximate number of months (33), children begin to combine words purposefully and in the word order dictated by their native language, as documented by Bloom and Beckwith in 1989 (Figure 14–2). Additional milestones of language development in the domain of morphology follow in Table 14–2.

Once children have solidified the link between a concept (e.g., a small, soft, furry animal that lives in my house) and a representation (e.g., cat), and once that bank of words reaches a critical mass, they begin to put these words together into meaningful combinations (Spelke & Tsivkin, 2001). As with the other hierarchies described here, children move through stages that begin with a single word, to the use of multiple words chunked into semantic relations, and then into full syntactic structures called sentences (Peters, 1995). Table 14–3 provides examples of meaningful combinations, also called semantic relations. Semantic relations are defined as the two- to three-word phrases that have a meaning that is not present when looking at each individual word (Bloom, Lahey, Hood, Lifter, & Fiess, 1980). In other words, the sum of the utterance is greater than its parts. A final developmental continuum demonstrating the complexity of children's work in their early years is the shift in their intentionality (Table 14–4), which is linked to their growing awareness that someone is paying attention to them, and that symbols can be used to achieve a goal (Bates, Camaioni, & Volterra, 1975; Bloom & Beckwith, 1989; Owens, 2004).

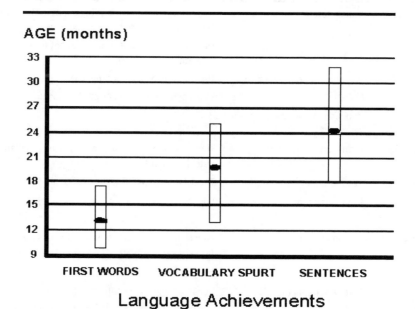

Language Achievements

Figure 14–2. Mean range of ages and ages of language development. Reprinted with permission from Bloom, L., and Beckwith, R. (1989). *Intentionality and language development.* Unpublished manuscript, Columbia University. doi:10.7916/D8KH0Z8N

Table 14–2. Brown's Stages of Morphological Acquisition

Age of Acquisition (Months)	Brown's Stage	Morphological Structure	Example
12–26	Stage I	One or two true words	"papa," "blankie"
27–30	Stage II	Present progressive	"singing"
		Articles "in" and "out"	"put it *in* the box"
		-s Plurals	"toy_s_"
31–34	Stage III	Irregular past tense	"fell"
		's Possessive	"Riley_'s_ bike"
		Uncontractible copula	"is it hot?"
35–40	Stage IV	Articles	"an," "the"
		Regular past tense	"talk_ed_"
		Third person regular, present tense	"he _rakes_ it"
41–46+	Stage V	Third person irregular	"she _does_"
		Uncontractible auxiliary	"_are_ they swimming?"
		Contractible copula	"_she's_ funny"
		Contractible auxiliary	"_they're_ going"

Source: Adapted from *"A first language: The early stages,"* by R. Brown, 1973 and *"Language disorders from infancy through adolescence: Listening, speaking, reading, writing, and communicating,"* by Paul, R. & Norbury, C. F., 2012.

Table 14–3. Semantic Relations

Two-Word Semantic Relations	Example
Agent + Action	Daddy go
Action + Object	Catch ball
Action + Locative	Sit chair
Entity + Locative	Cat bed
Possessor + Possession	Mommy bike
Attribute + Entity	Happy baby
Demonstrative + Entity	This book
Three-Word Semantic Relations	**Example**
Agent + Action + Object	Phoebe eat pasta
Agent + Action + Locative	Riley sleep crib
Agent + Object + Locative	Grammy key table
Action + Object + Locative	Get blanket bed

Source: Brown, 1973.

Table 14–4. Development of Intentionality

Stage	Behavior	Example
Non-Purposeful Communication		
Pre-Intentional	Behaviors are reflexive and express inner states (tired, hungry) and serve as signals for others. These behaviors are not directed to a specific person and there is no obvious expectation of an outcome.	Crying, cooing, posture changes, facial expressions
Unintentional-Intentional	Behaviors are intentional and goal orientated (reaching for a bottle), but are not conventionalized and recognized by both the speaker and listener. As above, these behaviors are not directed to a specific person and there is no obvious expectation of an outcome.	Fussing, reaching for or looking at an object
Purposeful Communication		
Non-Conventional Proto-Imperative	Non-conventional gestures, usually involving physical contact, are used with intent to affect a caregiver. The intention to communicate through behavior is confirmed when the child checks for the attention of the adult. The anticipation of an outcome is confirmed by persistence or frustration if the goal is not met. There is recognition that the caregiver provides the means to an end.	Tugging, pulling toward, pushing away
Conventional	Recognized or conventional vocalizations and gestures used to affect a caregiver's attention intentionally. There is a greater level of persistence.	Nodding, pointing, waving, alternating gaze, handing an object
Concrete	Recognizable symbols are used in a limited fashion. These symbols are used at some distance from the concept they represent. There is a range of intentions and they may be accompanied by vocalizations.	Requesting assistance or information, pointing, reaching, offering, signing
Symbolic Communication		
Abstract	Arbitrary symbols are used individually and in a limited fashion to represent the environment and the here and now. There is an understanding that words have referential value. There is still some use of idiosyncratic symbols. The use of gestures and vocalizations continues.	Symbols (words)
Formal	Words are combined in a rule-bound order. These combinations are used to talk about the *there and then*, and the concept represented by the symbol does not need to be present. The use of gestures and vocalizations fades and the primary means of communication is language.	Symbol (word) combinations

Source: Adapted from Bates, L., Camaioni, L., & Volterra, C. (1975). The acquisition of performatives prior to speech. *Merrill-Palmer Quarterly of Behavior and Development, 21*(3), 205–226; and Bloom L., & Beckwith, R. (1989). Intentionality and Language Development. Unpublished manuscript, Columbia University. In *Columbia Academic Commons* and *"Language disorders: A functional approach to assessment and intervention,"* by R. E. Owens, Jr., 2004, p. 89.

What these tables and figures tell us is that children are very, very busy in these early years as they work to acquire their native language by participating in the world around them. However, for a subset of children, this acquisition process is altered or delayed for various reasons that reflect their individual cognitive, motoric, sensory, and linguistic profiles, as well as various environmental, biological, cognitive, and behavioral factors as seen in Figure 14–3.

Specific disorders that contribute to these alterations or delays can include intellectual disability (ID), language learning disorder (LLD), autism spectrum disorder (ASD), specific language impairment (SLI), or other congenital or acquired impairments (American Speech-Language-Hearing Association [ASHA], n.d.; Rice, 2016). For these children, exposure to the language around them and participation in their world are not enough to support the acquisition of their native language and that is where you as an SLPA and as a member of the early intervention team become relevant. Your work should help children move to the next level in their acquisition process (Figure 14–4).

THE WORK OF INTERVENTION

An in-depth discussion and definition of language is well beyond the scope of this chapter; however, it is prudent to present a broad overview of what language is precisely because that is the tool with which you will be working in your role as an SLPA. Language can be viewed from many lenses: (a) language involves multifaceted relationships between communication, linguistic forms, and world knowledge

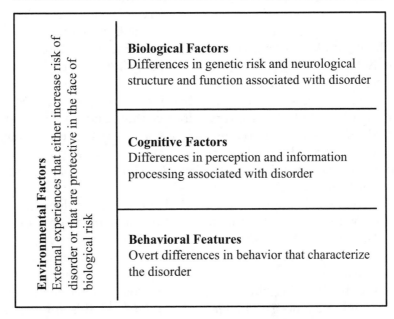

Figure 14–3. Factors affecting language development (Paul & Norbury, 2012, p. 10).

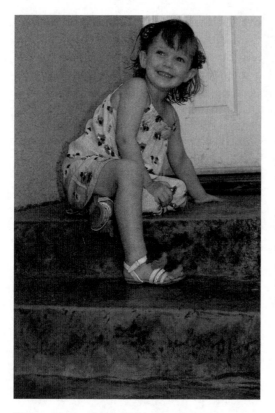

Figure 14–4. Child climbing stairs.

where you as the SLPA provide a bridge as the child moves up the language acquisition hierarchy.

This brings us to the definition of intervention itself. According to ASHA (2008) and Ukrainetz (2015), intervention is defined as intentional actions taken to accelerate, modify, or compensate for inadequate performance. It is further defined by Lahey and Bloom (1977) as the " . . . manipulation of the tangible non-linguistic, linguistic, and social context in ways designed to enhance the induction of regularities within and between these contexts" (p. 341). ASHA has identified four guiding principles that should serve as the foundation for early intervention:

1. Services should be family-centered and culturally responsive.
2. Services should be developmentally supportive and promote children's participation in their natural environments.
3. Services should be comprehensive, coordinated, and team-based.
4. Services should be based on the highest quality internal and external evidence that is available.
(ASHA, 2008, para. 5).

(Lahey & Bloom, 1977); (b) language is an indefinitely large system of meaning that is both created and exchanged (Halliday, 2003); and (c) language is a systematic conventionalized code of arbitrary signals agreed upon by a group (Lahey, 1988). Regardless of an individual's personal theory of language acquisition, one concept that unites all the theories is that language development is supported, at the very least, within human-to-human interaction (Bates et al., 1975; Eisenberg, 2004; Lightbrown & Spada, 2013). This means that there must be an interlocutor who responds to the child (Lightbrown & Spada, 2013). In intervention-based interaction, this implies a kind of mentorship

Specific to your role as an SLPA in early intervention, and under the supervision of a speech-language pathologist (SLP), you are expected to provide direct treatment to children as follows (ASHA, 2013):

1. Follow and implement documented treatment plans or protocols developed by your supervising SLP.
2. Document performance of the child (e.g., tallying data, preparing charts, records, graphs, language samples) and report this information to the supervising SLP.

3. Serve as an interpreter for children and their families who do no speak English.

In your role as an SLPA and as a language interlocutor for young children, the models described below will support your efforts and create a greater likelihood of success.

Zone of Proximal Development

The first model is called the *zone of proximal development* (ZPD), which was first identified by Vygotsky in 1978. The word *zone* refers to the space between what the child can currently do independently, and what the child will be able to accomplish independently in the near future, regardless of the task, as seen in Figure 14–5. The area of overlap defines your role as a bridge between the two different states. In your work as an SLPA, you may support a child in moving from labeling items to combining words into semantic relations (i.e., early word combinations), to generating three- to four-word phrases, to producing full, syntactically correct sentences (Gentner & Boroditsky, 2003). Likewise, you may support a child's transition from an individual picture description task, to retelling a short story, to creating a personal narrative with multiple characters, similar to the one my niece told me. There are various intervention techniques, which are expanded on later in this chapter, that can be used when working within a ZPD. One intervention technique is called *recasting*, where the SLPA adds an element (or elements) to a child's utterance (Proctor-Williams & Fey, 2007), as seen below:

Child: Doggie!

SLPA: Yes, a big doggie!

In this interaction, the SLPA has incorporated a word and concept the child has

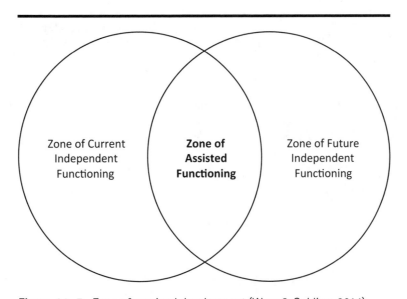

Figure 14–5. Zone of proximal development (Wass & Golding, 2014).

mastered and added a relevant descriptor that builds complexity onto the child's original utterance.

Caregiver–Mediated Instructional Practices

A second model that can be used to frame your intervention was defined by Dunst, Raab, and Trivette (2012) as caregiver-mediated instructional practices (CMIP; Figure 14–6). Although Dunst et al. identified parents as the caregiver in their conceptualization, for purposes of this chapter the role of the caregiver is being replaced by you, the SLPA. This model suggests that your intervention should reflect the interests of the child within everyday, meaningful, and familiar activities, as described in Table 14–5. These factors increase the likelihood of linguistic interactions between you and the child, which in turn increases the potential for further communicative and linguistic development (Dunst et al., 2012). In your role as an SLPA, you may interview the family to identify favorite and familiar activities of the child with whom you are working. You can also observe the child and her caregivers in a play session to gain better insight into the child's inter-

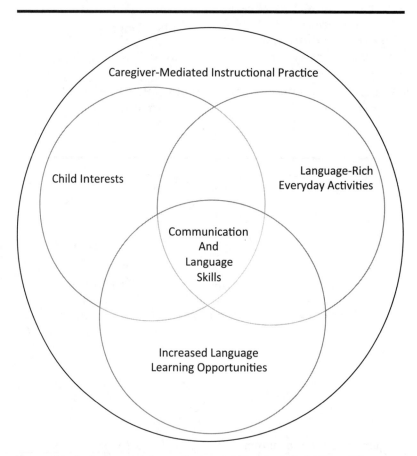

Figure 14–6. Language intervention model (Dunst et al., 2012, p. 13).

Table 14–5. Factors of Caregiver-Mediated Instructional Practices

Focus	Description
Child	Intervention targeting communicative and linguistic competence reflects the child's strengths and her personal and situational interests.
Activity	Intervention tasks increase naturalistic linguistic and communicative functioning in her environments.
	Intervention reflects her daily activities and incorporates tasks and objects that are relevant and familiar.
	Intervention allows for multiple communicative and linguistic learning opportunities within and across activities.
Methods	Intervention reinforces and sustains engagement with a positive affect and close attention to the child's interaction initiations.
	Intervention supports the development or refinement of reciprocal interactions between the SLPA and the child.
	Intervention follows the child's lead.

Source: Dunst et al., 2012.

action style. And finally, you can use this information to engage in intervention contexts that support the child's further language development.

Although this is good theoretical advice, it also has enormous practical value! As someone who has sat on the floor across from a 2½-year-old and attempted to entice her to engage in communication with a task that was too far removed from her daily life and much too artificial, I can attest that it does not always work. All my hard work in designing the session was met with a stony silence. However, when I stepped back and allowed this feisty toddler to guide the context and topic, our conversation took off with a bang! Going on a pretend shopping trip to Target for fruit and vegetables offered countless opportunities to use prepositions within phrases—put apple/grapes/broccoli in, take banana/strawberry/spinach out (Figure 14–7)—and I achieved the desired number of productions and she devel-

Figure 14–7. Toddler shopping for fruit.

oped greater mastery over prepositions. A final comment is that sometimes getting a child to engage is a bit like herding cats, but if you can bring her world into your intervention session, you are much more likely to be successful (Figure 14–8).

Figure 14–8. A herd of cats. Courtesy of Bing Images, free to share and use commercially.

Intervention Considerations

Competing Resources

One consideration central to language intervention, generally and specifically, is the notion of *competing resources* (Lahey & Bloom, 1994; Wallach, 2008; Wallach & Butler, 1994). When children's abilities are emerging or unstable, task demands have to be carefully crafted (Wallach, 2008). When there is a mismatch between abilities and demands, the child's resources have to compete for attention, and something must give. Paul and Norbury (2012) further explained this consideration as allowing new forms to express old communicative functions or allowing new communicative functions to be expressed

by an old form. Within an intervention context, this means that you must limit the task requirements. If you were working to expand a child's expressive vocabulary, it would be prudent to incorporate newly targeted words within a syntactic structure already well established in the child's repertoire. Conversely, if you were working toward an increase in utterance length, it would be best practice to incorporate familiar words into the longer, or more complex phrase (Paul & Norbury, 2012; Wallach, 2008).

Continuum of Naturalness

A final intervention consideration to be discussed is a continuum of naturalness as originally proposed by Fey (1986). This continuum describes three types of intervention that you will use in your role as an SLPA: (a) clinician-directed, (b) hybrid, and (c) child-centered (Cirrin & Gillam, 2008; Paul & Norbury, 2012; Owens, 2004; Roth & Worthington, 2015). Table 14–6 contains brief descriptions and examples of each intervention type.

There is not one single method or location on the continuum that is best for all children. What is needed is the best match among a specific child, a specific target, and the intervention approach (Kamhi, 1999; Paul & Norbury, 2012). For example, in the intervention context I described above, I made the wise decision to make a shift from a very clinician-directed and less natural context to a child-centered and more natural context. For that young girl, it was the right decision. However, with another child I work with, we sit at a table across from each other and engage

in a very structured literacy routine with very predictable syntactic demands. This young boy thrives in a structured context, and this more clinician-directed structure is the best match for the child and my targets. As you become more experienced and knowledgeable, differentiating the choices become easier, but it is always best to let the child guide your intervention decisions.

A final comment regarding the continuum of naturalness is that at every point along this continuum, best practices suggest that you be mindful of the ZPD as you target specific skills to ensure a smooth transition to the next skill level. Further, this continuum parallels the intervention model proposed by Dunst et al. (2012), but acknowledges that the nature of intervention should be individualized for each child and for each task or skill being targeted.

Table 14–6. Intervention Types on the Continuum of Naturalness

Type	Definition	Intervention Method	Example
Clinician-Directed	Highly structured: The clinician selects topics, materials, acceptable forms of response, and the method of reinforcement.	Drill	Picture identification, repetitive production of similar items. Targets specific forms.
Hybrid	Moderately structured and naturalistic: The clinician selects a narrow set of targets and materials that tempt the child.	Milieu language therapy. Focused stimulation.	Targets language development by modeling and highlighting specific forms.
Child-Centered	Naturalistic: The interests and preferences of the child dictate the topics, materials, and reinforcement method.	Indirect language stimulation.	Engagement in daily activities, facilitated play. Supports language development by responding to the child's utterances.

INTERVENTION STRUCTURE

Language Structure

Language is comprised of form, content, and use, as seen in Figure 14–9. These three domains have been expanded upon in Tables 14–7, 14–8, and 14–9. In addition to clarifying the three domains of language, these tables also provide a list of targets for intervention. For example, under the domain of *form*[1], potential targets can be seen in Table 14–10. Under the domain of *content*, potential targets can be seen in Tables 14–11 and 14–12.

In terms of words that can be incorporated into your intervention sessions, the domains of content and form can be viewed from a perspective of semantic relations as defined above. In other words, the sum of the utterance is greater than its parts (see Table 14–3 for examples of semantic relations). Table 14–13 lists words and word combinations that can be incorporated into your intervention sessions with children in the early stages of language development.

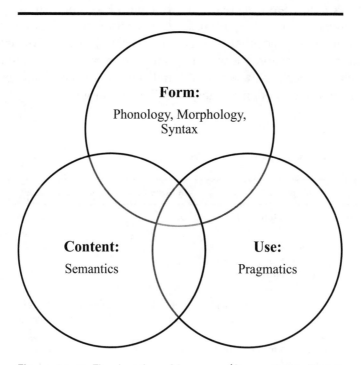

Figure 14–9. The domains of language (Owens, 2004; Paul & Norbury, 2012).

---

[1]Goals and intervention in the domain of phonology are addressed in Chapter 13 and thus will not be covered in this chapter.

Table 14–7. A Representation of Language Form (Phonology, Morphology, Syntax)

Categories of Spoken Form			
Language Domain	**Subdomain**	**Features**	**Example**
Phonology	Segmental	Phonemes	/b/, /p/, t/, /d/, . . .
		Syllables	/ba/, /pa/, /ta/, /da/, . . .
	Suprasegmental	Intonation	Phrase contour: rising, falling . . .
		Stress	
		Pause	
Language Domain	**Word Class**	**Word Type**	**Example**
Morphology	Substantive	Content Words	Verbs, Adjectives, Adverbs, Nouns
	Relational	Function Words	Prepositions, Conjunctions, Auxiliary Verbs, Articles, Pronouns
Language Domain	**Subdomain**	**Feature**	**Example**
Syntax	Word Order	Sentence Structure	Subject-Verb-Object, Subject-Object-Verb . . .
		Clauses	Coordinate, Subordinate
		Sentence Types	Active, Passive
	Inflection	Suffixes (ing, ed, ~s)	Verb: ~ing
			Noun: ~ist
			Adjective: ~able
			Adverb: ~ly

Source: Adapted from Lahey, 1988, p. 12.

Table 14–8. A Representation of Language Use (Pragmatics)

Categories of Language Use			
Language Use	**Subdomain**	**Features**	**Example**
Function	Personal/ Intrapersonal	Commenting	"Book funny."
		Vocal Play	"The seat belt goes 'click, click, click.'"
		Problem Solve	"Find socks?"
	Social/ Interpersonal	Request Object	"Give ball now!"
		Obtain Information	"Where is mommy?"
		Gain Attention	"I want down."
Language Use	**Subdomain**	**Features**	**Example**
Context	Nonlinguistic	Perceptual Support	Active listening, passive listening
		Adapt to Needs of Listener	Rate of speech, comprehension checks
		Social	Conversational Devices: Turn taking, initiating, terminating
			Status Relations: Politeness, direct and indirect requests
	Linguistic	Non-Contingent	N/A
		Contingent	Imitate
			Question
			Add Information

Source: Adapted from Lahey, 1988, p. 16.

Levels of Symbolism

Early intervention can be conceived of on a continuum of symbolic understanding and use (Owens, 2004). As detailed earlier, children move through a symbolic hierarchy that culminates with combining words in meaningful ways to express thoughts. It is likely that you will work with children who demonstrate no overt communication, those who use only vocalizations or gestures, and those who are beginning to put words together. As can be inferred, there are many states in this hierarchy, which implies many levels of intervention. Table 14–14 describes some of the intervention considerations and tasks related to a child's level of symbolic development.

Table 14–9. A Representation of Language Content (Semantics)

Categories of Language Content			
Language Domain	**Subdomain**	**Example**	
Object Knowledge	Specific Objects	Mother; father; specific siblings/friends/pets; specific familiar locations . . .	
	Object Classes	Animals, furniture, food, toys . . .	
Language Domain	**Subdomain**	**Feature**	**Example**
Object Relations	Reflexive	Existence/Disappearance	"Ball all gone."
	Interactions	Attribution Quantity	"Big pool." "Two cookies."
	Interclass	Action/State/Possession	"Drink milk." "Yummy cake." "Phoebe doll."
Language Domain	**Subdomain**	**Example**	
Event Relations	Temporal	Before, after	
	Causal	Because, since	
	Epistemic	Know, believe	

Source: Adapted from Lahey, 1988, p. 9.

Table 14–10. List of Potential Intervention Targets in the Domain of *Form*

Broad Target	Category	Example
Vocabulary	Content words	Adjectives, adverbs, nouns, verbs
	Function words	Prepositions, conjunctions, articles, pronouns, auxiliary verbs
Morphology	Plurals	Regular, irregular
	Verb tenses	Past, present, future
	Prefixes and suffixes	
Syntax	Word order	Subject-verb-object
	Clause types	Subordinate, coordinate, relative
	Sentence types	Passive, active, questions

Table 14–11. List of Potential Intervention Targets in the Domain of *Content*

Broad Target	Category	Example
Labeling	Objects, people	Toys, family members, friends
Combining words	Semantic relations	Existence, disappearance, re-occurrence, quantity, actions, possessions
	Events	Temporal (before, after), causation (because), states (knowing, being, having)

Table 14–12. List of Potential Intervention Targets in the Domain of *Use*

Broad Target	Category	Example
Language functions	Personal	Commenting, inner dialogue
	Social	Requesting, greeting, gaining attention, asking
Nonlinguistic	Implicit rules	Turn taking, initiating and ending interactions, polite behavior, tone of voice

Table 14–13. Semantic Relations That Can Be Incorporated into Intervention

Content	Relational Words	Object-Specific Relational Words	Substantive Words
Rejection	No		
Nonexistence/disappearance	No, all gone, away		
Cessation of Action	Stop, no		
Prohibition of action	No		
Recurrence of objects and actions	More, again, another		
Noting existence or object identification	This, there, that		
Actions on objects		Give, do, make, get, throw, eat, wash, kiss	
Actions of locating objects		Put, up, down, sit, fall, go	
Attributes or descriptions of objects		Big, hot, dirty, heavy	
Persons associate with objects			Personal names

Source: Lahey and Bloom, 1977, Appendix 14-A.

Table 14–14. Considerations and Goals Related to Symbolic Developmental Levels

Developmental Levels	Considerations	Intervention Tasks
Presymbolic/Nonsymbolic	Intervention should focus on the child's family and natural settings and contexts.	Expand the number of communicative functions.
		Increase the complexity of communicative functions.
		Support the transition from nonintentional to intentional communication.
		Replace unconventional communication with conventional communication.
Symbolic	Intervention should focus on increasing the child's communicative and linguistic competence.	Expand number of concepts expressed.
		Expand the length of utterances.
		Increase the complexity of utterances.
	Intervention should support greater communicative contexts.	Expand the child's communicative partners.
		Change the environment of the intervention.

Source: Owens, 2004.

INTERVENTION METHODS

As an SLPA, you will not be responsible for writing goals or specifying intervention targets (ASHA, 2013), but you will be implementing intervention defined and designed by your supervising SLP. Toward that end, Table 14–15 contains a list of intervention methods that can be used with children across contexts, diagnoses, and development levels. The decision to use one of these methods should be based on the child's unique characteristics and personality type, the intervention target, and your professional skill. It is important to note that these methods are not presented in an either/or fashion. There may be sessions where it is most advantageous to use more than one, or to adapt one based on a specific child's needs. Ultimately, it is your responsibil-

ity as an SLPA to engage the child and you may have to make a change in the moment. In your work in early intervention, it is never appropriate to blame the child for lack of engagement: you are the adult and the SLPA, and it is up to you to create a successful and productive intervention session.

Language Facilitation Methods

Additional language facilitation strategies not specific to a single intervention method can be found in the list below:

1. Ask open-ended questions to offer more opportunities for interaction to continue. Asking for a child's opinion allows him to share his thoughts and ideas. You can ask him to make a prediction about an outcome or an

Table 14–15. Intervention Methods

Drill	
Naturalness: Clinician-Directed	Definition: Uses discrete drill work in a highly controlled context in conjunction with relevant linguistic materials to increase the frequency of a language target with clear reinforcements.

Key Factors:

Intervention targets are broken down into a series of steps.

Targets are presented in a series of a high number of trials.

Reinforcements are consistent and reflect specific performance factors, such as "You used the sign for 'more'" and "That's right, the apple is IN the basket!"

Potential Session Structure:

Engage the child in a task with many pieces (Mr. Potato Head, a train set, setting a table) and require the child to produce a target, such as the preposition "on," before they can add a piece to the task.

Focused Stimulation	
Naturalness: Hybrid	Definition: The clinician arranges the intervention context so that the child is tempted to respond with utterances.

Key Factors:

Respond to all communicative acts (gestural, vocal, symbolic).

Refer to the here and now.

Allow processing time for the child.

Describe your actions and the child's actions.

Use short sentences with words of one or two syllables.

When possible, avoid the use of telegraphic speech, or short, ungrammatical phrases ("wash hand hot").

Potential Session Structure: This method can be used in any type of task or context.

Indirect Language Stimulation	
Naturalness: Child-Centered	Definition: Provides a simple model within the child's ZPD that links the child's behavior with a linguistic mapping of that behavior.

Key Factors:

Describe your own and the child's actions.

Imitate the behavior, communication, or language of the child.

Expand the child's utterance with additional grammatical detail and semantics.

Extend the child's utterance by restating the utterance with additional details.

Recast the child's utterance into a different type of utterance, such as a question or a negative statement.

Potential Session Structure: This method can be used in any type of task or context.

Incidental Training	
Naturalness: Child-Centered	Definition: Intervention occurs within unstructured situations. The child's interests and preferences frame the focus of the intervention.

Key Factors: Input by the SLPA should match or be slightly more complex or longer than the child's current level of communication or language.

Potential Session Structure:

Hide and find objects with accompanying comments.

While putting toys away, the SLPA differentiates between singular and plural nouns (block/blocks; doll/dolls; truck/trucks).

Table 14–15. *continued*

Enhanced Milieu Teaching	
Naturalness: Hybrid	Definition: The use of environmental arrangement to support the development of engagement. It is used to model, prompt, and cue new language forms.

Key Factors:

Choose materials of interest to the child.

Arrange the environment to elicit responses.

Wait expectantly for a response.

Expand the child's utterances.

Potential Session Structure: Establish an interactive routine that serves as the backdrop for your session.

Behavior Chain Interruption	
Naturalness: Clinician-directed	Definition: The intervention involves a break in an established routine.

Key Factors: The task must be familiar to the child.

Potential Session Structure:

Stop playing a favorite song.

Offer an empty crayon box for a drawing task.

Skip the child in a turn taking task.

Potential Session Structure: Establish an interactive routine that serves as the backdrop for your session.

Sources: Dunst et al., 2012; Hancock and Kaiser, 2006; Hart and Risley, 1975; Kaiser, Hancock, and Nietfeld, 2000; Owens, 2004, 2009; Paul and Norbury, 2012; Peterson, 2004; Proctor-Williams and Fey, 2007; Robertson and Weismer, 1999; Schuler and Prizant, 1987.

event or to solve a problem about a story or an aspect of a play schema (Tompkins, Zucker, Justice, & Binici, 2003).

2. Incorporate the O-W-L method into your intervention scenario. **O**bserve what the child is interested in. **W**ait for his response and look at the child expectantly. **L**isten closely to the child's gestures and utterances and go from there (Rhyner, Geuhther, Pizur-Barnekow, Cashin, & Chavie, 2012).

3. Follow the child's lead. Join in the child's activity, imitate the child, comment on what the child is doing, and use short, grammatically correct phrases to interpret what is going on in the context. Ask questions that build on what the child has already said (Dunst et al., 2012; Fey, Long, & Finestack, 2003).

4. Provide a running commentary of the child's actions. Do not require a response from the child and allow processing time between descriptions. Providing a language overlay onto the context offers multiple opportunities for the child to hear a new word or to hear a familiar word in a new context (Marzano, 2004).

5. Make indirect corrections *in the moment* during the play schema or literacy routine; however, corrections should be made with grammatically correct phrases (Fey, 2008; Owens, 2004).

6. Incorporate sensitive and positive contingent responses into the context (Kong & Carta, 2011).

Prompting

Using a least to most prompting hierarchy involves providing scaffolding with the least amount of prompting at the beginning and moving toward a greater amount of prompting over multiple trials. It is important to recognize that a child's compliance to a command, such as "Tell me what this is," is not communication, it is labeling. To determine an appropriate level of prompting, follow the following steps (Senner, n.d.) :

1. Identify an appropriate time to wait before providing a prompt. This time varies greatly between children, but it can be identified through careful observation.
2. Offer the communicative bid to the child, such as "Let's play with the Play-Doh."
3. Offer a contextual cue, such as looking at a specific item, and create an expectant pause.
4. Offer an indirect verbal cue, such as remarking, "Hmm, the Play-Doh is so hard to open." This indirect cue signals to the child that something is expected from them.
5. Move the item closer to the child to bring their attention to it.
6. Ask a question, such as, "Do you need help opening the Play-Doh?"
7. Provide a model, such as, "Tell me, 'open box.'"

Table 14–16. Topics in ASHA's Practice Portal

Topic	Link
Late Language Emergence	http://www.asha.org/Practice-Portal/Clinical-Topics/Late-Language-Emergence/
Intellectual Disability	http://www.asha.org/Practice-Portal/Clinical-Topics/Intellectual-Disability/
Spoken Language Disorders	http://www.asha.org/Practice-Portal/Clinical-Topics/Spoken-Language-Disorders/

ADDITIONAL SOURCES

Although you work under a supervising SLP who can answer your questions and support your early intervention, Tables 14–16 and 14–17 contain links to resources within ASHA that may be helpful in guiding your intervention. You will find that ASHA is a rich source of information for early intervention through its Practice Portal (Table 14–16) and Evidence Maps (Table 14–17).

CONCLUSION

In my work with children, I often think of a quote that beautifully represents what we do, "If you want to build a ship, don't assign men tasks and work, but rather, teach them to yearn for the vast and end-

Table 14–17. Topics in ASHA's Evidence Maps

Topic
Apraxia of Speech
Central Auditory Processing Disorder
Intellectual Disability
Late Language Emergence
Spoken Language Disorders

Note. ASHA Evidence Maps available at: https://www.asha.org/evidence-maps/

Figure 14–10. A ship in an immense sea. Courtesy of Bing Images, free to use and share commercially.

less immensity of the sea" (Bray, 2001) (Figure 14–10).

In the same vein, I work to convince children that language is their key to power and control, constructs that are often in short supply in the lives of children, more so in the lives of children with language impairments. With language, they can share their worlds and shape their futures, and in your role as an SLPA, you play a part in their journey. I urge you to take the theoretical and practical knowledge you gain through this chapter and the others in this book, and use it as you sit alongside children, talk to children, play with children, read with children, tell stories with children, learn from children, and have plain old fun with children. Whether you are using clinician-directed methods or incidental teaching, whether you are targeting labeling to increase vocabulary or more complex sentences to support the development of syntax, or whether the child is presymbolic or symbolic, be present in the moment, work in concert with the child and his world, and support the child's transition to the next level. As I wrote in the introduction, working with children in early intervention is wonderfully fun and I hope you will someday share those sentiments.

REFERENCES

American Speech-Language-Hearing Association. (2008). *Roles and responsibilities of speech-language pathologists in early intervention: Technical report* [Technical report]. Retrieved from http://www.asha.org/policy

American Speech-Language-Hearing Association. (2013). *Speech-language pathology assistant scope of practice.* Retrieved from https://www .asha.org/policy/sp2013-00337/#sec1.6.2

Bates, E. (2003). On the nature and nurture of language. In R. Levi-Montalcini, D. Baltimore, R. Dulbecco, F. Jacob, F., E. Bizzi, P. Calissano, & V. Volterra (Eds.), *Frontiers of biology: The brain of homo sapiens* (pp. 241–265). Rome, Italy: Instituto della Enciclopedia Italiana Fondata de Giovanni Trecanni.

Bates, E., Camaioni, L., & Volterra, V. (1975). The acquisition of performatives prior to speech. *Merrill-Palmer Quarterly, 21*(3), 205–226.

Bates, E., & Goodman, J. C. (1997). On the inseparability of grammar and the lexicon: Evidence from acquisition, aphasia, and real-time processing. *Language and Cognitive Processes, 12*(5/6), 507–584. doi:10.1080/0169 09697386628

Bloom, L., & Beckwith, R. (1989). Intentionality and language development. Columbia University [Unpublished manuscript]. doi:10.79 16/D8KH0Z8N

Bloom, L., Lahey, M., Hood, L., Lifter, K, & Fiess, K. (1980). Complex sentences: Acquisition of syntactic connectives and the relations they encode. *Journal of Child Language, 7*(2), 235–261. doi:10.1017/S0305000900002610

Bray, D. (2001). *A willful volunteer: Examining conscience in an unconscious world.* Lincoln, NE: iUniverse.

Brown, R. (1973). *A first language: The early stages.* London, UK. George Allen & Unwin.

Cirrin, F. M., & Gillam, R. B. (2008). Language intervention practices for school-age children with spoken language disorders: A systematic review. *Language, Speech, and Hearing in the Schools, 37,* S110–S137. doi:10.1044/0161-1461 (2008/012)

Dunst, C. J., Raab, M., & Trivette, C. M. (2012). Characteristics of naturalistic language intervention strategies. *Journal of Speech-Language Pathology and Applied Behavior Analysis, 5*(3–4), 8–16. doi:10.1037/h0100047

Eisenberg, S. (2004). Structured communicative play therapy for targeting language intervention in young children. *Communicative Disorders Quarterly, 26*(1), 29–35. doi:10.1177/15257 401040260010201

Fey, M. E. (1986). *Language intervention with young children.* Boston, MA: Allyn & Bacon.

Fey, M. E. (2008) The (mis-)use of telegraphic input in child language intervention. *Revista de Logopedia, Foniatria y Audiologia, 28*(4), 218–230. doi:10.1016/S0214-4603(08)70129-3

Fey, M. E., Long, S. H., & Finestack, L. H. (2003). Ten principles of grammar facilitation for children with specific language impairments. *American Journal of Speech-Language Pathology, 12,* 3–15. doi:10.1044/1058-0360(2003/048)

Gentner, D., & Boroditsky, L. (2003). Individuation, relativity, and early word learning. In M. Bowerman & S. C. Levinson (Eds.). *Language acquisition and conceptual development* (pp. 215–256). New York, NY: Cambridge University Press.

Goldberg, A. E., & Jackendoff, R. (2004). The English resultative as a family of constructions. *Language, 80*(3), 532–568. Retrieved from http:// www.jstor.org/stable/4489722

Halliday, M. A. K. (2003). *On language and linguistics.* In J. Webster (Ed.), *Collected works of M.A.K. Halliday* (Vol. 3). New York, NY: Continuum.

Hancock, T. & Kaiser, A. (2006). Enhanced milieu teaching. In McCauley, R., & Fey, M (Eds.) *Treatment of language disorders in children* (pp. 203–236). Baltimore, MD: Brookes.

Hart, B., & Risley, T. R. (1975). Incidental teaching of language in the preschool. *Journal of Applied Behavior Analysis, 8,* 411–420. doi:10.1901/ jaba.1975.8-411

Kaiser, A. P., Hancock, T. B, & Nietfeld, J. P. (2000). The effects of parent-implemented milieu teaching on the social communication of children who have autism. *Early Education and Development, 11*(4), 423–446. doi:10.1207/ s15566935eed1104 4

Kamhi, A. G. (1999). To use or not to use: Factors that influence the selection of new treatment approaches. *Language, Speech, and Hearing Services in the Schools, 30,* 92–98. doi:10.1044/ 0161-1461.3001.92

Kong, N. Y., & Carta, J. J. (2011). Responsiveness interaction interventions for children with or at risk for developmental delays. *Topics in Early Childhood Special Education, 33*(1), 4–17. doi:10.1177/0271121411426486

Lahey, M. (1988). *Language disorders and language development.* Needham, MA: Simon and Schuster.

Lahey, M., & Bloom, L. (1977). Planning a first lexicon: Which words to teach first. *Journal of Speech and Hearing, 42,* 340–350. doi:10.1044/ jshd.4203.340

Lahey, M., & Bloom, L. (1994). Variability in language learning disabilities. In G. P. Wallach, & K. G. Butler (Eds.). *Language learning disabilities in school-age children and adolescents: Some principles and applications* (pp. 354–372). Boston, MA: Allyn & Bacon.

Lightbrown, P. M., & Spada, N. (2013). *Oxford handbooks for language teachers: How languages are learned*. Oxford, UK: Oxford University Press.

Marzano, R. J. (2004). *Building academic background knowledge: Facilitator's guide*. Alexandria, VA: Association for Supervision and Curriculum Development. Retrieved from http://www.ascd.org/ASCD/pdf/site-ASCD/video/buildingacademic.pdf

Nadathur, P. (2017). *Causative verbs: Introduction to lexical semantics*. Retrieved from https://web.stanford.edu/~pnadath/handouts/ling130b-fall17/Nadathur-analytic-causatives.pdf

Owens, R. E. (2004). *Language disorders: A functional approach to assessment and intervention* (4th ed.). Boston, MA: Pearson Education.

Owens, R. E. (2009). *Language disorders: A functional approach to assessment and intervention* (5th ed.). Boston, MA: Pearson Education.

Paul, R., & Norbury, C. (2012). *Language disorders from infancy through adolescence: Listening, speaking, reading, writing, and communicating* (4th ed.). St. Louis, MO: Elsevier.

Peters, A. M. (1995). Strategies in the acquisition of syntax. In P. Fletcher & B. MacWhinney (Eds.) *The handbook of child language* (pp. 475–482). Oxford, UK: Blackwell.

Pinker, S. (1996). *Language learnability and language development*. Cambridge, MA: Harvard University Press.

Pinker, S. (1999). *Words and rules*. New York, NY: Perseus Book Group.

Peterson, P. (2004). Naturalistic language teaching procedures for children at risk for language delays. *The Behavior Analyst Today, 5*, 404–424. doi:10.1037/h0100047

Proctor-Williams, K., & Fey, M. (2007). Recast density and acquisition of novel irregular past tense verbs. *Journal of Speech, Language, and Hearing Research, 40*(4), 1029–1047. doi:10.1044/1092-4388(2007/072)

Rhyner, P. M., Guenther, K. L., Pizur-Barnekow, K., Cashin, S. E., & Chavie, A. L. (2012) Child caregivers' contingent responsiveness behaviors during interactions with toddlers within three day care contexts. *Communication Dis-*

orders Quarterly, 34(4), 232–241. doi:10.1177/1525740112465174

Rice, M. L. (2016). Specific language impairment, nonverbal IQ, attention-deficit/hyperactivity disorder, autism spectrum disorder, cochlear implants, bilingualism, and dialectal variants: Defining the boundaries, clarifying the clinical conditions and sorting out cases. *Journal of Speech, Language, and Hearing Research, 59*, 122–132. doi:10.1044/2015_JSLHR-L-15-0255.

Robertson, S., & Weismer, E. (1999). Effects of treatment on linguistic and social skills in toddlers with delayed language development. *Journal of Speech, Language, and Hearing Research, 42*, 1234–1248. doi:10.1044/jslhr.4205.1234

Roth, F., & Worthington, C. (2010). *Treatment resource manual for speech language pathology* (5th ed.). KY: Cengage Learning.

Schuler, A. L., & Prizant, B. M. (1989). Facilitating language: Prelanguage approaches. In D. J. Cohen & A. M. Donnellan (Eds.). *Handbook of autism and pervasive developmental disorders* (pp. 301–315). New York, NY: John Wiley.

Senner, J. E. (n.d.). *Least to most prompting*. Retrieved from http://www.talcaac.com/prompting.pdf

Smith, C. S. (1970). Jespersen's "move and change" class and causative verbs in English. In M. A. Jazayery, E. C. Polome, & W. Winter (Eds.) *Linguistic and literary studies in honor of Archibald A. Hill. Vol. 2: Descriptive linguistics* (pp. 101–109). The Hague, Netherlands: Mouton.

Spelke, E. S., & Tsivkin, S. (2001). Initial knowledge and conceptual change: Space and number. In M. Bowerman & S. C. Levinson (Eds.). *Language acquisition and conceptual development* (pp. 71–97). New York, NY: Cambridge University Press.

Tompkins, V., Zucker, T. A., Justice, L. M., & Binici, S. (2003). Inferential talk during teacher-child interactions in small-group play. *Early Childhood Research Quarterly, 28*(2), 424–436. doi:10.1016/j.ecresq.2012.11.001

Ukrainetz, T. A. (2015). *School-age language intervention: Evidence-based practices*. Austin, TX: Pro-Ed.

Vygotsky, L. S. (1978). *Mind in society: The development of higher psychological processes*. M. Cole, V. John-Steiner, S. Scribner, & E. Souberman (Eds.). Cambridge, MA: Harvard University Press.

Wallach, G. P. (2008). *Language intervention for school-age students: Setting goals for academic success.* St Louis, MO: Mosby/Elsevier.

Wallach, G. P., & Butler, K. G. (1994). *Language learning disabilities in school-age children and adolescents: Some principles and applications.* London, UK: Pearson Education.

Wass, R., & Golding, C. (2014). Sharpening a tool for teaching: The zone of proximal development. *Teaching in Higher Education, 19*(6), 671–684.

Wright, S. K. (2002). Transitivity and change of state verbs. *Berkeley Linguistics Society, 28,* 339–350. doi:10.3765/bls.v28i1.3849

CHAPTER 15

Language Intervention for Children

Margaret Vento-Wilson

Words are not vocal labels which have come to be attached to things and qualities already given in advance by Nature, or to ideas already grasped independently by the human mind. On the contrary, languages themselves, collective products of social interaction, supply the essential conceptual frameworks for . . . analysis of reality and, simultaneously, the verbal equipment for their descriptions of it. The concepts we use are creations of the language we speak.

—Saussure (1983, p. IX)

INTRODUCTION

Why do I work in a public elementary school with children with language disorders? It is a question I have often asked myself after long days of back-to-back sessions, seemingly endless and complex Individual Education Program (IEP) meetings, and hours of report writing that begin well after the students have gone home. However, the answer to that question can arrive, in the day's first session, in the form of a picture drawn by one of the students on my caseload, who believes —whole-heartedly—that he is as strong as a superhero and could save the world (and me!) if needed (Figure 15–1).

I work in this setting and with this population because the work is extraordinarily rewarding and because it matters deeply to the students on my caseload. I also work in this setting because I continue to be fascinated by the human capacity for language, and how we shape and are shaped by our language. Whether you are new to this population or very experienced in this work, I hope that in your role as a speech-language pathologist assistant (SLPA) you have the opportunity to work with a young superhero, who is not going to let a language learning disorder get in his way of saving the world.

LANGUAGE INTERVENTION WITH CHILDREN

Language intervention with children[1] is complex, far reaching, and encompasses a wide age range of ages, from about 6 to 18

Figure 15–1. Drawing by a student.

---

[1]For purposes of clarity, although the age range of the individuals discussed in this chapter moves from about first grade to twelfth grade, the term "children" will be used throughout.

years of age, or from first to twelfth grade (American Speech, Language, & Hearing [ASHA], 2001). In early intervention, one of the primary focuses is language acquisition, which supports the transition from the nonlinguistic state to the linguistic state (Pinker, 1996). Once children reside solidly in the linguistic world, the break between early intervention and language intervention emerges. As such, this chapter can be viewed as a continuation of the previous chapter on early intervention, but it is important to note that while the age of the children many change, the foundational principles of language intervention remain the same. As I have often reminded the students I teach at the university level, *language is language is language.*

Whether children are in the early stages of language acquisition, or developing and refining their language, it all comes down to supporting children's ability to use and produce the building blocks of language: semantics, syntax, and pragmatics (Roth, Paul, & Peirotti, 2006) (Figure 15–2).

As stated above, in our early intervention with children, the focus is on establishing an early lexicon, supporting the development of syntax, and expanding their ability to use language in social contexts (Bloom & Lahey, 1978); much of this intervention revolves around Brown's morphemes (Brown, 1973). As children continue to develop and move beyond the early years, however, intervention moves well beyond Brown's morphemes and can include any of the following (Nippold, Mansfield, Billow, & Tomblin, 2009):

- More advanced morphological markers
- Complex syntax
- Higher level vocabulary

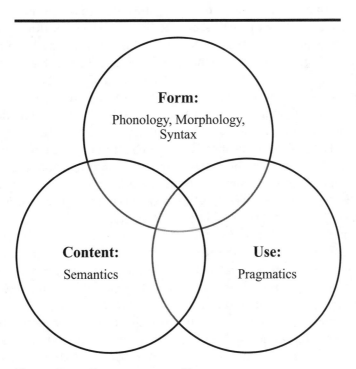

Figure 15–2. The components of language.

- Adjectival and adverbial markers
- Conjunctive and cohesive markers
- Noun phrase elaboration

Furthermore, in addition to the basic components of language described above, the following domains are well within the scope of practice for SLPAs because of the inherent links between language, reading, and writing (Pennington & Bishop, 2009; Sun & Wallach, 2014): spelling (Apel & Masterson, 2001), reading (Catts, Fey, Tomblin, & Zhang, 2002), and writing (Nelson, Van Meter, Chamberlain, & Bahr, 2001). A final comment with respect to the intervention for children with language learning disorders is the multifaceted relationships between all of the domains listed above. For example, intervention in vocabulary supports complex syntax (DeKemel, 2003), and syntax has been shown to be one of the underpinnings of reading comprehension (Brimo, Apel, & Fountain, 2017). In your work as an SLPA with children with language learning disorders, be confident that the skills you target build on each other in a cohesive manner that provides a bridge to the next step.

In this chapter, the term *language learning disorder* (LLD) will be used to describe the children you will work with as an SLPA (Wallach, 2008). This specific term is used to disambiguate the broad concept of a language impairment from the term *specific language impairment* (SLI), which is used for a specific type of language impairment. The term *language learning disorder* also differentiates this population from the special eligibility category of *speech-language impairment.*

This chapter explores and defines the following concepts: (a) foundational principles of language intervention, (b) legislative action and federal guidelines as they relate to the school-age population,

(c) broad intervention concepts, and (d) specific intervention practices that can be used across all domains of language. As a trained SLPA, you are qualified to work with these students and after reading this chapter, I hope you feel more confident and that the intervention feels less daunting than it may have initially.

LANGUAGE INTERVENTION FRAMEWORK

Language is defined as "a dynamic system that involves the ability to integrate knowledge of phonology, morphology, syntax, semantics, and pragmatics to create sentences within conversational, narrative, and expository discourse contexts" (Gillam & Ukrainetz, 2006, p. 62). Language development can be viewed as existing on several shifting paradigms: the oral-to-literate continuum, the narrative-to-expository continuum, and the change over time in the way language disorders are defined (Fey, Catts, Proctor-Williams, Tomblin, & Zhang, 2004; Sun & Nippold, 2012). In children, LLDs are often first revealed in their conversational contexts during the early stages of language development, but begin to manifest themselves in the comprehension and production of narratives and expository texts as they grow up (Gillam, McFadden, & vanKleek, 1995; Wallach & Butler, 1994; Wallach, Charlton, & Christie, 2014).

One concept deeply central to intervention with children with LLD is the need to maintain a view toward the horizon (Sun & Wallach, 2014). Over time, young children become students, who move through the K to 12 curriculum, who may or may not attend higher education, and who eventually shift into adulthood and gainful employment (Bashir, 1989). Also over time, speakers become readers and writers, with a parallel increase in linguistic and cognitive demands (Wallach, Charlton, & Christie, 2014). Children move from the concrete of the here and now to the more abstract *there and then* (Gillam & Ukrainetz, 2006). And finally, children move from the familiar world of stories and narratives to the demands of expository text, where the majority of learning occurs, with very different vocabularies and morphosyntactic structures (DeKemel, 2003; Gillam & Ukrainetz, 2006; Puranik, Lombardino, & Altmann, 2008). On a macro level, intervention must reflect the demands of each stage, while simultaneously supporting the transition to the next stage. However, on the micro level, the time spent with an individual child may be only at a single point, which underscores that need to always ask the question, "What's next for this child?"

FOUNDATIONAL PRINCIPLES OF LANGUAGE INTERVENTION

The definition of language intervention is defined as follows: intentional actions taken to accelerate, modify, or compensate for inadequate performance (Ukrainetz, 2006). In contrast to this concise and narrow definition, children with LLDs are a heterogeneous population whose unifying characteristics include challenges in understanding, acquiring, or using oral or written language (Cirrin & Gillam, 2008; Kamhi, 2014). These challenges are seen across semantics, syntax, and pragmatics, as well as across disability category (e.g., autism spectrum disorder [ASD], specific language impairment [SLI], intellectual disability [ID]). While the presentation of

these disorders varies considerably, the impact of reduced language abilities on the individual does not. LLDs are associated with decreases in educational outcomes, social interaction, and individual agency (Cohen, 2010; Lyons & Roulstone, 2018). As such, it is appropriate to discuss larger constructs useful in framing intervention for children with LLDs.

Systems Constructs

One foundational construct that can be applied to intervention with children is Bronfenbrenner's bioecological model (2006), which demonstrates the interaction between children and their environment, as seen in Figure 15–3.

This model provides a discrete separation between children and their linguistic micro-, meso-, exo-, and macrosystems; however, in reality the boundaries between each are very permeable, and children often move seamlessly among them. The model also suggests a list of systems and people that should be considered when intervening with children. Finally, this model involves several propositions describing the process of human development, with a tacit description of the process of language development that parallels human development:

. . . development takes place through processes of progressively more complex reciprocal interaction between an active . . . human . . . and the persons, objects, and symbols in its immediate . . . environment. To be effective, the interaction must occur on a fairly regular basis over extended periods of time . . . [as in] performing complex tasks, and acquiring new knowledge . . . (Bronfenbrenner & Morris, 2006, p. 797)

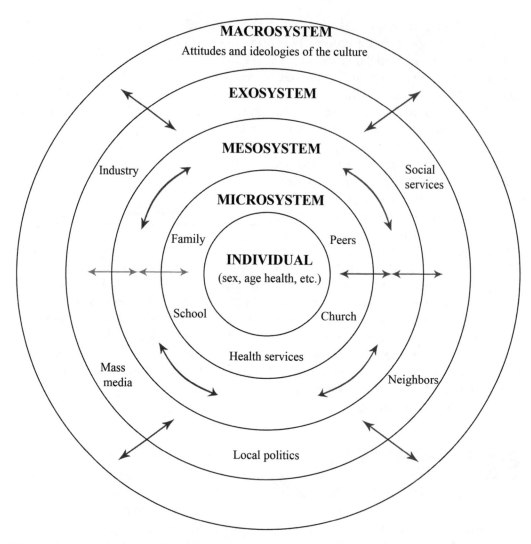

Figure 15–3. Bronfenbrenner's bioecological model. Courtesy of Bing Images, free to share and use commercially.

Of significance in this model is the relevance of approaching language intervention with a holistic perspective, involving multidirectional interactions among the child and his or her family, peers, the classroom, and the child's cultural and linguistic background (ASHA, n.d.-b.). For example, research has demonstrated that expressive language outcomes are very similar for clinician- and parent-delivered intervention (Law, Garrett, & Nye; 2004). Based on the underlying precepts of this model, language intervention with children is best implemented within naturalistic settings and contexts, and must be deeply connected to the demands and rigors of children's daily lives, regardless of the intervention setting (Dunst, Raab, & Trivette, 2012). Although this chapter is intended as a practice-based resource for language intervention with children, discussions of theoretical constructs have value in that,

> Theory underlies ... interventions, whether or not we acknowledge this openly, and the theory one adopts reflects what is believed to be important. One should be aware that approaches to intervention entail certain underlying theoretical assumptions, and theory and action should be consistent with each other. (Sutton, 2008, p. 60)

Considerations for *At-Risk* Children

Deeply related to Bronfenbrenner's bioecological model are multiple factors related to children's resilience and risk (Lyons & Roulstone, 2018). The term resilience is defined as the process of adapting positively when faced with adversity

or significant sources of stress (American Psychological Association, n.d.). Children defined as *at-risk* are those who are more likely then their peers to experience poor outcomes (Lyons & Roulstone, 2018). When looked at within an ecological model, resilience and the at-risk status can be impacted by children's internal capacity and by the capacity of their personal ecologies (Ungar, 2015). This suggests that protective factors, such as the ability to problem solve, and the presence of hope, agency, and positive relationships can mitigate negative effects (Lyons & Roulstone, 2018). However, there are also ecological factors that may contribute to poorer outcomes (Figure 15–4).

Statistics compiled by the National Center for Education Statistics (n.d.) and the United States Department of Education (n.d.) indicate that academic performance, retention and dropout rates, statewide assessment scores, and an eligibility

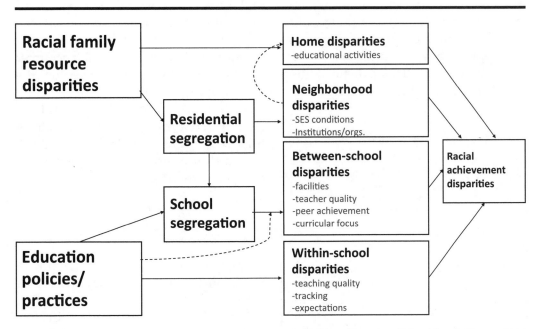

Figure 15–4. Factors contributing to poorer outcomes in children (Reardon, Kalogrides, & Shores, 2017 p. 46).

of LLDs or emotional disturbance (ED) as special education categories are related to poverty. Specific to language disorders, there are multiple factors that have been linked to greater likelihoods of LLDs, as described in Table 15–1 (Stanton-Chapman, Chapman, Bainbridge, & Scott, 2002).

In your role as an SLPA, you become part of the ecological system of the children with whom you work, and as such, you have an opportunity to support and mentor them, and provide a positive relationship as they make their way in the world.

Intervention Constructs

This next section discusses a valuable guideline in your intervention with children with LLDs: the distinction between performance and learning. As discussed by Kamhi (2014) and defined by Bjork (2004), *performance* should be viewed as the context-specific, short-term manifestation of a behavior, and *learning* can be viewed as an independent, long-term occurrence of a specified behavior. These two constructs parallel the distinct difference between what children can do in a

Table 15–1. List of Risk Factors Linked to LLDs

Individual–Level Risk Factors	Environmental Risk Factors
Male	Parental substance abuse
Very low birth weight	
Low 5-minute Apgar score	Poverty
	Lower maternal educational level
Lower maternal educational level	Child abuse or neglect
Earlier gestational age	Higher birth order

speech-language therapy session with a highly contrived context, and what they can do in naturalistic settings and in conversations involving spontaneous novel utterances. These constructs also parallel the difference between a set of narrow rules with predictable boundaries, and a broad-based set of rules that can be applied across unpredictable events (Kamhi, 2014). With respect to intervention with children with LLDs, this difference supports intervention in naturalistic settings with real-time demands. It also suggests that children benefit from repeated and varied opportunities and multiple contexts to acquire a new skill set (Yoder, Fey, & Warren, 2012).

SCHOOL-BASED ISSUES

There are multiple settings in which speech-language pathologists (SLPs), and SLPAs work: schools, private practice, and hospitals (ASHA, n.d.-e 2013, 2016, see Chapter 1 for a detailed description of the settings). Although SLPAs will encounter children with LLDs in each setting, the great majority of SLPs (53%) and SLPAs work in the K through 12 school-setting (ASHA, n.d.-c 2016), which mandates a brief overview of the major legislative acts that influence services in the schools for children with disabilities.

Legislation

Of primary importance to the work of SLPAs in the schools is the Individuals with Disabilities Education Act (IDEA) (P.L. 94-142), initially authorized in 1997 and reauthorized in 2004, which made a free and appropriate public education (FAPE) available to all children with disabilities determined to be eligible, and guaranteed protections for all students in (see Table 15–2 for a list of terms and their acronyms related to special education). Within the framework of FAPE is the explicit requirement that children with disabilities receive an education designed to meet their unique needs (IDEA, 2004). This legislation drives many of the service models observed in schools. A second legislative act, the No Child Left Behind (NCLB) (PL 107-110) (NCLB, 2001), was designed to support children with disabilities and those considered *at-risk* in their academic success. More recently, the Every Student Succeeds Act (ESSA) (P.L. 114-95) (2017) was enacted to further support critical protections and procedural safeguards for high-need and disadvantaged students. A final legislative act that relates to services in the schools is the Americans with Disabilities Act (ADA; 1990), prohibiting discrimination against individuals with disabilities and guaranteeing similar opportunities for these individuals to those of individuals with-

out disabilities in mainstream American life (ADA, n.d.).

While these legislative acts and terms can appear intimidating and confusing, in essence, they confirm that,

> Disability is a natural part of the human experience and in no way diminishes the right of individuals to participate in or contribute to society. Improving educational results for children with disabilities is an essential element of our national policy of ensuring equality of opportunity, full participation, independent living, and economic self-sufficiency for individuals with disabilities. (IDEA, n.d., para. 6)

Response to Intervention

As an SLPA in a school setting, it is likely you will be involved with the response to intervention (RtI) framework, also known as multi-tiered systems of support (MTSS). This framework supports instructional intensity across a continuum to support student learning (ASHA, n.d.-d.; Ehren, Lenz, & Deshler, 2014; Ehern & Nelson, 2005; Scott, Witt, Connell, & Koenig, 2005; Wixson, Lipson, & Valencia, 2014). Rather than being based on a *wait to fail* paradigm, RtI is grounded in the concept of *prevention* that is intended to address culturally and linguistically diverse inequities that have persisted in special education in the United States (Wixson, Lipson, & Valencia, 2014). According to ASHA (n.d.-d., para. 1), RtI and MTSS include the following (Figure 15–5):

- Universal screening
- High-quality instruction
- Intervention matched to student need

Table 15–2. List of Terms Related to Special Education Legislation

Abbreviation	Expanded Term
ADA	American with Disabilities Act
ESSA	Every Student Succeeds Act
FAPE	Free and Appropriate Public Education
IDEA	Individuals with Disabilities Education Act
IEP	Individualized Education Plan
NCLB	No Child Left Behind Act

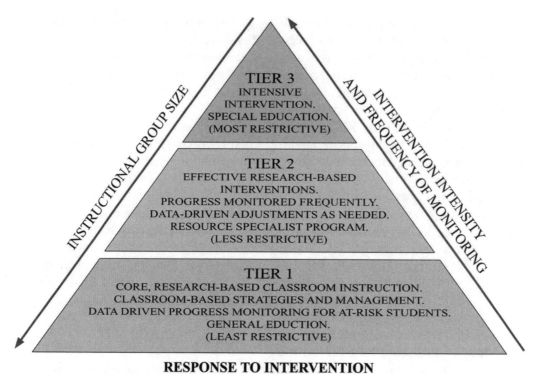

RESPONSE TO INTERVENTION
MULTI-TIERED SYSTEM OF SUPPORT

Figure 15–5. Model of response to intervention or multi-tiered system of support.

- Frequent progress monitoring
- Use of child response data to make educational decisions

Specific to your role as an SLPA you may be involved in the following tasks:

- Collaborating with general education teachers to support students identified as at-risk,
- Consulting with general education teachers to meet the needs of students identified as at-risk,
- Conducting small group instruction in the general education classroom for students (with and without an IEP) with similar needs. (Ehren, Lenz, &

Deshler, 2014; Wixson, Lipson, & Valencia, 2014).

Individualized Educational and 504 Plans

The information detailed in the preceding paragraphs leads to a discussion of Individual Education Plans (IEPs) and 504 Plans, which drive the services delivered in the schools. An IEP is a plan or program developed specifically for a child with a disability that ensures specialized instruction and services (DO IT, n.d.). These plans were designed to ensure appropriate accommodations supporting academic success and access to the learning environment for children with disabilities (DO IT, n.d.). A 504 Plan is based on Section 504 of the Rehabilitation Act of 1973, a federal civil rights law written to end discrimination against individuals with disabilities (Disability Rights Education & Defense Fund, n.d.). Children qualify for IEPs or 504s based on federal special education eligibility categories that are identified and specified through a comprehensive assessment, as detailed in Table 15–3.

Table 15–3. Federal Special Education Eligibility Categories

Disability	Definition
Autism (Aut)	A disability that significantly affects verbal and nonverbal communication and social interactions.
Deafness (DEAF)/ Hearing Impairment (HI)	Deafness: A severe hearing impairment that impairs a child's ability to process spoken linguistic information with or without amplification and that adversely affects educational performance. Hearing Impairment: A category that includes both individuals who are hard of hearing and those who are deaf.
Deaf-blindness (DB)	Concomitant hearing and visual impairments that cause complex communication needs that cannot be accommodated in special programs designed solely for children with deafness of children with blindness.
Emotional Disturbance (ED)	A condition exhibited over a long period of time that adversely affects educational performance. Examples of conditions include pervasive depression, anxiety, schizophrenia, or an inability to maintain relationships with peers or adults.
Established Medical Disability (EMD)	A disabling medical condition or congenital syndrome re special education services. This category applies only to children ages 3-5 years.
Intellectual Disability (ID)	Subaverage general cognitive abilities manifested in the developmental period that coexist with significant deficits in adaptive behavior affecting a child's educational performance.
Multiple Disabilities	A combination of concomitant impairments causing severe educational needs that cannot be accommodated in special education programs designed solely for one of the impairments.
Orthopedic Impairment (OI)	Severe orthopedic impairment that adversely affecting a child's educational performance.
Other Health Impairment (OHI)	Having limited strength, alertness, or vitality due to an acute or chronic health problem(s) that significantly affect a child's educational performance.
Specific Language Impairment (SLI)	Communication or language disorders that adversely affect a child's educational performance, such as stuttering or disorders of the speech-sound system, articulation, voice, or language.
Specific Learning Disability (SLD)	A disorder in one or more of the basic psychological processes related to understanding or using oral or written language that manifests in reduced abilities in listening, thinking, speaking, reading, writing, spelling, or performing math calculations.
Visual Impairments (VI)	Visual impairments that, even with correction, adversely affect a child's educational performance.

Source: Adapted from *California Department of Education (CDE): CALPADS primary disability category codes,* by CDE, n.d. Retrieved from https://www.cde.ca.gov/ta/tg/ca/disablecodes.asp

As an SLPA working with children with LLD, at least some of your work will involve the goals and services detailed in IEPs, examples of which can be found in Appendices 7-A and 7-D from Chapter 7. Although your supervising SLP is responsible for the development and implementation of the goals and services addressed in each child's IEP, it would be wise to familiarize yourself with the structure and language of IEP forms to ensure appropriate delivery of intervention. Even if you do not work in a school setting, it is likely that many of the children on your caseload will have an IEP that can be shared with your supervising SLP by the parents, and can be used to inform and guide your intervention decisions with those children. A final recommendation is to review the national database on Common Core State Standards CCSS (http://www.corestandards.org), or your state-specific site, which may provide a rich source to guide your intervention.

SETTING-SPECIFIC INTERVENTION

As was discussed in Chapter 1, in your role as an SLPA, you will be conducting your intervention in multiple settings, such as private clinic, schools, rehabilitation settings, and hospitals, and in each of these settings, there are multiple service delivery models, such as those listed below (ASHA, n.d.-c.; Cirrin et al., 2010):

- Direct Services:
  - Individual or group therapy session
    - Pull-out
    - Push-in
- Indirect Services:
  - Consult or collaborative
    - Push-in

In more recent years, inter-professional collaborative practice (IPP) has been validated as an evidence-based practice (ASHA, n.d.-f.; Cirrin et al., 2010) and its use has increased. This approach gives SLPAs opportunities to learn with, from, and about their colleagues to improve outcomes for the children with whom you work (ASHA, n.d.-c). As an SLPA in a school, this may involve co-teaching in the different settings (Table 15–4).

All professionals can experience the benefits of collaboration. For example, teachers (e.g., general, special, and resource) may become more competent in

Table 15–4. A Description of the Continuum of Settings in the Schools

Setting	Definition
General Education Classroom	The majority of the classrooms in a school. Most children in these classrooms receive generalized instruction across all curricular topics.
Resource Specialist Program Classroom (RSP)	A classroom supporting children who have been identified in an IEP and whose academic needs cannot be met solely in the general education classroom. Children receive sheltered learning on various subjects to support greater access to the curriculum, but spend the majority of their day in a general education classroom.
Special Day Class	A self-contained classroom providing specialized and intensive services to children identified in an IEP, and whose academic needs cannot be met in either the RSP setting or the general education classroom.

Source: Understanding Special Education, n.d.

providing appropriate language supports, while SLPAs may become more competent in linking their intervention to relevant classroom content (Cirrin & Gillam, 2008; Davies, Shanks, & Davies, 2004). In clinical, hospital, or private practice settings, you may collaborate with audiologists, physical therapists, occupational therapists, nurses, and social workers (Johnson, 2016). This service delivery of IPP includes: (a) parallel, supplemental, primary, and co-teaching; (b) consulting with team members; (c) modeling targeted skills; and (d) greater inclusion of the child's peers to the benefit of all. When collaborating with colleagues SLPAs can model interactive teaching styles and support their colleague(s) by introducing listening, speaking, reading, and writing activities into instructional tasks, while ensuring that the tasks are structured to support children with LLDs (ASHA, 2013; Farber & Klein, 1999). In light of this recommendation, two concepts must remain in the forefront of all decisions: (1) children are all individuals with unique needs and (2) targeting different skills requires unique contexts (Cirrin et al., 2010).

LANGUAGE INTERVENTION

Language intervention with children mandates broad considerations because of the wide age range and the heterogeneity of language disorders. As far as the field of speech-language pathology has come in the past fifty years, there are still no published guidelines or hard and fast rules governing intervention for children with language disorders (Cirrin & Gillam, 2008). Fortunately, there are evidence-based practices that have been shown to be effective at the micro and macro levels (Cirrin et al., 2010). However, just as important as identifying what language intervention with children is, it is important to identify what it is not. This chapter does not detail disorder-specific language intervention (e.g., ASD, TBI, ID), but provides broad guidelines for intervention with children. Regardless, it would not be unexpected that many of the intervention concepts presented here would be appropriate for children with LLDs and comorbidities.

Broad Intervention Concepts

This section of the chapter describes and discusses evidence-based intervention practices you can implement in your work with children, presented in a hierarchy that moves from broad to specific.

Language intervention with children encompasses form, content, and use, because language disorders exert influence over characteristics of phonology, morphology, syntax, semantics, and pragmatics (Paul & Norbury, 2012). This influence can result in deficits observed in (a) phonological memory, awareness, and production at the word and sentence levels (Pennington & Bishop, 2009); (b) use of morphological markers (Eisenberg, 2007; Moyle, Karasinski, Weismer, & Gorman, 2011); (c) comprehension of embedded and relative clauses, passive voice, and negation (Eisenberg, 2007; Paul, 2000); and (d) production of varied and complex vocabulary (Catts et al., 1999). From a broad perspective, effective language intervention can be framed through the inclusion of critical elements that can be implemented regardless of age, disorder (e.g., SLI, TBI, ASD), or language domain (i.e., form, content, use) (Ukrainetz, 2006).

Just as a rudder serves to guide a sailboat through the unfamiliar waters, familiarity with guiding intervention principles supports more effective intervention with the children on your caseload (Figure 15–6).

Although there are many guiding principles out there, the following broad principles provide a solid framework, as described by Paul and Norbury (2012):

1. Use of curricular-based instruction.
   Although you may not be in a school setting, considering the academic demands placed on children supports their success across all other contexts of their daily lives (Nelson, 2010; Wallach, 2010). This requires familiarity with the demands of academic language and the CCSSs (Appendix 15–A.) Whether the overarching goal is vocabulary acquisition or use of cohesive language, the CCSSs allow you to gain a better understanding of the demands. The CCSSs can be found here: http://www.corestandards.org

2. Integration of oral and written language.
   Because oral and written language exist on a continuum, they cannot be truly separated in intervention (Wallach, 2008, 2014). Just as children look different across the age span, so too does intervention integrating oral and written language. Integration of the two language modalities can be accomplished by providing varied activities that cross from oral language tasks (talking about the meaning of a word) to incorporating target words in a short story or poem that you and the children write together.

3. Focus on metacognitive, metalinguistic, and metapragmatic activities.
   Talking and thinking about language are *metaskills* (Wallach, Charlton, & Christie, 2009). The word *meta* is an ancient Greek term that means *beyond*.

Figure 15–6. Sailboat in the ocean. Courtesy of Bing Images, free to use and share commercially.

In the world of language, *meta* means going beyond the use of language as a function of communication and to focus on underlying structures (Wallach, Charlton, & Christie, 2009). By modeling and practicing specific language structures and then taking those structures outside of the production, the focus can shift to the explicit rules of language (Wallach, 2010). Defining a sentence form and how it differs from another is an example of a metatask. Stating the unspoken rules about what one cannot say is another.

4. For SLPAs in schools, collaborative participation in response to intervention (RTI).

RTI uses tiered instruction to support children with learning needs (Ardoin, Witt, Connell, & Koenig, 2005). For example, you can co-teach with the RSP or general education teacher in their setting to attenuate or prevent failure of children at-risk for LLDs.

With these four principles in mind, intervention can be further guided by the following list of skill formats (Table 15–5; Ukrainetz, 2006).

Scaffolding is an instructional strategy that supports children's independent use of language-processing skills and strategies (Nelson, 2005). It is related to the socially-mediated learning process identified by Vygotsky and the zone of proximal development (ZPD), which is "the distance between the level of performance a child can achieve independently and the higher level that same child can achieve with effective social mediation" (Nelson, 2005, p. 328). Scaffolding techniques are as follows (Scott & Balthazar, 2015):

- Manipulating the length of the stimuli (clauses, sentences)
- Ensuring familiarity with the content (grade level, curriculum, vocabulary)
- Modulating the difficulty of the stimuli (abstractness, information density)
- Including visual supports (written modality, key words)
- Paying close attention to the amount and quality of linguistic facilitations (modeling, expansions, extensions)

The process of intervention can be further framed through these three approaches (Paul & Norbury, 2012):

Table 15–5. Intervention Skill Formats

Skill	Task Structure
Hierarchical Skill Intervention	Target skills one at a time within a hierarchy, moving from simple, contrived tasks in the therapy setting to naturalistic activities with minimal to no prompting or correcting.
Skill Stimulation	Practice skills using simple tasks with minimal to no prompting or correcting.
Enrichment and Task Assistance	Target skills in naturalistic life activities with prompts and corrections as needed.
Contextualized Skill Intervention	Target several skills at a time within a mix of naturalistic and contrived contexts, with prompting and correction as needed.

1. Clinician-Directed:
   The clinician identifies a skill to be targeted, selects the materials or manipulatives to use, and determines the success or failure of an outcome. The use of drills is common in this context.

2. Child-Centered:
   The clinician provides appropriate scaffolding to support the child's ZPD in a particular skill. In this model, the child has a voice in the selection of targets, in selecting manipulatives and materials, and in the determination of outcome. The use of play or conversational interaction is common in this context.

3. Hybrid:
   The clinician shifts between the two previous structures according to the situation, the child's performance, and the task demands.

A final set of principles relates to grammatical intervention for children with SLI. However, these principles are evidence-based and sufficiently broad so as to support increases in the overall behavioral, communicative, academic, and social performance of children across contexts, age, and population (Fey, Long, & Finestack, 2003):

1. The primary focus of grammatical intervention should be to support children's increased mastery over comprehension and use of morphology and syntax, in the naturalistic context of the oral and written modalities of conversation, narratives, exposition, and additional text-based genres. However, research has demonstrated that discrete, explicit instruction can be an appropriate method in specific situations.

2. Based on our understanding that grammatical deficits rarely exist independent of deficits in the other domains of language, grammatical intervention should never be addressed in isolation.

3. Intermediate level goals that support language acquisition and development, rather than specific language forms, are more effective because of the possibilities of triggering shifts in a grammatical system (Bates, Thal, & MacWhinney, 1991).

4. Children must exhibit a readiness for a specific targeted form, as demonstrated by an emergence of this form in specific contexts, regardless of whether the emerging form is produced with errors.

5. Manipulating intervention contexts (e.g., social, physical, linguistic) increases the number of opportunities to address specific grammatical targets. An example is when a clinician becomes less cooperative in a conversation, which creates an expectation for children to "fill in the spaces."

6. Appropriate contexts for intervention can be developed by capitalizing on different genres of text and incorporating a written modality. For example, narratives often use more past tense, informational discourse uses more present tense, and higher level grammatical forms (e.g., passives, adverbial clauses) are seen more often in written texts.

7. Manipulating the target within discourse to draw attention to specific forms. For example, change loudness, pitch, and word length for increased salience.

8. Sentence recasts are an effective method of systematically contrasting the less mature form produced by

children with the more mature forms produced by adults.

9. Modeling well-formed sentences to support comprehension of both function and content words.

10. Eliciting imitation of targeted forms allows children to practice with forms that are difficult to produce. It also encourages children to use words in the natural contexts of phrases or sentences, and develops a better understanding of the relationships between forms.

Specific Language Intervention Models

The R.I.S.E.+ Model

The first specific intervention framework discussed is based on repeated opportunities for practice and learning with a focus on appropriate levels of *Repeated opportunities, Intensive schedule, Systematic support, and Explicit skill focus* (Ukrainetz, 2015). This model, called R.I.S.E+, is described in Table 15–6.

Repeated opportunities are necessary to gain mastery over a concept, although the actual number of opportunities is highly individualized. Intensity refers to the number of interactions between the child and the intervention, or the more holistic concept of session length and frequency. Systematic support refers to efforts of the SLPA to support success of the child in the session and includes: (a) modifying the environment, (b) being aware of pause time when waiting for a response, and (c) providing scaffolding within an appropriate hierarchy. Explicit skill focus refers to the instruction provided by the SLPA and can involve: (a) drill-based work, (b) strategic highlighting, and (c) a clear focus on a specified skill (Ukraintez, 2015).

In addition to the concepts described above, effective intervention should include prompting, modeling, guidance, and explanation (Ukrainetz, 2015). The modeling can be presented in the form of developmentally appropriate recasts and expansions, where the clinician either simply restates what the child says or

Table 15–6. Continuum of R.I.S.E.+ for Intervention and Instruction

Feature	Intervention Contexts
Repeated Opportunities	Few—some—many
Intensity of Scheduling	Clinic or Classroom—Group or Individual
	Occasional—Regular—Frequent
	Short—Medium—Long
Systematic Support	Little—Some—Significant
Explicit Skill	Implicit—Explicit—Metalinguistic or Metacognitive
+ The Learner Factor	Passive attention or minimal engagement—Motivated attentive engagement—Motivated, self-directed, and sustained engagement

Source: Ukrainetz, 2015, p. 58.

expands on it, as seen in the exchanges below:

Recast

Child: We *goed* to the store after school and *finded* the kind of cake she likes.

SLPA: Oh, you *went* to the store and *found* that cake? Your mother must have been happy.

Expansion

Child: Got the special cake.

SLPA: Oh, you finally got the cake your mother likes?

Recent research by Venker et al. (2015) found that the use of telegraphic speech, which omits function words and grammatical morphemes, might have a negative impact on the development and refinement of syntax. As such, restating utterances with the correct morphosyntactic form reflects best practices (Kamhi, 2014) as seen in the exchange below:

Child: Basketball school friend.

SLPA: Oh, you played basketball with a friend? That must have been fun!

The final but important factor in the R. I. S. E.+ model is the learner factor. One of the greatest challenges in intervention is developing and maintaining the engagement, motivation, and buy-in of the child. This engagement is supported by evidence (ASHA, Evidence-Based Practice, n.d.-a) and can be mediated by the following: (a) using relevant activities, (b) creating authentic interactions between the SLPA and the child, (c) allow-ing the child to make choices throughout the session, and (d) providing clear task expectations (Ukrainetz, 2015).

Literature-Based Units

Literature-based units is a contextualized language intervention based on books, reading, and discussion (Gillam & Ukrainetz, 2006). A description of the intervention follows.

Intervention Components:

1. Functional activities:
   The individual needs of children are addressed through an oral context.
2. Thematic unity:
   Activities are linked thematically, progressing from an initial reading of a story to a final parallel story generation. Thematic intervention provides structure, builds coherence, supports extended learning, and varies activities.
3. Whole-part-whole:
   The intervention begins with a piece of literature and ends with generating a parallel story. Activities are selected to target specific goals and objectives.

Many methods can facilitate language when working with literature-based units. Table 15–7 lists a series of facilitation devices that can be embedded in your intervention with storybooks.

Some final recommendations for your intervention with children who have LLDs follow (Ukrainetz, 2015):

- Relate the known to the unknown.
- Modify the complexity of the task and content.
- Make connections between ideas, content, and task.

Table 15-7. Facilitation Methods

Linguistic Facilitation	
Syntactic Expansion:	Child: Her lived in the Netherlands.
The production of a syntactically correct form that parallels the student's production.	Clinician: Yes, she lived in the Netherlands.
Semantic Expansion:	Child: Her lived in the Netherlands.
The production of a parallel form of the student's production with additional information.	Clinician: Yes, she lived in the Netherlands during World War II.
Recast:	Child: Her lived in the Netherlands.
The production of a parallel form with an altered syntactic structure.	Clinician: Right, Anne Frank lived in the Netherlands.
Prompt:	Child: Her lived in the Netherlands.
A question or comment that elicits a correction in a previous syntactically incorrect sentence.	Clinician: Who did she live with?
	Child: She lived in the Netherlands with her family.
Elaboration:	Child: Her lived in the Netherlands.
A question that elicits an expansion of a previous response.	Clinician: Whom did she have in her family?
	Child: She lived in the Netherlands with her parents and her sister.
Vertical Structure:	Child: Her lived in the Netherlands.
A question that elicits additional information. The clinician incorporates the new response with the question to form a more complex structure.	Clinician: Why did she stay in the Netherlands?
	Child: Because they couldn't leave.
	Clinician: She stayed in the Netherlands because she couldn't leave? How terrible!
Response Facilitations	
Model:	Clinician: Anne Frank was hidden by Miep Gies and her family.
A model of a targeted form or word.	
Question:	Clinician: What happened to Anne Frank when the Nazi's came to the Netherlands?
A question used to elicit a targeted structure.	
Prompt:	Clinician: Anne Frank was . . .
The use of pause, repetition of the child's utterance, or a statement to elicit the targeted structure.	
Regulatory Facilitations	
State the Goal/Target:	Clinician: We are going to work on pronouns and passive verbs and we are going to use those to talk about "The Diary of Anne Frank."
Explicit statement of what the child will be working on.	
Compare or Contrast:	Clinician: Anne Frank lived with her family and Miep Gies lived with her family too.
Highlighting differences or similarities between words or forms.	
Informative Feedback:	Child: Anne Frank hid Miep Gies and her family.
Explicit feedback on accuracy.	Clinician: No, Anne Frank was hidden by Miep Gies and her family. Those two sentences have two very different meanings.

Source: Gillam & Ukrainetz, 2006.

- Call attention to specific aspects of the text.
- Incorporate graphic organizers in the tasks.
- Model the process.

Instructional Discourse

Instructional discourse is an intervention process based on strategic conversations between children and clinicians (Culatta, Blank, & Black, 2010). Instructional discourse is highly valuable because it can be used with both written and oral texts and across levels. The primary goals of this intervention are to support access and strengthen comprehension of a specific text by modifying the demands. Strategies that can be used include: (a) engaging in exploratory discussion; (b) establishing an emotional link between children and the text; (c) acknowledging and elaborating on comments, questions, and contributions of the children; (d) encouraging all participants to engage; and (e) providing scaffolding and multiple response options.

Additional supports to consider are graphic organizers, also called thinking maps and concept diagrams. These are visual displays demonstrating relationships among concepts, terms, and facts that help children make sense of information (Kim, Vaugn, Wanzek, & Wei, 2004). Figure 15–7 shows examples of thinking maps.

In information discourse intervention, graphic organizers can help identify cohesive structures, intertopic relationships, and support overall organization. Informational discourse requires an emphasis on vocabulary. Supporting children in the development of a mental schema about words increases comprehension and allows them to apply their new word knowledge in future contexts (DeKemel, 2003). Linking words to synonyms and antonyms, giving examples, and creating semantic maps (Beck, McKeown, & Kucan, 2002), are some methods used to target vocabulary (Figure 15–8).

Instructional strategies to support connections between ideas and content might relate (a) the familiar to the unfamiliar, (b) past experiences to the current text, (c) previously read text to the current text, (d) the concrete to the abstract, (e) the remote to the immediate, and (f) the implicit to the explicit (Culatta et al., 2010).

CONCLUSION

This chapter ends with recommendations for how best to implement the many theoretical constructs, principles, and intervention practices it described. The first is to remain informed and current on evidence-based practices; this is the best way to instill confidence in the children and families. The second is to be mindful of the worlds the children come from, the challenges they face daily because of their LLDs, and the importance of holistic approaches to intervention. A third recommendation is to build and maintain authentic, caring relationships with these children and their families—it is truly worth the effort. A final recommendation is to recognize that as much theoretical knowledge and practical experience you may have or may gain in your role as an SLPA, it is likely that you have not had the lived experience of LLDs. This lived experience gives the children and their families a level of expertise and validity that should solidify their relevance in the intervention process. And finally, I charge you to go forth and do good work,

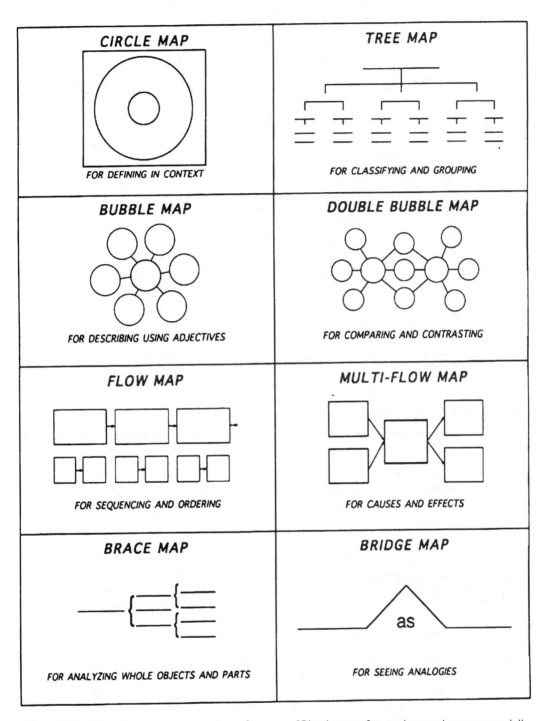

Figure 15–7. Examples of graphic organizers. Courtesy of Bing Images, free to share and use commercially.

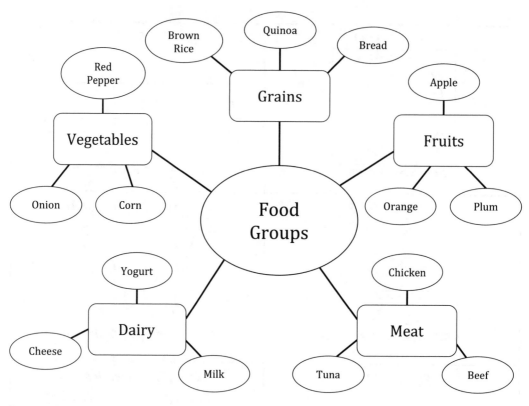

Figure 15–8. Example of graphic organizer or semantic map.

because what we do matters deeply to all the children we work with, not just those who are superheroes.

REFERENCES

American Psychological Association. (n.d.). *The road to resilience.* Retrieved from http://www.apa.org/helpcenter/road-resilience.aspx

American Speech-Language-Hearing Association (ASHA). (n.d.-a). *Evidence-based practice.* Retrieved from https://www.asha.org/Research/EBP/Evidence-Based-Practice/

American Speech-Language-Hearing Association (ASHA). (n.d.-b). *Cultural competence* (Practice portal). Retrieved from https://www.asha.org/Practice-Portal/Professional-Issues/Cultural-Competence/

American Speech-Language-Hearing Association (ASHA). (n.d.-c). *Collaboration and teaming.* Retrieved from https://www.asha.org/Practice-Portal/Clinical-Topics/Intellectual-Disability/Collaboration-and-Teaming/

American Speech-Language-Hearing Association (ASHA). (n.d.-d). *Response to intervention.* Retrieved from https://www.asha.org/slp/schools/prof-consult/RtoI/

American Speech-Language-Hearing Association (ASHA). (n.d.-e). *Employment settings for SLPs.* Retrieved from https://www.asha.org/Students/Employment-Settings-for-SLPs/

American Speech-Language-Hearing Association (ASHA). (n.d.-f). *Interprofessional education/interprofessional practice (IPE/IPP).* Retrieved from https://www.asha.org/practice/interprofessional-education-practice/

American Speech-Language-Hearing Association (ASHA). (2001). *Roles and responsibilities of speech-language pathologists with respect to reading and writing in children and adolescents* [Position statement]. Retrieved from http://www.asha.org/policy

American Speech-Language-Hearing Association (ASHA). (2013). *Speech-language pathology assistant scope of practice* [Scope of practice]. Retrieved from http://www.asha.org/policy

American Speech-Language-Hearing Association (ASHA). (2016). *Schools survey report: SLP caseload characteristics trends 1995–2016.* Retrieved from https://www.asha.org/uploaded Files/2016-Schools-Survey-SLP-Caseload-Characteristics-Trends.pdf

Americans with Disabilities Act (ADA). (n.d.). *Information and technical assistance on the American with disabilities act.* Retrieved from https://www.ada.gov/ada_intro.htm

Apel, K., & Masterson, J. J. (2001). Theory-guided spelling assessment and intervention: A case study. *Language, Speech, and Hearing Services in Schools, 32,* 182–195. doi:10.1044/0161-1461(2001/017)

Ardoin, S. P., Witt, J. C., & Connell, J. E., & Koenig, J. L. (2005). Application of a three-tiered response to intervention model for instructional planning, decision making, and the identification of children in need. *Journal of Psychoeducational Assessment, 4,* 362–380. doi:10.1177/073428290502300405

Bashir, A. S. (1989). Language intervention and the curriculum. *Seminars in Speech and Language, 10*(3), 181–191.

Bates, E., Thal, D., & MacWhinney, B. (1991). A functionalist approach to language and its implications for assessment and intervention. In T. M. Gallagher (Ed.), *Pragmatics of language: Clinical practice issues* (pp. 133–161). San Diego, CA: Singular. doi:10.1007/978-1-4899-7156-2_5

Beck, I. L., McKeown, M. G., & Kucan, L. (2002). *Bringing words to life*: Robust vocabulary instruction. New York, NY: Guilford Press.

Bjork, E. (2004). *Research on learning as a foundation for curricular reform and pedagogy.* Paper presented at the Reinvention Center Conference, Washington, DC. Retrieved from http://reinventioncenter.miami.edu/Conference/2004Conference/2004ConferenceDetails.html#ElizabethBjork

Bloom, L., & Lahey, M. (1978). *Language development and language disorders.* New York, NY: Wiley. doi:10.7916/D8QZ2GQ5

Brimo, D., Apel, K., & Fountain, T. (2017). Examining the contributions of syntactic awareness and syntactic knowledge to reading comprehension. *Journal of Research in Reading, 1,* 57–74. doi:10.1111/1467-9817.12050

Bronfenbrenner, U., & Morris, P. A. (2006). The biological model of human development. In R. M. Lerner (Ed.), *Handbook of child psychology* (6th ed., Vol. 1, pp. 792–828; Editors-in-chief: W. Damon & R. M. Lerner). Hoboken, NJ: Wiley.

Brown, R. (1973). *A first language: The early stages.* London, UK: George Allen & Unwin.

California Department of Education. (n.d.). *CALPADS primary disability category codes.* Retrieved from https://www.cde.ca.gov/ta/tg/ca/disablecodes.asp

Catts, H. W., Fey, M. E., Tomblin, J. B., & Zhang, X. (2002). A longitudinal investigation of reading outcomes in children wit language impairments. *Journal of Speech, Language, and Hearing Research, 45*(6), 1142–1157.

Cirrin, F. M., & Gillam, R. B. (2008). Language intervention practices for school-age children with spoken language disorders: A systematic review. *Language, Speech, and Hearing in the Schools, 37,* S110–S137.

Cirrin, F. M., Schooling, T. L., Nelson, N. W., Diehl, S. F., Flynn, P. F., Staskowski, M., . . . Adamczyk, D. F. (2010). Evidence-based systematic review: Effects of different service models on communication outcomes for elementary school-age children. *Language, Speech, and Hearing in Schools, 41,* 233–264. doi:10.1044/0161-1461(2009/08-0128)

Cohen, N. J. (2010). The impact of language development on the psychosocial and emotional development of young children. *Language Development and Literacy* [PDF document]. Retrieved from http://www.child-encyclopedia.com/sites/default/files/textes-experts/en/622/the-impact-of-language-development-on-the-psychosocial-and-emotional-development-of-young-children.pdf

Common Core State Standards. (n.d.). *Common core state standards initiative: Preparing America's students for college and career.* Retrieved from http://www.corestandards.org

Culatta, B., Blank, M., & Black, S. (2010). Talking things through: Roles of instructional processing of expository texts. *Topics in Language Disorders*, 308–322.

Davies, P. Shanks, B., & Davies, K. (2004). Improving narrative skills in young children with delayed language development. *Educational Review, 53*(3), 271–286. doi:10.1080/0013191042000201181

DeKemel, K. (2003). *Intervention in language arts: A practical guide for speech-language pathologists.* St Louis, MO: Mosby/Elsevier.

Disabilities, Opportunities, Internetworking, and Technology [DO IT]. (n.d.) *What is the difference between and IEP and a 504 Plan?* Retrieved from https://www.washington.edu/doit/what-difference-between-iep-and-504-plan

Disability Rights Education & Defense Fund (DREDF). (n.d.). *Doing disability justice: Section 405 of the Rehabilitation Act of 1973.* Retrieved from https://dredf.org/legal-advocacy/laws/section-504-of-the-rehabilitation-act-of-1973/

Dunst, C. J., Raab, M., & Trivette, C. M. (2012). Characteristics of naturalistic language intervention strategies. *Journal of Speech-Language Pathology and Applied Behavior Analysis, 53*(4), 8–16.

Ehren, B. J., Lenz, B. K. B. H., & Deshler, D. (2014). Adolescents who struggle with 21st Century literacy. In C. A. Stone, E. R. Silliman, B. J. Ehren, & G. W. Wallach (Eds.), *Handbook of language and literacy: Development and disorders* (pp. 619–636). London, UK: Guilford Press.

Ehren, B. J., & Nelson, N. W. (2005). The responsiveness to intervention approach and language impairment. *Topics in Language Disorders, 25*(2), 120–131.

Eisenberg, S. (2007). How can I say that better? In T. Ukrainetz (Ed.), *Contextualized language intervention: Scaffolding preK-12 literacy achievement* (pp. 7–58). Austin, TX: Pro-Ed.

Every Student Succeeds Act (ESSQA). (2015). (2017). In *Current Events in Context.* Retrieved from http://www.abc-clio.com/current/

Farber, J. G., & Klein, E. R. (1999). Classroom-based assessment of a collaborative intervention with kindergarten and first-grade students. *Language, Speech, and Hearing Services in the Schools, 30,* 83.91. doi:10.1044/0161-1461.3001.83

Fey, M. E., Catts, H. W., Proctor-Williams, K., Tomblin, J. B., & Zhang, X. (2004). Oral and written story composition skills of children with language impairment. *Journal of Speech, Language, and Hearing Research, 47,* 1301–1318. doi:10.1044/1092-4388(2004/098)

Fey, M. E., Long, S. H., & Finestack, L. H. (2003). Ten principles of grammar facilitation for children with specific language impairments. *American Journal of Speech-Language Pathology, 12,* 3–15. doi:10.1044/1058-0360(2003/048)

Gillam, R., McFadden, T. U., & van Kleeck, A. (1995). Improving narrative abilities: Whole language and language skills approaches. In M. E. Fey, J. Windsor, & S. F. Warren (Eds.), *Language intervention: Preschool through the elementary years* (pp. 145–182). Baltimore, MD: Paul H. Brookes.

Gillam, R. B., & Ukrainetz, T. A. (2006). Language intervention through literature-based units. In T. Ukrainetz (Ed.), *Contextualized language intervention* (pp. 7–58). Eau Claire, WI: Thinking Publications.

Individuals with Disability Education Act (IDEA). (n.d.). *About IDEA.* Retrieved from https://sites.ed.gov/idea/about-idea/

Johnson, A. (2016). *Interprofessional education and interprofessional practice in communication sciences and disorders* [PDF document]. Retrieved from http://www.asha.org/uploadedFiles/IPE-IPP-Reader-eBook.pdf

Kamhi, A. G. (2014). Improving clinical practices for children with language and learning disorders. *Language, Speech, and Hearing Services in the Schools, 45,* 92–103. doi:10.1044/2014_LSHSS-13-0063

Kim, A. H., Vaughn, S., Wanzek, J., & Wei, S. (2004). Graphic organizers and their effects on the reading comprehension of students with LD: A synthesis of research. *Journal of Learning Disabilities, 37,* 105–118. doi:10.1177/00222194040370020201

Law, J., Garrett, X., & Nye, C. (2004). The efficacy of treatment with developmental speech and language delay/disorder: A meta-analysis. *Journal of Speech, Language, and Hearing Research, 44*(4), 924–943.

Lyons, R., & Roulstone, S. (2018). Well-being and resilience in children with speech and language disorders. *Journal of Speech, Language, and Hearing Research, 61,* 324–344. doi:10.1044/2017_JSLHR-L-16-0391

Moyle, M. J., Karasinksi, C., Weismer, S. E., & Gorman, b. K. (2011). Grammatical morphology in school-age children with and without language impairment: A discriminant function analysis. *Language, Speech, and Hearing in Schools, 42,* 550–560. doi:10.1044/0161-1461 (2011/10-0029)

National Center for Education Statistics. (n.d.). *Trends in high school drop out and completion rates in the United States.* Retrieved from https://nces.ed.gov/programs/dropout/

Nelson, N. W. (2005). The context of discourse difficulty in classroom and clinic: An update. *Topics in Language Disorders, 25*(4), 322–331.

Nelson, N. W. (2010). *Language and literacy disorders: Infancy through adolescence.* San Antonio, TX: Pearson Education.

Nelson, N. W., Van Meter, A. M., Chamberlain, D., & Bahr, C. M. (2001). The speech-language pathologist's role in a writing lab approach. *Seminars in Speech and Language, 22,* 209–219. doi:10.1055/s-2001-16148

Nippold, M. A., Mansfield, T. C., Billow, J. L., & Tomblin, J. B. (2009). Syntactic development in adolescents with a history of language impairments: A follow-up investigation. *American Journal of Speech-Language Pathology, 18,* 241–251. doi:10.1044/1058-0360(2008/08-0022)

No Child Left Behind Act. (n.d.). NCLB. Retrieved from https://www2.ed.gov/policy/elsec/leg/esea02/index.html

Paul, R. (2000). Understanding the "whole" of it: Comprehension assessment. *Seminars in Speech and Language, 21*(3), 10–17.

Paul, R., & Norbury, C. F. (2012). *Language disorders from infancy through adolescence: Listening, speaking, reading, writing, and communicating.* St. Louis, MO: Elsevier Mosby.

Pennington, B., & Bishop, D. (2009). Relations among speech, language, and reading disorders. *Annual Review of Psychology, 60,* 283–306. doi: 10.1146/annurev.psych.60.110707.163548.

Pinker, S. (1996). *Language learnability and language development.* Cambridge, MA: Harvard University Press.

Puranik, C. S., Lombardino, L. J., & Altmann, J. P. (2008). Assessing the microstructure of written language using a retelling paradigm. *American Journal of Speech-Language Pathology, 17,* 107–120. doi:10.1044/1058-0360(2008/012)

Reardon, S.F., Kalogrides, D., & Shores, K. (2017). *The Geography of Racial/Ethnic Test Score Gaps* (CEPA Working Paper No.16–10). Retrieved from Stanford Center for Education Policy Analysis: http://cepa.stanford.edu/wp16-10

Roth, F. P., Paul, D. R., & Pierotti, A. (2006). *Let's talk: For people with special communication needs.* Retrieved from https://www.asha.org/public/speech/emergent-literacy.htm

Saussure, F. D. (1983). *Course in general linguistics.* Illinoi: Open Court Classics.

Scott, C. Bathazar, C. M. (2015). The role of complex sentence knowledge in children with reading and writing difficulties. *Perspectives on Language and Literacy, 39*(3), 18–30.

Scott, P. A., Witt, J. C., Connell, J. E., & Koenig, J, L. (2005). Application of a three-tiered response to intervention model for instructional planning, decision making, and the identification of children in need. *Journal of Psychoeducational Assessment, 23*(4), 362–380. doi:10.1177/073428290502300405

Stanton-Chapman, T. L., Chapman, D. A., Bainbridge, N. L., & Scott, K. G. (2002). Identification of early risk factors for language impairment. *Research in Developmental Disabilities, 23,* 390–405.

Sun, L., & Nippold, M. A. (2012). Narrative writing in children and adolescents: Examining the literate lexicon. *Language, Speech, and Hearing in Schools, 43,* 2–13. doi:10.1044/0161-1461(2011/10-0099)

Sun, L., & Wallach, G. P. (2014). Language disorders are learning disabilities: Challenges on the divergent and diverse paths to language learning disability. *Topics in Language Disorders, 34*(1), 25–38. doi:10.1097/TLD.0000000000000005

Sutton, A. (2008). Language acquisition theory and AAC intervention. *Perspectives on Augmentative and Alternative Communication, 17*(2), 56–61. doi:10.1044/aac17.2.56

Ukrainetz, T. A. (2006). *Contextualized language intervention.* Eau Claire, WI: Thinking Publications.

Ukraintez, T. A. (2015). Assessment and intervention within a contextualized skill framework. In T. Ukrainetz (Ed.). *School-age language intervention: Evidence-based practices.* Austin, TX: Pro-Ed.

Understanding Special Education. (n.d.). *Special education terms and definitions.* Retrieved from http://www.understandingspecialeducation.com/special-education-terms.html

Ungar, M. (2015). Practitioner review: Diagnosing childhood resilience—A systemic approach to the diagnosis of adaptation in adverse social and physical ecologies. *The Journal of Child*

Psychology and Psychiatry, 56(1), 4–17. doi:10.11 11/jcpp.12306

United States Department of Education. (n.d.). *Education for homeless children and youths (EHCY) program.* Retrieved from https://nche .ed.gov/downloads/ehcy_profile.pdf

Venker, C. E., Bolt, D. M., Meyer, A., Sindberg, H., Weismer, S. E., & Tager-Flusberg, H. (2015). Parent telegraphic speech use and spoken in preschoolers with ASD. *Journal of Speech, Language, and Hearing Research, 58*(6), 1733–1746. doi:10.1044/2015_JSLHR-L-14-0291

Wallach, G. P. (2008). *Language intervention for school-age students: Setting goals for academic success.* St Louis, MO: Mosby/Elsevier.

Wallach, G. P. (2010). It was a dark and stormy night: Pulling language-based learning disabilities out of the drifting snow. *Topics in Language Disorders, 30,* 6–14.

Wallach, G. P. (2014). Improving clinical practice: A school-age and school-based perspective. *Language, Speech, and Hearing Services in the Schools, 45,* 127–136. doi:10.1044/2014_LSHSS-14-0016.

Wallach, G. P., & Butler, K. G. (1994). *Language learning disabilities in school-age children and adolescents: Some principles and applications.* London, UK: Pearson Education.

Wallach, G. P., Charlton, S., & Christie, J. (2009). Making a broader case for the narrow: Where to begin. *Language, Speech, and Hearing Services in Schools, 40,* 201–211. doi:10.1044/0161-1461(2009/08-0043)

Wallach, G. P., Charlton, S., & Christie, J. (2014). The spoken-written comprehension connection. In C. A. Stone, E, R. Silliman, B. J. Ehren, & G. P. Wallach (Eds.). *Handbook of language & literacy: Development and disorders* (pp. 485–501). New York, NY: Guilford Press.

Wixson, K. K., Lipson, M. Y., & Valencia, S. W. (2014). Response to intervention for teaching and learning in language and literacy. In C. A. Stone, E. R. Silliman, B. J. Ehren, & G. P. Wallach (Eds.), *Handbook of language & literacy: Development and disorders* (pp. 637–653). New York, NY: Guilford Press.

Yoder, P., Fey, M., & Warren, S. (2012). Studying the impact of intensity is important but complicated. *International Journal of Speech-Language Pathology, 14,* 410–413. doi:10.3109/17549507.2012.685890

APPENDIX 15–A
Examples of Common Core State Standards

Strand	Grade	Standard	Description
Speaking and Listening	3	Comprehension and Collaboration English Language Arts:	Engage effectively in a range of collaborative discussions (one-on-one, in groups, and teacher-led) with diverse partners on *grade 3 topics and texts*, building on others' ideas and expressing their own clearly.
	6	Presentation of Knowledge and Ideas English Language Arts:	Present claims and findings, sequencing ideas logically and using pertinent descriptions, facts, and details to accentuate main ideas or themes; use appropriate eye contact, adequate volume, and clear pronunciation.
	9–10	Comprehension and Collaboration English Language Arts:	Initiate and participate effectively in a range of collaborative discussions (one-on-one, in groups, and teacher-led) with diverse partners on grades 9–10 topics, texts, and issues, building on others' ideas and expressing their own clearly and persuasively.
Language	4	Conventions of Standard English Literacy:	Demonstrate command of the conventions of standard English grammar and usage when writing or speaking.
	8	Vocabulary Acquisition and Use Literacy:	Determine or clarify the meaning of unknown and multiple-meaning words or phrases based on *grade 8 reading and content*, choosing flexibly from a range of strategies.

continues

Strand	Grade	Standard	Description
Language *continued*	11–12	Knowledge of Language Literacy:	Apply knowledge of language to understand how language functions in different contexts, to make effective choices for meaning or style, and to comprehend more fully when reading or listening.
History/ Social Studies	6–8	Craft and Structure Literacy	Determine the meaning of words and phrases as they are used in a text, including vocabulary specific to domains related to history/social studies.
	9–10	Integration of Knowledge and Ideas	Integrate quantitative or technical analysis (e.g., charts, research data) with qualitative analysis in print or digital text.
Writing	6–8	Writing	Write informative/explanatory texts, including the narration of historical events, scientific procedures/experiments, or technical processes.
	11–12	Writing Literacy	Introduce precise, knowledgeable claim(s), establish the significance of the claim(s), distinguish the claim(s) from alternate or opposing claims, and create an organization that logically sequences the claim(s), counterclaims, reasons, and evidence.

Source: Common Core State Standards, n.d. Copyright 2010. National Governors Association Center for Best Practices and Council of Chief State School Officers. All rights reserved.

CHAPTER 16

Incorporating Play and Literacy in Treatment

Sara M. Aguilar

Play is a child's work.

Jean Piaget
(prominent developmental psychologist)

Children learn about the world they live in through play. It provides them with a way to learn, experiment with, and use new information. Beginning in infancy with basic games, such as peek-a-boo, play goes on to assume a critical role in a child's physical, emotional, social, and cognitive-linguistic development. It is commonly believed that most of a child's linguistic knowledge develops in the context of play. The American Speech-Language-Hearing Association (ASHA) suggests that speech-language therapy within the context of play "provides both the children and their caregivers with more objects and actions to share in interactions and provides a context for enhancing the child's communication skills" (ASHA, 2008, Areas to Screen, Evaluate, and Assess, para. 2). As such, the ability to incorporate play into treatment sessions is an important skill for a speech-language pathology assistant (SLPA).

DEVELOPMENT OF PLAY

As you consider how to incorporate play into treatment, it is important to understand how play develops. A child's play begins with reflexive behaviors that initially lack inherent intentionality, such as crying, cooing, and smiling (Schwartz, 2004). When these behaviors are met with meaningful reactions from caregivers, they are treated as communicative acts. With time, these behaviors mature into

more complex cognitive processes, including representational thought, imagination, exploration, analysis, and problem solving. As such, the stages in a child's cognitive development will be reflected in that child's play. Based on Piaget's work, we know that children engage in four stages of cognitive development: sensorimotor, preoperational, concrete operational, and formal operational (Table 16–1).

The ability to engage in representational thought is a cognitive skill that typically emerges by 18 months, during the sensorimotor period of cognitive development. This period is often associated with *practice play*, Piaget's earliest classification of play (Casby, 2003). During practice play, children explore objects in an egocentric manner as they learn about the world through their physical senses (e.g., mouthing objects, banging and throwing objects). Later in this stage, children begin to engage in simple cause and effect actions, such as physically moving toward

Table 16–1. Piaget's Stages of Cognitive Development

Age	Stage	Characteristics	Language Behaviors
Birth to 2 years	Sensorimotor	Reflexive behaviors and motor learning and progress rapidly, learning object permanence, means-end behaviors, and so on.	Reflexive vocal behaviors (e.g., crying and cooing) and develop into using true words when referents are not present (e.g., child says "Daddy" even when he is not present).
2 to 7 years	Preoperational	Most rapid stage of language learning; develops representational thought and learns to solve physical problems.	Engages in make believe and starts to comprehend and express temporal concepts (e.g., past, future).
7 to 11 years	Concrete Operations	Learns to categorize and organize information; begins to be a logical thinker.	Develops conversational skills; uses logic to complete tasks.
11 to 15 years	Formal Operations	Learns to be an abstract thinker, tests mental hypotheses.	Uses verbal reasoning to produce "if . . . then" statements.

Source: Adapted from Casby, 2003.

a desired object, finding a toy obscured by an object, and pulling a string to get a toy located at the end of the string (Westby, 1980).

Representational thought serves as a foundation for children to later develop *symbolic play*. Symbolic play is associated with the preoperational period of cognitive development and includes the symbolism involved with the acquisition of true language behaviors (Westby, 1980). The presence of symbolic play indicates that a child understands that an object or entity can be used to represent something distinct from itself. For example, a child demonstrates this knowledge when using a shoebox to represent a doll's bed. This basic symbolism, used first in play, later serves as a foundation for children's understanding of the more abstract symbols involved with language, such as the words used to represent objects and ideas. For instance, a pattern of sounds such as "*b-e-d*" represents *a piece of furniture used for sleeping*. Overall, symbolic play and language share the underlying ability to engage in symbolism. In fact, observation of a child's symbolic play behaviors helps determine that child's level of functioning relative to the skills required for the development of language.

The remaining stages of cognitive development identified by Piaget are concrete operations and formal operations. These stages are associated with more advanced types of play. During the concrete operations stage, children learn to categorize and organize information. Later, in the formal operations stage, children engage in abstract thought and begin to test mental hypotheses during play (Wadsworth, 2004).

One way to better understand a child's level of play and representational abilities is through careful observations,

using a research-based tool, such as Westby's (1980) Symbolic Play Scale. Westby's play scale was developed out of observational research conducted on children who were typically developing and those with intellectual impairments. Interestingly, Westby found that both groups of children progressed through the same sequence of play stages. Westby's Symbolic Play Scale was originally published as an appendix in her landmark 1980 article, "Assessment of Cognitive and Language Abilities Through Play," and the scale is now easily located using an online Web search. A description of the 10 stages of symbolic play, as depicted by Westby (1980), is summarized in Appendix 16–A. This summary can be used as an observational tool to determine a child's representational abilities, which in turn can guide the creation of developmentally appropriate treatment environments and materials. In addition, knowledge of the sequence of symbolic play allows you to engage in appropriate data collection to document children's progression through the stages of play.

PLAY IN SPEECH-LANGUAGE TREATMENT

Play can be incorporated in treatment as a platform for intervention approaches that focus on language form (i.e., phonology, morphology, syntax, semantics), and use (i.e., pragmatics). Play is a natural context for all children, since it gives them an opportunity to interact and experiment with their surroundings. Children develop language during social interactions. Hence, play in treatment provides opportunities for meaningful social scenarios that encourage language. During play scenarios, a child's communication acts elicit appropriate social responses from you, the child's communication partner. Clinicians can then expand on, and enhance, a child's communication acts to support her or him in becoming a competent language user.

Intervention in the context of play requires the provision of appropriate language input and skillful selection of materials and activities, including imaginative play scenarios, toys, and books. At its core, play in treatment should be a fun, child-directed experience and involve adult guidance and scaffolding to encourage children to experiment with new language forms to understand, describe, and manipulate the world around them.

Because play involves spontaneous and fluid interaction with a child's surroundings, clinicians must ensure that treatment is organized and systematic as intervention becomes more naturalistic and less structured (Norris & Hoffman, 1990). Without an organized and systematic approach, play in treatment merely becomes play. The balance between the spontaneity of play and the organization and methodology of intervention is a delicate one to achieve and maintain. To achieve this balance, it is critical that you work with your supervising speech-language pathologist (SLP) to (a) carefully determine a child's level of play, (b) create opportunities for meaningful communication, (c) provide effective scaffolding, and (d) select appropriate materials for use during play.

Determining the Level of Play

The first step in using play in treatment is to identify a child's current level of play and developmental abilities. You can identify where a child is functioning on the continuum of play by observing that child's behaviors, consulting with your supervising SLP, and using a play scale such as the one discussed above (Westby, 1980; Appendix 16–A). During observations, be aware that children typically engage in activities and interact with toys to the extent of their developmental level. In other words, an activity will be abandoned as soon as play reaches the capacity of that child's knowledge of the actions and relationships that can be performed or established with a particular toy. Consider this excellent example provided by Norris and Hoffman (1990):

> The child rocks a baby doll and then abandons the activity, failing to recognize that the doll's hair can be brushed, her hat can be worn, she can be placed in a stroller and taken for a walk, etc. (p. 74)

Once a child has reached her or his level of knowledge about a given situation (i.e., the relationship between objects or the actions that can be performed on objects, etc.), it is your job as the clinician to extend that child's current knowledge to new learning opportunities. Norris and Hoffman (1990) suggest the following in relation to the scenario above:

> If the child rocks the doll and begins to abandon it, the SLP might extend the child's understanding at that moment by making the child aware of some other object in relationship to the doll. The SLP can point to the doll's hair, refer to its state of messiness, and guide the child to brush the doll's hair while referring to all of the relation-

ships between the doll and the brush ("The doll's hair is messy—it has to be brushed—you're brushing her hair—now it's looking prettier—don't brush it too hard"). (p. 74)

The actions and the accompanying language help the child to organize information about the doll in relationship to the brush that was not previously understood.

Creating Communication Opportunities

Once you have extended opportunities for play, you can create the opportunity for a child to become a communicator in that environment by helping the child to: (a) understand how to control and/or manipulate activities and (b) formulate the language involved in the completion of such tasks. Norris and Hoffman (1990) point out that "the goal is not to *teach* language, but rather to provide for active experiences with the use of language so that language may *emerge*" (p. 78). One way to accomplish this is to develop a set of *communication temptations* (Wetherby & Prutting, 1984). Although originally intended to be used in the assessment of children on the autism spectrum, communication temptations can be helpful in developing play scenarios for any young child.

Communication temptations are situations devised specifically to lure a child into initiating communicative acts (Wetherby & Prutting, 1984). For instance, you can present the child with a jar of bubbles, open it and blow a few bubbles, capture one and encourage the child to pop it, then tightly close the lid on the bubble jar and hand it to the child. Next, without prompting or cueing, simply wait for

the child to produce a communicative signal for help. Once the child initiates communication through vocalization, gesture, or some other means, you can respond naturally by opening the bottle and repeating the blowing and popping action with the child. After repeating this scenario a few times, you can add an additional communication temptation by bringing the bubble wand up to your lips, waiting to blow the bubble with an expectant look on your face. Once the child produces a communicative signal, you should respond naturally by blowing the bubbles. This communication temptation scenario may be adapted to a number of activities, including balloons, wind-up toys, and peek-a-boo.

The key to creating this type of communication opportunity is to consistently view a child's behaviors as communicative (i.e., request, comment, command, question, protest, etc.) and follow through on that child's communicative act by responding in an appropriate and meaningful way. As such, play interactions should be led by the child, meaning that your goal is to focus on responding to the child's behaviors (e.g., "Oh, you want to roll the ball!") rather than requesting behaviors from the child (e.g., "What's that?" or "Say *ball*."). When you treat a child's behavior as a communicative act it creates the opportunity to expose that child to more complex communication acts. For instance, a child's utterance of *ball* may have been merely produced as a label, but when you interpret it as a request (e.g., "You want the ball?") and provide that child with an appropriate consequence (e.g., giving the ball to the child), the child is immediately exposed to this new and more complex communication act.

Scaffolding Communication

After extending play and creating communication opportunities, you can also clarify any additional information needed by the child's communication partner (whether that is another child, you as the clinician, an adult, a doll, etc.). This can be done by modeling the language required to express the missing information and providing support as the child attempts to engage in this more complex communication act. In this way, you are partnering with the child to assist in the communication of more complex information. This is referred to as *scaffolding* (Cazden, 1988). Much like the scaffolding used in the construction of a building, therapeutic scaffolding temporarily provides adult support to a child who is learning how to perform increasingly complex communication acts. Adult support ensures the opportunity to practice using language at a higher level than a child would produce independently. The amount of adult support is adjusted as the child becomes more proficient with the targeted language forms independently. Table 16–2 outlines various approaches to supporting the development of complex communication acts. The techniques listed in Box 16–1 may also be helpful during play activities.

Box 16–1

- **Self-talk:** The clinician watches the child's play and then engages in the same behavior, but while describing her or his own actions. For example, the child is playing with a tea set and the clinician begins playing with the set, stating things like, "I'm making tea. I am going to pour some tea for everyone. The tea is so yummy, but hot."
- **Parallel talk:** The clinician describes the child's behaviors during play. For example, during the above play activity with a tea set, the clinician says, "You are making tea and pouring it into each glass. Oh, the tea must be yummy, but hot."
- **Expansion:** The clinician rephrases the child's utterance but uses a grammatically correct version. For example, if the child in the above example says, "Tea hot," the clinician can expand by saying, "Yes, the tea is hot."
- **Extension or expatiation:** Similar to expansion (above), but the clinician rephrases the child's utterance, adding additional semantic information. For example, if the child said "Tea hot," the clinician could say, "Yes, we should be careful to sip the tea slowly."
- **Recast:** The clinician reformulates the child's utterance into a different form, such as a question. For example, if the child says, "Drink tea," the clinician can say, "Are you drinking the tea?" or "Should I drink the tea?"

Source: Adapted from Roth and Paul (2007, pp. 165–166).

Table 16–2. Scaffolding Approaches

Scaffolding Approach	Description	Example
Cloze procedures	Child and adult collaborate in creating a message. Adult omits words from phrases/sentences to allow child to provide missing information.	Adult: "Baby is tired, so she will go to _____." Child: "Bed"
Gestures and pantomime	Nonlinguistic physical cues that encourage child to produce language.	Adult: "She's tired. What should she do?" (tilting head and placing it on hands) Child: "Sleep"
Relational terms	Cues child to provide more information.	Child: "She need blanket" Adult: "So she can . . . " Child: "Go bed"
Preparatory sets	Highlights important information for child, including appropriate communication acts for particular contexts.	"You can't just take the blanket, you have to *ask* baby for it."
Constituent questioning	Encourages child to produce important details about and relationships between agents, actions, objects, and locations.	Adult: "What does baby need?" Child: "Blanket" Adult: "What does she need the blanket for?" Child: "Baby go sleep"
Comprehension questions	Monitors child's level of understanding during play.	"Why did she cry?" "Why isn't she sleeping?" "What happens next?"
Summarization or evaluation	Encourages child to summarize or evaluate information about play activity and provides additional opportunity to practice communicating the message.	"Tell mommy what the baby did."
Binary choices	Provides child with choices for communicating a message.	"You can ask nicely—'I want blanket, please' or you can be mean—'Give me the blanket!'"
Turn-taking cues	Indirectly requests more information from child.	Child: "I want blanket." Adult: "I want the blanket . . . " (with expectant pause and look) Child: "I want blanket." Adult: "Yeah?" (with rising intonation)
Phonemic cues	Provides child with beginning sound or syllable to support child's production.	Adult: "I need the bl___." Child: "-anket"

Source: Adapted from Norris & Hoffman, 1990.

Selecting Toys and Materials for Play

Another important consideration in incorporating play in treatment relates to the actual toys and materials that you use during intervention sessions. Selection of toys should be driven by the anticipated outcome(s) targeted in your treatment session and informed by the child's interests and preferences. Before selecting toys you must first ask yourself, "What do I want the child to do or say?" Table 16–3 lists examples of language opportunities that can be targeted using particular toys. However, be sure to cautiously manage the treatment environment. It is a good idea to provide options, but be careful not to overwhelm the child with too many choices. It is also helpful to keep some toys visible but out of reach of the child to encourage the child to initiate comments and requests.

In addition, toys used in treatment must be safe for a child at a particular age (Schwartz, 2004). Clinicians should consult a toy's packaging for age recommendations; however, if packaging is not available, a good resource is the United States Consumer Product Safety Commission (2013). Be sure to take appropriate precautions when working with children who have developmental delays and may continue to mouth toys past the typical age of development. Chapter 6 discusses additional procedures in ensuring toys and materials are properly cleaned for use in treatment.

Lastly, Lahey and Bloom's (1977) article is an excellent resource for determining what language input to provide to a child during play. These authors suggest that clinicians focus on using words that frequently occur in the child's environment rather than more specific and less frequently used vocabulary. For example,

it is better to say *car* rather than *Toyota* and *money* instead of *quarter*. Using more general terms is valuable because they may be used in a wider variety of situations. In addition, some words express multiple meanings, allowing a child to use a single utterance in multiple ways. A good example of one such word is *no*, which can be used to reject, deny, or express disappearance.

SHARED READING AS PLAY

Young children with language disorders are more likely to experience academic difficulties later in life, particularly in the area of literacy, as spoken and written language have a close and interdependent relationship (Catts & Kamhi, 2005). It is common for children with a language impairment to experience difficulties learning to read and write, just as children who face difficulty with reading and writing often have problems with spoken language. Furthermore, the relationship between spoken and written language is established early in a child's development and continues to grow throughout childhood and into adulthood. ASHA (2001) points out that individuals engaging in early speech-language intervention can play a significant role in the prevention of future literacy problems. Table 16–4 lists various approaches to early literacy intervention that have been shown to effectively prevent future literacy problems. As an SLPA, you may be asked to engage in tasks to support literacy development. To do so effectively, you need to work with your supervising SLP to (a) incorporate print referencing into treatment sessions and (b) select appropriate books for use during shared reading activities.

Table 16–3. Activities, Toys, and Language Opportunities

Activity/Toy	Language Opportunities
Peek-a-boo	• Joint attention (fundamental skill required for language development) • Turn-taking • Cause/effect: child learns to anticipate your reappearance • Model/encourage language routines: "Where is (child's name)? Is he under the table? There you are!"
Blocks	• Cause/effect relationships: stack blocks, then knock them down • Model/encourage language routines: "Uh, oh! Fall down! Oh no!" • Color/size concepts: label and request blocks of different colors, shapes, and sizes • Prepositions: support child' in understanding and/or using prepositions (e.g., "Let's put it on top")
Cars	• Cause/effect: Expand understanding of cause and effect by first stacking blocks, then using a car to knock down blocks • Model/encourage language routines: *ready, set, go!*; *crash!*; *stop/go*; *go fast/go slow* • Expand utterance: *yellow car*; *big car*; *fast car* • Sabotage: present a car with a broken wheel and see how child reacts to it. • Encourage/model language: "Oh, no!" "What happened?" "It's broken!" "Let's fix it!"

Bubbles	• Expand utterances:
	  ○ Actions: *open/close bubble,*; *blow bubble, pop bubble*
	  ○ Adjectives: *big bubble, small bubble, red bubble (with colored bubbles)*
	• Request recurrence: *more bubbles*

Puzzles	• Child identifies puzzle pieces when you request them: "Give me the _____." • Encourage child-initiated requests • Teach vocabulary for the puzzle pieces (e.g., farm animals, shapes) • Turn-taking

Puppets	• Feeding puppet
	  ○ Teach food vocabulary
	  ○ Identify/request foods: "Feed him the banana" "What do you want to feed him?"
	  ○ Use puppet to model language: "I want more grapes! Yum, yum, yum! I like grapes!"

Balls (various sizes, textures, weights, etc.)	• Expanding utterances:
	  ○ Actions: *roll ball, bounce ball, throw ball*
	  ○ Prepositions: *ball in, ball out, ball on, ball off*
	  ○ Adjectives: *small ball, red ball, bumpy ball*

Table 16–4. Approaches to Early Literacy Intervention

Type of Approach	Description of Approach	Examples
Joint book reading	Shared reading between adult and child in which adult and child jointly explore content, language, and illustrations. Adult produces models by commenting on what is being read or pictured and asks questions about the book.	• Asking questions that can be answered by either looking at pictures or using information read in book (e.g., "Who is hiding under the table?" [pointing to picture of a bear under the table]) • Asking questions that require child to go beyond what is shown in pictures or given in text (e.g., "What will happen next?")
Environmental print awareness	Understanding the meaning of common symbols/knowledge and that print communicates meaning.	• Community signs (STOP, EXIT, etc.) • Logos (restaurants, brands, etc.)
Conventions of print	Teaching children about book handling and other common features of print and reading.	• Front-to-back direction of book reading • Left-to-right reading orientation • Meaning of punctuation (exclamations, etc.)
Phonemic awareness/ phonological processing skills	Drawing attention to sounds and encouraging sound play and sound recognition during reading.	• Alliteration in books • Nursery rhymes and other books with rhyming
Alphabetic principle/letter knowledge	Recognition of letters and their corresponding sounds.	• Labeling letters • Drawing attention to words

Source: Adapted from ASHA, 2001.

Print Referencing

Print knowledge is an area of preliteracy development that involves a child's exposure to and basic understanding of written language (Storch & Whitehurst, 2002). It has received attention as a form of early literacy intervention that is associated with later success in word recognition and spelling (National Early Literacy Panel, 2004). Print referencing is an evidence-based approach for increasing print knowledge during the emergent literacy period (typically 3–5 years old) (Justice & Ezell, 2000, 2002; Justice,

Kaderavek, Xitao, Sofka, & Hunt, 2009; Lovelace & Stewart, 2007). Print knowledge includes understanding the organization and functions of print in text (i.e., book title, author's name, speech bubbles, etc.), alphabet knowledge (i.e., names and features of letters), and emergent writing (i.e., expressing meaning through writing). The theory behind print referencing is that fostering a child's learning about print and literacy increases that child's awareness of, and interest in, print during shared reading activities.

Print referencing involves adult-generated cues that guide a child to notice salient features and functions of written language during shared storybook reading (Justice & Ezell, 2004). The cues may be either verbal or nonverbal. Verbal cues include commenting about print, asking questions about print, and making requests of the child regarding print. Nonverbal cues include drawing attention to print by pointing to text and tracking text with a finger. Table 16–5 has examples of how to use print referencing cues in the context of shared storybook reading.

Selecting Appropriate Books for Shared Reading

Books with *print salience* lend themselves to a print referencing approach (Zucker, Ward, & Justice, 2009). Print salience refers to books that contain exciting print fea-

tures that draw a child's attention to print in books. Examples of print-salient features include: (a) bright colors, (b) interesting font changes, (c) visible speech (e.g., speech bubbles that connect illustrations and characters to text), (d) visible sounds (e.g., "meow" near a picture of a cat), and (e) environmental labels on illustrations (e.g., the word *candy* on a box). These qualities invite readers to explore, discuss, and interact with print in a meaningful way, thereby making the act of reading a rich and exciting experience rather than a passive and possibly tedious routine.

Print referencing and the use of books with print-salient material should be implemented strategically to encourage children's understanding of the forms and functions of print while introducing new vocabulary and concepts. Be mindful, though, to create a positive and fun

Table 16–5. Print Referencing Cues

Type of Cue	Examples
Questions about print	• "Do you know what this letter is called?" • "There are words in the bear's speech bubble! What do you think he is saying?" • "Which word says *bear*?" • "What do you think this says?"
Requests of child	• "Show me where I start reading on this page." • "Look at the letters in this word. Show me one that is in your name." • "Help me read this word." • "Find the letter *C*."
Comments about print	• "This is the title of the book. It tells us what this book is called." • "This word in the title says *bear*." (points to word) • "That says *Eric Carle* (points to author's name). He's the author of this book." • "Uppercase *C* is the same shape as lower case *c*."
Nonverbal cues	• Point to words and letters • Point to the first word on page (to show where you begin reading) • Track print left to right

Source: Adapted from Zucker, Ward, & Justice, 2009.

atmosphere that encourages children's exploration of books and fosters enjoyment of reading.

REFERENCES

American Speech-Language-Hearing Association. (2001). *Roles and responsibilities of speech-language pathologists with respect to reading and writing in children and adolescents.* Retrieved from http://www.asha.org/policy

American Speech-Language-Hearing Association. (2008). *Roles and responsibilities of speech-language pathologists in early intervention: Guidelines.* Retrieved from http://www.asha.org/policy

Casby, M. W. (2003). The development of play in infants, toddlers, and young children. *Communication Disorders Quarterly, 24*(4), 163–174.

Catts, H., & Kamhi, A. (2005). *Language and reading disabilities.* Boston, MA: Pearson Education.

Cazden, C. B. (1988). *Classroom discourse: The language of teaching and learning.* Portsmouth, NH: Heinemann.

Justice, L. M., & Ezell, H. K. (2000). Enhancing children's print and word awareness through home-based parent intervention. *American Journal of Speech-Language Pathology, 9*(3), 257–269.

Justice, L. M., & Ezell, H. K. (2002). Use of storybook reading to increase print awareness in at-risk children. *American Journal of Speech-Language Pathology, 11*(1), 17–29.

Justice, L. M., & Ezell, H. K. (2004). Print referencing: An emergent literacy enhancement strategy and its clinical applications. *Language, Speech, and Hearing Services in Schools, 35,* 185–193.

Justice, L. M., Kaderavek, J. N., Xitao, F., Sofka, A., & Hunt, A. (2009). Accelerating preschoolers' early literacy development through classroom-based teacher-child storybook reading and explicit print referencing. *Language, Speech, and Hearing Services in Schools, 40*(1), 67–85.

Lahey, M., & Bloom, L. (1977). Planning a first lexicon: Which words to teach first. *Journal of Speech & Hearing Disorders, 42*(3), 340–350.

Lovelace, S., & Stewart, S. R. (2007). Increasing print awareness in preschoolers with language impairment using non-evocative print referencing. *Language, Speech, and Hearing Services in Schools, 38*(1), 16–30.

National Early Literacy Panel. (2004, November). *The National Early Literacy Panel: A research synthesis on early literacy development.* Paper presented at the National Association of Early Childhood Specialists, Anaheim, CA.

Norris, J. A., & Hoffman, P. R. (1990). Language intervention within naturalistic environments. *Language, Speech, and Hearing Services in Schools, 21,* 72–84.

Roth, F., & Paul, R. (2007). Communication intervention. In R. Paul & P. Cascella (Eds.), *Introduction to clinical methods in communication disorders* (pp. 157–178). Baltimore, MD: Paul H. Brookes.

Schwartz, S. (2004). *The new language of toys: Teaching communication skills to children with special needs* (3rd ed.). Bethesda, MD: Woodbine House.

Storch, S. A., & Whitehurst, G. J. (2002). Oral language and code-related precursors to reading: Evidence from a longitudinal structural model. *Developmental Psychology, 38,* 934–947.

United States Consumer Product Safety Commission. (2013, June 15). *Safety education.* Retrieved from http://www.cpsc.gov/

Wadsworth, B. J. (2004). *Piaget's theory of cognitive and affective development* (5th ed.). Boston, MA: Pearson Education.

Westby, C. (1980). Assessment of cognitive and language abilities through play. *Language, Speech, and Hearing Services in Schools, 11,* 154–168.

Wetherby, A. M., & Prutting, C. A. (1984). Profiles of communicative and cognitive social abilities in autistic children. *Journal of Speech and Hearing Research, 27,* 364–377.

Zucker, T. A., Ward, A. E., & Justice, L. M. (2009). Print referencing during read-alouds: A technique for increasing emergent readers' print knowledge. *Reading Teacher, 63*(1), 62–72.

Summary of Play Stages

Stage	Typical Age of Acquisition	Description	Examples
I	9–12 months	■ Development of object permanence ■ Means-ends behaviors ■ Uses some toys appropriately/ ceases to mouth/bang all toys ■ Vocalizations begin to function as requests or commands	■ Child finds toy covered by scarf ■ Moves to desired object/ pulls string to attain toy at end of string ■ Rolls car on table (rather than putting it in his or her mouth)
II	13–17 months	■ Explores toys ■ Understands that adults are entities who can act upon objects ■ Single words emerge but are context dependent ■ Communication becomes increasingly intentional (gestures/vocalizes to request, command, gain attention, initiate interactions with others, protest, label)	■ Identifies part of toy responsible for operation and attempts to physically activate it (push, pull, turn, pound, shake) ■ Child seeks help from adult when unable to operate toy independently
III	17–19 months	■ Representational abilities begin to emerge (pretend play) ■ Autosymbolic play emerges ■ Begins to exhibit tool use ■ True verbal language emerges ■ Marked growth in vocabulary; a variety of words used for various functions and semantic roles	■ Child pretends to sleep, eat, etc. ■ Finds toy hidden out of view ■ Obtains toy with use of a stick
IV	19–22 months	■ Symbolic play extends beyond himself or herself ■ Word combinations used to express semantic relations (possessive relation is most common) ■ Child has combined sensorimotor concepts and has acquired internalized action schemas and is now able to refer to objects and individuals who are not physically present	■ Child pretends doll is sleeping ■ Child says, "my baby," "my car," etc.

continues

Stage	Typical Age of Acquisition	Description	Examples
V	22–24 months	■ Child engages in pretend play scenarios about other individuals ■ Simple sequences emerge (not yet able to perform more complex realistic sequences) ■ Emergence of present progressive -*ing*, plural and possessive –*s* ■ Begins to use short sentences to describe what is presently occurring ■ Communicative acts begin to include simple interrogatives, often lacking proper syntactic form	■ Child plays house and pretends to be mommy ■ Child puts food in bowl, then uses a spoon to feed doll; stacks blocks, then knocks them down ■ With rising intonation, child says, "The doggy sleepy" in order to ask, "Is the doggy sleepy?"
VI	2½ years	■ Child begins to depict less-common events ■ Child's role in play changes quickly ■ Associative play begins to emerge (though parallel play remains most common) ■ Uses language to analyze experiences ■ Begins to provide syntactically and semantically appropriate answers to "who," "whose," "what," "where," and "what . . . do" questions ■ Begins to ask "why" questions, especially in response to negative statements, but may not yet understand adult's answer to "why" questions	■ Child engages in pretend play involving doctor/sick child, or teacher/student ■ Child switches from being teacher to child often with little indication or warning ■ Child asks, "Where the doggy is?" ■ Child participates in the same activity as another individual but plays independently (without working together cooperatively)
VII	2 ½ -3 years	■ Begins to link several play schemas in a sequence ■ With the use of sequences, the child begins to talk about past and future events using past and future verb tenses ■ Play becomes increasingly associative	■ Child pretends to make a pizza, bake it, cut it, serve it, and wash the dishes ■ Child says, "He ate pizza." and "He will eat pizza."

Stage	Typical Age of Acquisition	Description	Examples
VIII	3–3½ years	■ Plays with less realistic toys, which involves abstraction in order to identify similarities and differences between real and pretend objects ■ Descriptive vocabulary increases ■ Begins to take another's perspective and develops the metalinguistic ability to think about and talk about language ■ Dolls are given personalities and begin to participate in play scenarios	■ Child plays with doll house, barn ■ Child uses blocks to construct enclosures (house, fence, etc.) ■ Child pretends a row of chairs is a bus ■ Child provides dialogue during play
IX	4 years	■ Child begins to consider future events and solve problems for novel events ■ Child begins to use modal verbs: *can, may, might, could, would, will* (these will not be mastered until 10–12 years) ■ Child begins to use conjunctions, including *and, but, if, so, because*	■ Child begins to consider and verbalize, "What would happen if . . . ?" or "If I do this, then . . . " ■ Child builds increasingly elaborate structures with blocks and other 3D objects ■ Uses dolls to test out hypotheses ("What would happen if . . . ")
X	5 years	■ Child begins to plan out sequences and play scenarios in advance ■ Identifies what will be required to carry out planned play scenarios ■ Play becomes more imaginative and the child is able to manage more than one event at a time ■ Child begins to use relative and subordinate clauses in order to link two or more prepositions ■ Child begins to use relational terms, including *then, when, first, while, next, before, after* (these will not be mastered until 12 years)	■ Child states that she will be the mother and while she is feeding the baby, her other children clean their room and daddy works in the yard ■ Child produces phrases such as, "I'm the princess who lives in the castle."

Source: Based on Westby, 1980.

CHAPTER 17

Autism Spectrum Disorder (ASD)

Jodi Robledo

Autism isn't something a person has, or a "shell" that a person is trapped inside. There's no normal child hidden behind autism. Autism is a way of being. It is pervasive: It colors every experience, every sensation, perception, thought, emotion, and encounter, every aspect of existence. It is not possible to separate the autism from the person—and if it were possible, the person you'd have left would not be the same person you started with.

Sinclair, 1993, p. 1, as cited in Kluth, 2010, p. 3

As a speech-language pathology assistant (SLPA), you will have the opportunity to work with individuals with autism spectrum disorder (ASD). According to the Centers for Disease Control and Prevention, one of every 59 school-aged children have been diagnosed with ASD (CDC, 2018). It is four to five times more common in boys than in girls and can be found in all cultures across the world. Researchers believe that the cause or causes of ASD involve both genetic and environmental factors. Current research continues to search for both its cause and a cure for ASD, as well as evidence-based practices to support individuals with ASD across the life span.

This chapter gives you a general overview of the definitions and common characteristics of ASD and foundational supports to benefit individuals with ASD. The goal is not to simply present a list of deficits that distinguish individuals with ASD from those without ASD. Rather, the goal is to present you with information to guide your learning regarding the individuals with ASD whom you will support. Remember this famous saying about ASD: "if you know one individual with autism, then you know one individual with autism" (Stephen Shore, as cited in Kolarik, 2016, p. 479). As professionals, we must continue to learn and grow in relationship with and understanding of the individuals we support. As the disability rights movement reminds us, it is imperative that we work with individuals, rather than work on them.

DEFINITIONS OF AUTISM SPECTRUM DISORDER

Clinical Definitions

Within a medical (or clinical) model, autism is described as a spectrum disorder, meaning that individuals will range in intensity of characteristics. According to the fifth edition of the *Diagnostic and Statistical Manual of Mental Disorders* (*DSM-5*; American Psychiatric Association [APA], 2013), individuals with ASD display persistent deficits in social communication and social interaction across multiple contexts, as well as restricted, repetitive patterns of behavior, interests, and activities. Severity is described in three levels: Level 1 requiring support, Level 2 requiring substantial support, and Level 3 requiring very substantial support. In addition, the *DSM-5* specifies that symptoms must be present in the early developmental period; cause clinically significant impairment in social, occupational, or other important areas of current functioning; and are not better explained by intellectual disability or global developmental delay.

Challenges within the category of social communication and social interaction may include challenges with reciprocity; reduced sharing of interests, emotions, or affect; challenges with initiation or response to social interactions; challenges with nonverbal communication (e.g., eye contact, understanding and using gesture and facial expressions); and deficits in developing, maintaining, and understanding relationships.

Challenges within the category of restrictive, repetitive patterns of behavior, interests, and activities may include stereotyped or repetitive motor movements, object use, or speech; insistence on sameness (e.g., inflexible adherence to routines, ritualized patterns of verbal or nonverbal behavior); highly restricted, fixated interests that are abnormal in intensity or focus; and hyperreactivity or hyporeactivity to sensory input or unusual interests in sensory aspects of the environment.

Educational Definition

The category of autism was added to the Individuals With Disabilities Education Act (IDEA) in 1990 under PL 101-476 (Hall,

2009; Knoblauch & Sorenson, 1998). To receive supports and services from special education, individuals must meet the following three criteria: they must be eligible in a disability category as defined in IDEA, there must be an adverse impact on educational performance, and there must be an actual need for special education and related services to achieve a free and appropriate public education. Autism is specifically defined in IDEA as a developmental disability significantly affecting verbal and nonverbal communication and social interaction, repetitive activities, stereotyped movements, resistance to environmental change or change in daily routines, and unusual responses to sensory experiences. Generally, autism is evident before age 3 years and adversely affects an individual's educational performance (Hall, 2009).

An Insider's Perspective

I think that much of the characteristics of autism is a result of not being able to cope with the neurological impairment which autistic people seem to have. I expect that withdrawal of an autistic person into his own world is a result of the impairment. I also believe that an autistic person's inability to cope makes them less able to concentrate and therefore to learn. I hope this evaluation by an autistic individual will help other people to understand that we are intelligent even though we may not always appear to be. (Hale & Hale, 1999, p. 60)

I believe that autism results when some sort of mechanism that controls emotion does not function properly,

leaving an otherwise relatively normal body and mind unable to express themselves with the depth that they would otherwise be capable of. (Williams, 1992, p. 203)

I believe Autism [sic] is a marvelous occurrence of nature, not a tragic example of the human mind gone wrong. In many cases, Autism [sic] can also be kind of genius undiscovered. (O'Neil, 1999, p. 14)

Although clinical and educational definitions are most commonly associated with the definition of ASD, they leave out one of the most important aspects of truly understanding what ASD is—the perspective and experiences of individuals with ASD—the true experts. One important aspect of including an insider's perspective is that we can better understand how ASD affects individuals in different ways—that no two people with ASD experience it the same way. As we move on to explore the common characteristics of ASD, we must remember that individuals will vary greatly in the intensity or type of characteristic and that if we are truly hoping to understand the individuals we support, we must understand their strengths and challenges.

COMMON CHARACTERISTICS

Although no two individuals experience ASD in the same way, there are nonetheless, common characteristics that many individuals with ASD share. These include social differences, communication differences, sensory differences, movement differences, and learning differences, compared to typically developing individuals, as well as unique passions, interests, and rituals. Common characteristics presented in this chapter include both the clinical description and insiders' perspectives.

Social Differences

I can't speak for other kids, but I'd like to be very clear about my own feelings. I did not ever want to be alone. And all of those child psychologists who said, "John prefers to play by himself" were dead wrong. I played by myself because I was a failure at playing with others. (Robison, 2007, p. 211)

Some people have said that autistic people don't care about friendships. That wasn't true at all for me. I tried to make as many friends as possible . . . I just want to say that people mean more than anything to me. I always try to be as friendly as I can to people I meet. However, I still need to work more on my social skills. They are not as good as a lot of people's. (McDonnell, 1993, p. 363)

Challenges with social relationships and interactions have been paramount to the definition of ASD since it was first described. In 1943, Leo Kanner suggested that social impairment was the defining component of autism (Heflin & Alaimo, 2007; Kanner, 1943; Waterhouse, Fein, & Modahl, 1996). Social challenges associated with ASD are well documented within the literature (Attwood, 1998; Baron-Cohen, 1989; Bellini, 2008; Brown & Whiten, 2000; Dawson & Fernald, 1987; Rogers, 2000; Travis, Sigman, & Ruskin, 2001; Wing & Gould, 1979).

The major social challenges of ASD are nonverbal communication, social initiating, social reciprocity, social cognition, behavior associated with perspective taking and self-awareness, and social anxiety and withdrawal (Bellini, 2006, 2008).

Nonverbal Communication

Individuals with ASD often have difficulty reading the body language and nonverbal cues of others. Many individuals with ASD also report that they can attend better to the speaker when they are looking away from the person's face (Robledo, Strandt-Conroy, & Donnellan, 2012). However, in avoiding direct eye contact, individuals may miss nonverbal communication. Individuals with ASD may struggle to read and understand subtle social signals or to decode what they experience as social secrets (Kluth, 2009, 2010). Other individuals with ASD report that they also have trouble using nonverbal communication such as gestures, body language, and facial expressions (Kluth, 2009, 2010).

Social Initiation

Individuals with ASD experience two common categories of social initiation challenges: there are those who rarely initiate interactions with others and those who initiate frequently but inappropriately (Bellini, 2006, 2008). Individuals in the first category often demonstrate fear, anxiety, or apathy regarding social interactions. Within the second category, individuals may initiate often but might do so by interrupting, repeating phrases or questions, or violating other social rules or norms when initiating. In addition, some individuals with ASD may attempt to initiate, but others might not recognize their attempts to be social or interact.

Social Reciprocity

Challenges associated with social reciprocity involve the give-and-take, turn-taking, mutuality, and back-and-forth exchanges of social interactions. Many individuals with ASD engage in one-sided conversations, forgetting to ask the perspective of their social partner (Bellini, 2008). Individuals with ASD may fail to jointly attend, meaning they are not always able to shift their attention in unison to an object, event, or person when their social partner does. Many individuals with ASD report that they have difficulty keeping up with the rhythm or pace of conversation and struggle to know when it is appropriate to jump into a conversation. Others report challenges with knowing when to terminate an interaction, often reporting difficulty determining the social cues that signal the end of a conversation. Knowing how to appropriately terminate an interaction can also be challenging. An individual with ASD may walk away, change topics, or hang up the phone before the social partner believes the conversation is finished.

Social Cognition

Researchers have suggested that many social challenges displayed by individuals with ASD stem from difficulties with social cognition (Baron-Cohen, 1989; Bellini, 2006, 2008). Social cognition refers to understanding the thoughts, intentions, motives, and behaviors of ourselves and others (Flavell, Miller, & Miller, 1993), as well as the social norms, customs, and values of the surrounding culture (Resnick, Levine, & Teasley, 1991). Challenges related to difficulty with social cognition can include difficulty analyzing social situations, understanding the jokes or humor of others, or incorrectly interpreting the intentions of others (Bellini, 2008).

Perspective Taking and Self-Awareness

Individuals with ASD often make socially inappropriate comments, have challenges expressing sympathy for others, have difficulty maintaining personal hygiene or personal space, or may fail to talk about or acknowledge the interests of others (Bellini, 2008). Difficulty with taking the perspective of another has been described as lacking a theory of mind (Baron-Cohen, 1989). However, we must consider that some of these problems might reflect an inability to show concern and care, rather than a lack of perspective taking or self-awareness. Some individuals with ASD report being so attuned to the feelings of others that they themselves can feel emotional distress just by being around others who are in distress (Kluth, 2009).

Social Anxiety and Performance Fears

Individuals with ASD may experience social anxiety, or intense fears of social situations (Bellini, 2008). Due to intense fears, they might avoid interacting with peers and might engage in solitary activities instead. It is important to remember that many of these individuals do want to engage in social interactions, but a lack of social skills or intense fears might be holding them back.

Communication Challenges

My speech really just bulges out of my mouth like a balloon, and the real thoughts in my head just keep on a direct line. The direct line and the balloon are related, but they do not correspond, and the more the balloon bulges, the less sense it makes, until it bursts, leaving nearly all my thoughts scattered, and me wild with anger and shame. (Blackman, 1999, p. 135)

There are, on occasion, still times when I want to talk, but I can't. I can try and try and try, but I can't talk. There is a fear holding me back. I do not know what it is I am afraid of, I only know that it is a feeling of fear unlike any other feeling of fear I have ever known. It is not that I do not want to talk, it is that I am unable to at that moment. (McKean, 1994, p. 39)

I am very fortunate that my friends and family are people who know me very intimately. Many times I feel as if oral communication is overrated. Much of how I express myself is through my eyes. Those close to me are easily able to tell if I am sick, tired, or happy, by just looking at my face. My expressions are not always appropriate yet my eyes are the windows to my soul. (Rubin, in Biklen, 2005, p. 89)

For most individuals with ASD, there are no problems with the physical form or function of the mouth, vocal cords, or other parts of the anatomy involved in speech and communication. Nonetheless, challenges with both nonverbal and verbal communication are a defining characteristic of ASD. Approximately 33% to 50% of individuals with ASD do not develop functional speech (Noens & van Berckelaer-Onnes, 2005). If an individual with ASD does use speech, there may be impairments in the ability to initiate or sustain conversations (Paul & Sutherland, 2005).

The quality or tone of voice of an individual with ASD may be monotone, singsong, flat, husky, or unusual sounding. Fay (1980) described that the prosody, pitch, or volume in speech may be unusual. Intonation may be mechanical, wooden, or arrhythmic. This can be problematic because others may believe that the individual is cold, aloof, or odd.

Individuals with ASD may also use immediate or delayed echolalia (Fay, 1980; Prizant & Rydell, 1993). Immediate echolalia refers to repeating sounds or speech that the individual has just heard. Delayed echolalia refers to repeating sounds or speech that the individual has heard in the past. There is great debate as to the purpose of echolalia, and some researchers believe it serves different functions for individuals (Prizant & Rydell, 1993). Some have described it as attempts to communicate with those around them or as self-stimulatory or calming, whereas others have called echolalia "words of annoyance" that are not volitional and have little meaning.

Individuals with ASD have also reported difficulty processing speech, spanning all aspects of speech (Kluth, 2009, 2010). Many report that they hear bits and pieces of a conversation and have trouble processing and understanding the general message of the speaker. In addition, individuals with ASD often have trouble with figurative language idioms, metaphors, jokes, slang, and sarcasm (Kluth, 2009).

A review by Hall (2009) summarized common communication challenges associated with ASD. Challenges with pronoun use has been reported, in terms of using the third person when individuals are talking about themselves (Scheuermann & Webber, 2002). Gender is commonly confused in the speech of individuals with ASD, with words such as *he, she,* or *it* used incorrectly. Difficulty with word boundaries and a tendency to comprehend phrases as single chunks of speech are also common (Fay, 1980). Using bound morphemes and answering *Wh*-questions can present challenges for individuals with ASD (Koegel & Koegel, 1995), and they may have a greater capacity for learning nouns over verbs.

Sensory Differences

The unmodulated sensory input often overwhelmed me, causing me mental torture, and I would begin feeling mentally confused and sluggish. My head would feel fogged so that I could not think. My vision would blur, and the speech of those around me would become gibberish. My whole body buzzed. The slight tremor that always plagued me would worsen. My hands would feel detached from my body, as if they were foreign objects. I would be paralyzed, unable to comprehend my own movements unless I could see them. I could not tell where my hand started and the table ended, or what shape the table was, or even if it was rough or smooth. I felt like I was in a cartoon world. (Hawthorne, as cited in Gillingham, 2000, pp. 21–22)

Individuals with ASD report a variety of sensory differences, compared to typically developing individuals. Some are hypersensitive and others are hyposensitive to sensory stimulation, and reports indicate that any of their senses can be affected (i.e., smell, touch, vision, taste, temperature, hearing, vestibular system, and proprioception) (Gillingham, 2000). The impact of sensory differences in the everyday life of an individual with ASD should not be underestimated and is an area in need of support. A description of each area of sensory differences will focus heavily on the experience of individuals with ASD to give you a rich understanding of how these differences affect them.

Tactile Sensitivity

Individuals with ASD can experience the sensation of touch in different ways (Robledo et al., 2012). Some may crave and seek out touch, whereas others may avoid any kind of touch. Some individuals seek out deep-pressure touch, like a firm hug or handshake, but pull away from light or soft touch. Unexpected touch can startle many individuals with ASD and should be avoided. Many individuals report avoiding activities or situations where touch may become unbearable. Sean Barron and Temple Grandin described their experiences with tactile sensitivity:

I felt acutely uncomfortable sitting upright in the bathtub, so I didn't enjoy taking a bath in the least. I absolutely hated the way my bottom felt against the tub, and I couldn't make myself think about something else so I wouldn't feel it. When I tried to sit normally it felt "squishy" and I was extremely sensitive to this feeling. I couldn't shake it off. It was the same feeling I used to have when I couldn't stand to touch our rug with my bare feet. To make it more bearable, I shifted most of my weight onto one side so that only a part of me came into contact with the bathtub. When they insisted I "sit right," it only compounded the problem. (Barron & Barron, 1992, p. 96)

"I'll miss you, Temple." She walked quickly to my side and kissed my cheek. I ached to be enfolded in her arms, but how could she know? I stood rigid as a pole trapped by the approach avoidance syndrome of autism. I drew back from her kiss, not able to endure tactile stimulation—not even loving, tactile stimulation. (Grandin & Scariano, 1986, p. 65)

Individuals with tactile sensitivities also describe challenges with personal hygiene such as brushing teeth and hair. Some report avoiding certain fabrics or preferring to wear similar clothing again and again, or both. Tactile sensitivities have also been reported for eating, and many individuals with ASD seek or avoid particular food textures, which limit their diet.

Auditory Sensitivities

Auditory input typically causes anxiety for individuals with ASD. Donna Williams (1992, 1994) and Temple Grandin (1995) explained that hearing certain sounds created painful experiences. For Williams (1992), the tone of people's voice disturbed her. Grandin (1992) said her hearing felt "like having a hearing aid with the volume control stuck on super loud" (p. 107) and expressed that "sudden loud noises hurt my ears like a dentist's drill hitting a nerve" (p. 107). She described her dislike for environments that had many different noises, "such as shopping centers and sports arenas. High pitched continuous noise, such as bathroom vent fans or hair dryers, are annoying" (p. 2).

Lucy Blackman (1999) described her auditory differences:

Because other people's sound processing was alien to me, I had no idea that sound should not be like a pressure-cooker lid. I put my hands to my ears for loud sudden noises, but the continuous clamor of everyday life was only relieved by movement. Even in the classroom there was visual stimulation and noise, which combined with my own breathing and a buzzing effect that I think was my own inner ear. (p. 51)

Matt Ward explained that sudden loud noises were very stressful:

Especially things like gunshots, loud motors, and brass bands. My mom took me through a drive-thru car wash once when I was in grade school and I was terrified. The brushes sounded to me like the sound of intense machine gunfire, but I could not communicate well enough to explain why I got so upset. (Robledo et al., 2012, p. 4)

Other individuals with ASD noted that, at times, they had an inconsistent ability to process auditory input. Darren White explained a "trick which my ears played was to change the volume of sounds around me. Sometimes when other kids spoke to me I could scarcely hear them and sometimes they sounded like bullets" (White & White, 1987, p. 225). Donna Williams (1992) said that she sometimes needed people to repeat a particular sentence several times because she heard the message in bits. She stated that her mind segments sentences into words, leaving her with a strange and sometimes unintelligible message. She described it as a "bit like when someone plays around with the volume switch on a TV," (p. 69). In fact, she described that she would sometimes turn the sound up and down on the television, breaking up people's voices while keeping the picture intact. This seemed to imitate the difficulty she sometimes had hearing people consistently.

Visual Sensitivities

Individuals with ASD have described several different types of visual differences, including unique interactions with colors, lighting, stimulation or pain caused by visual stimuli, and challenges with eye contact.

Sean Barron described his intrigue with colors and the positive emotions he felt when comparing colors for hours at a time (Barron & Barron, 1992). Donna Williams (1992) said her early memories included spending hours looking at bright spots of color that made her laugh. Years later she learned that the spots of color were air particles of reflected light, which her hypersensitivity to color and light allowed her to see.

Other individuals with ASD experienced colors quite differently. Darren White described a situation where he received a bike as a Christmas present. He explained that he could not look at the yellow color on his bike because it was too painful. Extra red was added to make the color look orange and that color "blurred upwards making it look like it was on fire" (White & White, 1987, p. 226). He also could not see blue clearly because it "looked too light and it looked like ice" (p. 227).

Many individuals report sensitivity to lights, particularly fluorescent light. A participant in Robledo et al. (2012) pointed out:

There are certain types of light I cannot tolerate—they make me nervous . . . If I am in a hall and it is too bright, I can't handle it, I have to put a sun hat on. Fluorescent light absolutely turns my stomach into knots. It does a trip on my nervous system. (p. 5)

Other colors and patterns have also been reported as problematic.

A common visual characteristic in ASD is a lack of eye contact (Kluth, 2009; Robledo et al., 2012). Individuals with ASD shared their perspective on lack of eye contact related to visual sensitivity:

When I concentrated on the sound, I felt my eyes and nose shutting off. I could never do everything together at the same time. That is, I could not see you and at the same time hear you. My sense of hearing was always sharper than my sight. This is the reason I never used my eyes to interact with anybody. Psychologists call it "lack of eye contact." The result was the knowledge of a fragmented world perceived through isolated sense organs. (Mukhopadhyay 2000, p. 74)

Sometimes, eye contact literally is painful for me to achieve. This has become easier for me to achieve however with those in my life with whom I am extremely comfortable. There are certain days, though, where eye contact is not something I am able to achieve, regardless of who the person is. (Rubin, in Biklen, 2005, p. 89)

Olfactory Sensitivities

Individuals with ASD report sensitivities to smell. Some smells may be unbearable, whereas others are pleasing. Intense smells such as perfume or air fresheners may be highly distracting for individuals with ASD. It is important to note that many of these smells do not bother individuals without ASD. Therefore, it is critical to examine the environment for potential sensory triggers.

Other Areas of Sensitivities

Additional sensitivities that individuals with ASD report include taste, temperature, pain, vestibular system, and proprioception (Gillingham, 2000). It is critical to become aware of the particular sensitivities an individual with ASD may experience. Variables such as emotion, fatigue, and hunger can greatly affect a person's ability to regulate their sensory system.

Movement Differences

I often can't control my body and make jerky weird movements. I believe the problem is with purposeful movement. Sadly we cannot even move from one place to another when we want to. We compensate by going where a movement takes us and actually use our weird movements to get where we want to go. For example, when I want to move from one area on the keyboard to another I will jerk and have my hand land where I want it to. Movements appear as mental retardation when we can't get our bodies to follow directions. Movement disorders make it appear that we don't understand what is being asked or we are being noncompliant. (Rubin et al., 2001, p. 426)

I cannot seem to tell my right from my left although I know my right from my left. I cannot seem to find my mouth upon command. I have trouble finding where my nose is when I am asked. I find that my breath will not come when I am asked to blow or when I am asked to take a deep breath. I am unable to draw through a straw. I have trouble sticking out my tongue. I cannot seem to spit the water out when brushing my teeth. I cannot purse my lips when I want to drink out of a bottle. I don't seem to get the message to wave or to smile when I should be responding to someone or something. My autism seems to be apparent in my random use of my hands and feet. My habit of biting is a symptom of my being nonverbal and is mostly due to frustration. (Hale & Hale, 1999, p. 60)

They asked him to point at his body parts, but the boy could not do it. Not that he was ignorant of the parts of the human body, but he was unable to point and identify them in his own self. Pointing at objects was difficult too, as he pointed only at the letters on the board and could not generalize it with the other things. Then the doctors asked the other way around. They touched his legs and hands and so on. They asked him to point on the board. This he did with ease. (Mukhopadhyay, 2000, p. 26)

At times, individuals with ASD may move their bodies in ways that seem atypical to individuals without ASD. They might rock, or flap, or jump, or repeatedly touch an object. We might assume that these behaviors are communicative attempts to interact or volitional behaviors that demonstrate a diminished cognitive ability. Movement differences are the least understood characteristic of ASD. However, many researchers (Leary

& Donnellan, 2012; Torres et al., 2013) indicate that our understanding of these movement differences will not only help us better support individuals with ASD, but will also play a significant role in objectively measuring and standardizing ASD—its treatment and the tracking of an individual's changes over time.

Donnellan, Leary, and Robledo (2006) have defined a movement difference as a difference, interference, or shift in the efficient, effective utilization and integration of movement; a disruption in the organization and regulation of perception, action, posture, language, speech, thought, emotion, and/or memory. Movement differences are manifested in a wide range of behaviors, including the more easily identifiable activities such as unusual gait and posture, constant physical movement, or repetitive rocking. Other movement differences tend to become evident at transition points:

- Starting—difficulty initiating
- Executing—difficulty with the rate, rhythm, target, and so on of movement
- Continuing—difficulty staying on track, not taking alternative paths, and so forth
- Stopping—difficulty terminating a movement; the tendency to perseverate; getting stuck in one sensory mode (e.g., staring into space)
- Combining—difficulty adding a sensory mode or a movement (e.g., listening to someone speak while watching his or her gestures and facial expression, doing two things at once)
- Switching—difficulty letting go of one perception or movement and initiating a new one.

Many individuals without ASD also experience movement differences from time to time. However, these movement differences (e.g., intensity, duration, rhythm, rate, frequency, timing) are exacerbated in individuals with ASD, affecting their ability to communicate, relate, and function in their communities.

Learning Differences

I think in pictures. Words are like a second language to me. I translate both spoken and written words into full-color movies, complete with sounds, which run like a VCR tape in my head. When somebody speaks to me, his words are instantly translated into pictures. (Grandin, 1995, p. 19)

All of the previous described characteristics of ASD can affect an individual's ability to learn. Many individuals with ASD report experiencing learning challenges similar to those with learning disabilities, such as difficulty with input, organization, memory, generalization, and output (Kluth, 2009). Many individuals excel at tasks involving concrete thinking and have more difficulty with abstract thinking, awareness, and judgment. It is critical to remember that lack of cognitive ability might not be the area of challenge. Rather, an individual may not be performing academically due to other challenges of ASD, such as sensory sensitivities, movement differences, or communication skills.

Individuals with ASD also have learning strengths, including precocious and highly developed text reading and word recognition. In addition, many display advanced skill when memorizing chunks of language, including songs, have excellent mathematical skills, or can write beautiful poetry.

Passions, Interests, and Rituals

People with autism like routines, and if those routines are broken it does not mean that we don't understand what is happening it just means that it is harder for us than most to stop our brains from spinning off into their regular patterns. (Rubin, in Biklen, 2005, p. 88)

Intense passions, fascinations, and restricted interests are a key feature of ASD (Kluth, 2009). Some may have only a few interests over their life, while for others interests are more variable. The most common topics of fascination across individuals with ASD are trains, cars, transportation systems, machines, weather, natural disasters, geography, animals, drawings, music, pop stars, and television shows (Hippler & Klicpera, 2004; Mercier, Mottron, & Belleville, 2000).

Strict adherence to specific rituals is common in individuals with ASD. These might involve how objects, space, and time are arranged or organized or may involve repetitive types of behavior. Passions, restricted interests, and rituals clearly serve a specific purpose for individuals with ASD. As such, it is critical to understand the role these play in their lives.

FOUNDATIONAL SUPPORTS

Individuals with ASD can be successful in any and every environment. The following section highlights some foundational strategies and supports to support individuals with ASD. Although there are numerous methodologies and packaged programs available to support individuals with ASD, this section focuses on foundational supports that should be involved in every interaction and intervention.

Inclusion and Collaborative Teaming

Inclusion supports and benefits all learners. It stresses interdependence and independence, views all students as capable and complex, values a sense of community, and promotes civil rights and equity (Doyle, 2008; Falvey, Givner, & Kimm, 1995; Kluth, 2010; Sapon-Shevin, 2007; Udvari-Solner, 1997; Villa & Thousand, 1995). For individuals with ASD, access to the least restrictive environments will help them learn and grow. Opportunities to practice and learn from typically developing peers are invaluable for individuals with ASD. Supporting them requires a collaborative team approach. Professionals, parents, peers, and the individuals themselves should all be on the same page when designing supports across the life span.

Relationships and Belonging

Developing, maintaining, and facilitating relationships and belonging are critical for building community for individuals with ASD. Relationships with parents, therapists, teachers, peers, and others should guide all supports for individuals with ASD. When they feel they are in a safe, supportive, and trusting relationship, learning and growth occurs. Collaboration and connection with families and other individuals with ASD are key—they are the true experts in ASD.

Social Communication Supports

As many individuals with ASD struggle to communicate and interact socially, communication and social support must be at the forefront of any intervention. It is critical to take the perspective of the individual with ASD and focus on what communication and social skills are important and meaningful to his or her life. Fitting students with ASD into packaged communication or social skills programs does not take into account their individual variability. Our challenge is to determine what supports and strategies work best for each individual with ASD. It is a difficult yet fruitful task.

Sensory and Movement Supports

Understanding each individual's unique sensory system and patterns of movement is critical for truly offering personalized supports and accommodations. This requires that you get to know the individuals you work with by listening and observing. As you become more familiar with and build a relationship with each individual, you can partner as a team to discover the best accommodations, modifications, and adaptations to fit the individual needs of the person you support.

Positive Behavior Supports

It is important to remember that individuals with ASD are trying their best to behave appropriately. Often what looks on the surface like a problem behavior is actually a manifestation of a sensory or movement problem, physical discomfort, inability to communicate effectively, or inability to understand what is being asked and per-

form the required task (Kluth, 2010). Be sure you spend ample time teaching and reinforcing desired behaviors. When trouble does arise, use strategies that are respectful and promote learning and growth. Behavioral support should not be about control; rather, it should be about collaboratively teaming up to support dreams.

Learning and Environmental Supports

By understanding the many characteristics of ASD, you can help create environments and supports that will enable individuals with ASD to function effectively. Think about the sensory systems of the individuals with ASD whom you support—what types of sensory sensitivities do they have and in what ways can they be accommodated in the environment? Individuals with ASD often report that they learn best when materials are presented clearly and visually. Active learning that provides visuals, examples, manipulatives, and interaction will be most successful. Do not forget to use your most valuable resource: the individuals with ASD. Elicit their perspective on ways they might prefer to receive support. Be creative and flexible in all supports.

CONCLUDING THOUGHTS

This chapter presents a general overview of ASD, including definitions, characteristics, and foundational supports. Effective support requires true understanding of each and every individual that you work with. As SLPAs, your growth in understanding will come from working with, listening to, and knowing individuals with ASD in your daily practice.

REFERENCES

American Psychiatric Association. (2013). *Diagnostic and statistical manual of mental disorders* (5th ed.). Washington, DC: Author.

Attwood, T. (1998). *Asperger's syndrome: A guide for parents and professionals.* Philadelphia, PA: Kingsley.

Baron-Cohen, S. (1989). The autistic child's theory of mind: A case of specific developmental delay. *Journal of Child Psychology and Psychiatry, 30,* 285–297.

Barron, J., & Barron, S. (1992). *There's a boy in here.* New York. NY: Simon & Schuster.

Bellini, S. (2006). Social challenges of children and youth with autism spectrum disorders. In E. Boutot & B. Myles (Eds.), *Autism spectrum disorders: Foundations, characteristics, and effective strategies* (pp. 201–222) Upper Saddle River, NJ: Pearson.

Bellini, S. (2008). *Building social relationships: A systematic approach to teaching social interaction skills to children and adolescents with autism spectrum disorders and other social difficulties.* Shawnee Mission, KS: Autism Asperger Publishing.

Biklen, D. (2005). *Autism and the myth of the personal one.* New York, NY: New York University Press.

Blackman, L. (1999). *Lucy's story: Autism and other adventures.* Brisbane, Australia: Book in Hand.

Brown, J., & Whiten, A. (2000). Imitation, theory of mind and related activities in autism: An observational study of spontaneous behavior in everyday contexts. *Autism: The International Journal of Research and Practice, 4,* 185–205.

Centers for Disease Control and Prevention. (2018). *Prevalence and characteristics of autism spectrum disorder among children aged 8 years —Autism and Developmental Disabilities Monitoring Network, 11 Sites, United States, 2014.* Retrieved from https://www.cdc.gov/mmwr/volumes/67/ss/ss6706a1.htm

Dawson, G., & Fernald, M. (1987). Perspective taking ability and its relationship to the social behavior of autistic children. *Journal of Autism and Developmental Disorders, 17,* 487–489.

Donnellan, A., Leary, M., & Robledo, J. (2006). I can't get started: Stress and the role of movement differences for individuals with the autism label. In G. Baron, J. Groden, G. Groden, & L. Lipsitt (Eds.), *Stress and coping in autism* (pp. 205–245). Oxford, UK: Oxford University Press.

Doyle, M. (2008). *The paraprofessional's guide to the inclusive classroom: Working as a team* (3rd ed.). Baltimore, MD: Brookes.

Falvey, M., Givner, C., & Kimm, C. (1995). What is an inclusive school? In R. Villa & J. Thousand (Eds.), *Creating an inclusive school* (pp. 1–12). Alexandria, VA: ASCD.

Fay, W. (1980). Aspects of language. In W. Fay & A. Schuler (Eds.), *Emerging language in autistic children* (pp. 51–85). Baltimore, MD: University Park Press.

Flavell, J., Miller, P., & Miller, S. (1993). *Cognitive development* (3rd ed.). Upper Saddle River, NJ: Prentice-Hall.

Gillingham, G. (2000). *Autism: A new understanding!* Edmonton, Canada: Tacit.

Grandin, T. (1992). An inside view of autism. In E. Schopler & G. B. Mesibov (Eds.), *High functioning individuals with autism* (pp. 105–126). New York, NY: Plenum.

Grandin, T. (1995). *Thinking in pictures: And other reports from my life with autism.* New York, NY: Doubleday.

Grandin, T., & Scariano, M. (1986). *Emergence: Labeled autistic.* Novato, CA: Arena.

Hale, M., & Hale, C. (1999). *I had no means to shout!* Bloomington, IN: 1st Books.

Hall, L. (2009). *Autism spectrum disorders: From theory to practice.* Upper Saddle River, NJ: Pearson.

Heflin, L., & Alaimo, D. (2007). *Students with autism spectrum disorder: Effective instructional practices.* Upper Saddle River, NJ: Pearson.

Hippler, K., & Klicpera, C. (2004). A retrospective analysis of the clinical case records of "autistic psychopaths" diagnosed by Hans Asperger and his team at the University Children's Hospital, Vienna. In U. Frith & E. Hill (Eds.), *Autism: Mind and brain* (pp. 21–42). Oxford, UK: Oxford University Press.

Kanner, L. (1943). Autistic disturbances of affective contact. *Nervous Child, 2,* 217–230.

Kluth, P. (2009). *The autism checklist: A practical reference for parents and teachers.* San Francisco, CA: Jossey-Bass.

Kluth, P. (2010). *'You're going to love this kid!' Teaching students with autism in the inclusive classroom* (2nd ed.). Baltimore, MD: Brookes.

Knoblauch, B., & Sorenson, B. (1998). IDEA's definition of disabilities. *ERIC Digest.* Reston,

VA: ERIC Clearinghouse on Disabilities and Gifted Education.

Koegel, R., & Koegel, L. (1995). *Teaching children with autism: Strategies for initiating positive interactions and improving learning opportunities.* Baltimore, MD: Brookes.

Kolarik, J. (2016). In their own words: Stories from CIP. In M.P. McManmom (Author), *Autism and learning differences: An active learning teaching toolkit* (pp.455-482). Philadelphia, PA: Jessica Kingsley.

Leary, M. R., & Donnellan, A. M. (2012). *Autism: Sensory-movement differences and diversity.* Cambridge, WI: Cambridge Book Review Press.

McDonnell, J. (1993). *News from the border.* New York, NY: Ticknor & Fields.

McKean, T. (1994). *Soon will come the light.* Arlington, TX: Future Horizons.

Mercier, C., Mottron, L., & Belleville, S. (2000). Psychosocial study on restricted interest in high-functioning persons with pervasive developmental disorders. *Autism, 4,* 406–425.

Mukhopadhyay, T. R. (2000). *Beyond the silence.* London, UK: National Autistic Society.

Noens, I., & van Berckelaer-Onnes, I. (2005). Captured by details: Sense-making, language and communication in autism. *Journal of Communication Disorders, 38,* 123–141.

O'Neil, J. (1999). *Through the eyes of aliens: A book about autistic people.* Philadelphia, PA: Jessica Kingsley.

Paul, R., & Sutherland, D. (2005). Enhancing early language in children with autism spectrum disorder. In F. Volkmar, R. Paul, A. Klin, & D. Cohen (Eds.), *Handbook of autism and pervasive developmental disorders* (3rd ed., pp. 925–945). New York, NY: John Wiley.

Prizant, B., & Rydell, P. (1993). Assessment and intervention strategies for unconventional verbal behavior. In J. Reichle & D. Wacker (Eds.), *Communication approaches to challenging behavior: Integrating functional assessment and intervention strategies* (pp. 263–297). Baltimore, MD: Brookes.

Resnick, L., Levine, J., & Teasley, S. (1991). *Perspectives on socially shared cognition.* Washington, DC: American Psychological Association.

Robinson, J. (2007). *Look me in the eye: My life with Asperger's.* New York, NY: Crown.

Robledo, J., Strandt-Conroy, K., & Donnellan, A. (2012). An exploration of sensory and movement differences from the perspective of individuals with autism. *Frontiers in Integrative Neuroscience, 6,* 1–13.

Rogers, S. (2000). Interventions that facilitate socialization in children in autism. *Journal of Autism and Developmental Disabilities, 30,* 399–409.

Rubin, S., Biklen, D., Kasa-Hendrickson, K., Kluth, P., Cardinal, D., & Broderick, A. (2001). Independence, participation, and the meaning of intellectual ability. *Disability and Society, 16,* 425–429.

Sapon-Shevin, M. (2007). *Widening the circle: The power of inclusive classrooms.* Boston, MA: Beacon.

Scheuermann, B., & Webber, J. (2002). *Autism: Teaching does make a difference.* Belmont, CA: Wadsworth/Thomson Learning.

Sinclair, J. (1993). Don't mourn for us. *Our Voice, 1*(3). Retrieved from http://ani.autistics.org/don't_mourn.html

Torres, E., Brincker, M., Isenhower, R., Yanovich, P., Stigler, K., Numbereger, J., . . . Jose, J. (2013). Autism: The micro-movement perspective. *Frontiers in Integrative Neuroscience, 7,* 1–26.

Travis, L., Sigman, M., & Ruskin, E. (2001).Links between social understanding and social behavior in verbally able children with autism. *Journal of Autism and Developmental Disorders, 31,* 119–130.

Udvari-Solner, A. (1997). Inclusive education. In C. Grant & G. Ladson-Billings (Eds.), *Dictionary of multicultural education* (pp. 141–144). Phoenix, AZ: Oryx.

Villa, R., & Thousand, J. (1995). *Creating an inclusive school* (pp. 1–12). Alexandria, VA: ASCD.

Waterhouse, L., Fein, D., & Modahl, C. (1996). Neurofunctional mechanisms in autism. *Psychological Review, 103,* 457–489.

White, G. B., & White, M. S. (1987). Autism from the inside. *Medical Hypothesis, 24,* 223–229.

Williams, D. (1992). *Nobody nowhere.* New York, NY: Avon.

Williams, D. (1994). *Somebody somewhere.* New York, NY: Times Books.

Wing, L., & Gould, J. (1979). Severe impairments of social interaction and associated abnormalities in children: Epidemiology and classification. *Journal of Autism and Developmental Disorders, 9,* 11–29.

CHAPTER 18

Augmentative and Alternative Communication

Margaret Vento-Wilson

Just as a dance couldn't be possibly be a dance unless people moved to it, so language doesn't become communication until people grow to express it back. It has to be a two-way exchange.

—Staehely, 2000, p. 1

The position statement of the American Speech-Language-Hearing Association (ASHA) asserts that, "communication is the essence of human life and that all people have the right to communicate to the fullest extent possible" (ASHA, 2001, Position Statement, para. 2). For people with significant congenital or acquired complex communication needs (CCNs), this directive presents greater challenges and increased complexity than for those for whom communication occurs through typical development and normal channels. Approximately .03% to 1.3% of the United States population experiences communication impairments that impede their ability to produce and/or comprehend spoken, written, or signed language (ASHA, n.d.-a.; Beukelman & Mirenda, 2013). These percentages translate into a conservative estimate of two million individuals who are unable to use speech or handwriting as a means to communicate about their daily needs (ASHA, n.d.-a; Sigafoos, Schlosser, & Sutherland, 2013). Fortunately, through the effective intervention of trained professionals, including speech-language pathology assistants

(SLPAs), at least some of these communication barriers may be overcome through the use of assistive technology (AT) or augmentative and alternative communication (AAC; ASHA, n.d.-a; "What is Assistive Technology," 2013).

Research conducted by ASHA in 2016 revealed that 45% of SLPs surveyed provided services to individuals with AAC needs, with the occurrence being slightly higher in hospitals than in school settings. In health care settings, SLPs surveyed reported that 66% of referrals received were for patients who were likely AAC candidates, with the majority of these referrals being from pediatric hospitals (ASHA, 2002). Further, in a recent analysis of caseload distribution in hospitals, SLPs reported spending approximately 3% of their clinical, adult-focused service time with clients using AAC and approximately 6% of their clinical, pediatric-focused service time with children in AAC (ASHA, 2017). In the school setting, between the years of 2000 to 2016, the percentage of school-based SLPs with nonverbal students or students using AAC ranged between 48% and 62% (ASHA, 2016). Given the high level of need these figures represent, it is very likely that as an SLPA, you will encounter individuals with AAC needs in your employment and training settings.

As an SLPA, you will be expected to be knowledgeable and competent in AAC concepts and implementation practices. As discussed in Chapter 1 (Defining Roles: SLPAs), in the area of service delivery, ASHA specifically states that, provided training, supervision, and planning as appropriate, one of the tasks that may be delegated to an SLPAs is to, "program and provide instruction in the use of AAC devices." (ASHA, 2013, Responsibilities

within the Scope of SLPAs, para. 1). The following list provides a general description of the potential roles of an SLPA in AAC intervention (ASHA, 2010; Beukelman, Ball, & Fager, 2008):

- Support of multi-modality intervention
- Prepare low-tech materials
- Integrate low- and high-tech materials into developmental, restorative, or compensatory intervention
- Instruct communication partners in AAC use
- Maintain AAC technology
- Serve as a liaison between AAC commercial companies and related AAC personnel

This chapter provides an overview of AAC concepts and practices. While this topic may initially seem daunting, as you read about and become more familiar with AAC, you may find that this challenging topic offers an opportunity for you to grow as an SLPA and that AAC intervention can, and often does, have a profound effect on the lives of your clients. The journey you are undertaking by reading this chapter is very similar to the journey your clients undertake, whether they come to you as toddlers with CCNs, or as adults who have suffered an abrupt or gradual, but nonetheless devastating, loss of speech and language. With the appropriate guidance and support, they too will evolve from a novice AAC user into an experienced AAC user, with the ability to maintain and develop relationships and remain relevant and involved with their world (Light, Parsons, & Drager, 2002). Augmentative and alternative communication offers your clients the opportunity to more fully experience that quintessential tool of language, "which is so tightly woven into human experience that it is scarcely possible to imagine life without it" (Pinker, 1994, p. 17).

ASSISTIVE TECHNOLOGY

Assistive technology (AT) can be defined broadly as an item, piece of equipment, or system used as a means to preserve, enhance, or improve the functional capabilities of an individual (Bugaj & Norton-Darr, 2010). Examples of AT include the use of eyeglasses, hearing aids, enlarged handles on kitchen utensils, walkers, wheelchairs, and Braille codes on elevator buttons ("What is Assistive Technology," 2013). Other examples of AT that many people are familiar with today is the use of speech-to-text and the use of reminders on smartphones. Specific to communication, AT can include the use of a broad range of AAC devices or systems (Parette & Sherer, 2004).

AUGMENTATIVE AND ALTERNATIVE COMMUNICATION

The term *AAC* is defined as a system that can be used to temporarily or permanently compensate for the impairments and activity and participation limitations and restrictions of individuals with severe expressive or receptive difficulties with speech, language, or communication (ASHA, n.d.-a; Branson & Demchak, 2009; Davidoff, 2017). Augmentative and alternative communication is also defined as a dynamic, multimodal communication continuum that evolves based on a user's growth and development, the situation, and the communication partner. Its ultimate purpose is to minimize barriers to successful communication and increase communicative competence (Barker, Akapa, Brady, & Theirmann-Bourque, 2013; Blackstone, Williams, & Wilkins, 2007; Calculator & Black, 2009). Before delving further into a discussion of AAC, it is essential to have an understanding of the distinctions between the terms *speech*, *language*, and *communication*.

Speech is the individual sounds and sound patterns of any given language. It is a vocal production that is comprehended auditorily. *Language* is symbolic and is used to covey messages through a rule-governed system, which involves syntax, semantics, phonology, morphology, and pragmatics. Language can occur independently of speech, as with American Sign Language (ASL; Figure 18–1), to communicate, either in addition to or instead of spoken language. *Communication* is the act of conveying a message that establishes a shared understanding between the message sender and the message receiver. Communication can occur without speech or language, such as when two people who speak different languages use gestures or pictures to ask or answer a question. For people with deficits in the production or comprehension of speech, language, or communication, AAC offers the opportunity to create intelligible and comprehensible messages through a combination of symbols, and then to use those symbols with their communication partners in multiple settings and circumstances (ASHA, n.d.-a; Barker et al., 2013; Blackstone, Williams, & Wilkins, 2007; Calculator & Black, 2009).

"I   pledge   allegiance   to   the flag   of

the United States   of   America and   to

the Republic for which it stands, one nation under

God,   indivisible,   with   liberty

and   justice   for   all."

Figure 18–1. The Pledge of Allegiance in American Sign Language. Courtesy of Bing Images, free to share and use commercially.

476

Foundational AAC Concepts

In 2007, Blackstone, Williams and Wilkins published six principles specific to AAC research and practice. The list reflects extensive collaborative work between AAC users and their families, practitioners, researchers, faculty from universities, policy makers, and AAC developers and manufacturers. The list can be seen in Table 18–1 (Blackstone, Williams, & Wilkins, 2007, p. 192). It is beneficial to keep these principles in mind as you navigate your intervention with AAC users and their families and caregivers.

A second foundational concept integral to AAC intervention is the participation model (Beukelman & Mirenda, 2013) (Figure 18–2), which ASHA has endorsed as a valuable framework for AAC intervention. It is based on a premise of supporting individuals who use AAC in communicating, functioning, and participating in communicative contexts in the same manners as their typically-developing peers of the same chronological age. The participation model requires professionals to identify barriers relating to opportunity (i.e., policy, practice, knowledge, skill, attitude) and access (i.e., natural abilities, environmental, AAC systems). Identifying these barriers has the potential to reduce their frequency and level, as well as to increase the participation of AAC users broadly and across contexts (Beukelman & Mirenda, 2013). The participation model aligns with ASHA's zero-exclusion policy for AAC services (Brady et al., 2016) and the World Health Organization's (2014) International Classification of Functioning (ICF), as seen in Figure 18–3.

AAC Users

AAC users are a heterogeneous group of individuals, whose only shared links are the presence of CCNs and an inability to use oral language as their primary source

Table 18–1. Augmentative and Alternative Communication (AAC) Principles

1. People who rely on AAC participate actively in AAC research and practice.

2. Widely accepted theoretical constructs are specifically addressed in the design and development of AAC technologies and instructional strategies.

3. AAC technologies and instructional strategies are designed to support and foster the abilities, preferences, and priorities of individuals with complex communication needs, taking into account strengths, challenges, and motor, sensory, cognitive, psychological, linguistic, and behavioral skills.

4. AAC technologies and instructional strategies are designed so as to recognize the unique roles communication partners play during interaction.

5. AAC technologies and instructional strategies enable individuals with complex communication needs to maintain, expand, and strengthen existing social networks and relationships and to fulfill societal roles.

6. AAC outcomes are realized in practical forms, such as guidelines for clinical practice, design specifications, and commercial products. The social validity of these outcomes is determined by individuals with complex communication needs, their family members, AAC manufacturers, and the broader community.

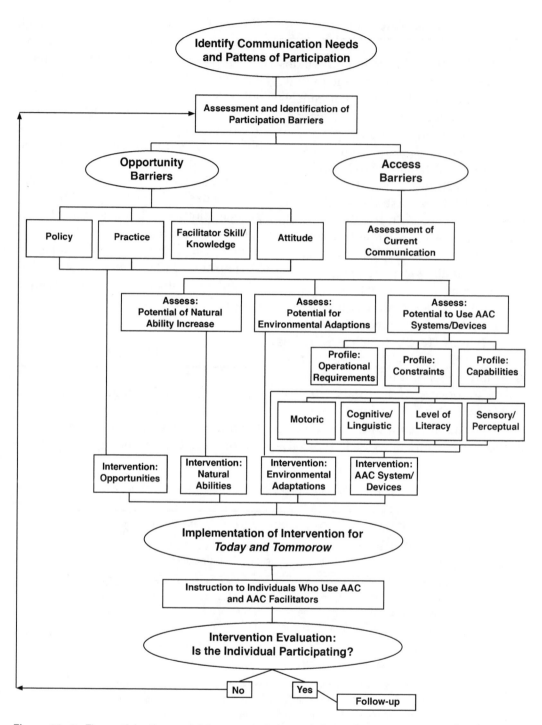

Figure 18–2. The participation model for augmentative and alternative communication (AAC).

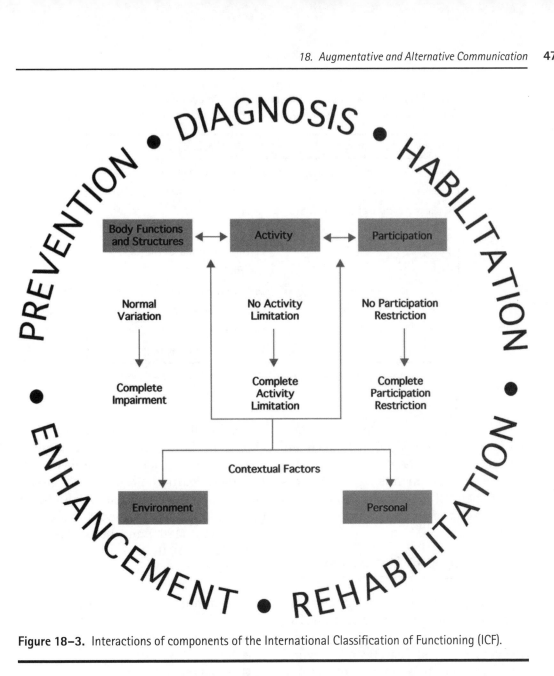

Figure 18–3. Interactions of components of the International Classification of Functioning (ICF).

of communication (ASHA, n.d.-a; Blackstone, Williams, & Wilkins, 2007; Branson & Demchak, 2009; Davidoff, 2017). An additional factor that contributes to the need for AAC is challenging communicative behavior that (a) is unacceptable in society, (b) involves the use of unusual or reflexive movement, (c) fatigues the user, (d) is so unconventional or idiosyncratic that only familiar communicators can interpret them, (e) is inefficient, or (f) is potentially harmful to the user (ASHA, n.d.-a). Complex communication needs requiring the use of AAC can be congenital or acquired. Common congenital and acquired impairments that can cause CCNs, necessitating the needed for AAC, are listed in Table 18–2. When working with individuals with CCNs, it is vital to keep in mind that these impairments do

Table 18–2. Common Congenital and Acquired Impairments That May Benefit From Augmentative and Alternative Communication (AAC)

Congenital Impairments	Acquired Impairments
Autism spectrum disorder (ASD)	Acquired apraxia of speech (AOS)
Cerebral palsy (CP)	Amyotrophic lateral sclerosis (ALS)
Childhood apraxia of speech (CAS)	Aphasia
Intellectual disability (ID)	Cancer
Deaf/blind	Cerebral vascular accident (CVA)
	Dysarthria
	Locked-in syndrome
	Multiple sclerosis (MS)
	Primary progressive aphasia (PPA)
	Traumatic brain injury (TBI)

Sources: ASHA, n.d.-a; Beukelman & Mirenda, 2013; Hux, Weissling, & Wallace, 2008.

not always suggest a concomitant cognitive impairment (Fried-Oken, Beukelman, & Hux, 2012). As Chapter 4 (Professional Conduct) recommends, practitioners should view all individuals as unique in their needs, preferences, and abilities.

Purpose of AAC Intervention

When working with individuals with CCNs, it is important to be mindful of the primary purpose of AAC intervention, which extends significantly beyond the directive to find a technical solution to communication problems (Light & McNaughton, 2012). Augmentative and alternative communication intervention involves language organization, strategies, and techniques, and also the emotional and social issues that surround receptive and expressive language impairments (Cress, 2004). The broadly stated and humanistic purpose of AAC intervention is to enable people to engage efficiently and effectively with others in a

variety of situations and contexts of their choice. It allows users to participate in conversations at home and in their communities, learn their native language, and to initiate and maintain relationships (Light, Parsons, & Drager, 2002). According to Light (1988) and Beukelman and Mirenda (2013), the purposes of communicative interaction are:

- Communication of wants and needs,
- Information transfer,
- Social closeness,
- Social etiquette, and
- Communication with oneself or engagement in inner dialogue.

In order to fully accomplish these goals and support communicative interaction, AAC intervention needs to incorporate not just the AAC user, but must also consider and integrate family members and other communicative partners— AAC cannot be taught or used in isolation (Cress, 2004).

Myths About AAC Use

One of the basic theoretical underpinnings of AAC is that all individuals have the right to communicate, regardless of the method, and regardless of a perceived ability to communicate. Although the effectiveness of AAC has been demonstrated through an extensive body of literature (ASHA, n.d.-a; Beukelman & Mirenda, 2013; Light, & McNaughton, 2012b), there is a high level of misunderstanding about its assessment and intervention among related professionals, family members, and even users themselves. Table 18–3 identifies some of the more commonly encountered myths and provides research-based data that dispel them and offers support for the use of appropriate AAC assessment and intervention. Although this table highlights many of the myths regarding AAC use, various researchers have indicated that a minimal level of speech comprehension and the ability to use distal gestures, such as pointing, may be suggestive of greater success in AAC use (ASHA, n.d.-a). For individuals with congenitally based CCNs, it is never too early to introduce AAC into comprehensive communication and language intervention (Cress & Marvin, 2003; Romski & Sevcik, 2005). Similarly, for individuals with acquired CCNs, early introduction of compensatory AAC strategies can support remaining verbal comprehension and expression abilities (Hux, Weissling, & Wallace, 2008).

AAC Components

AAC should be thought of as an integrated communication system comprised of several primary components or modes rather than a single device: symbols, aids, strategies, and techniques (ASHA, n.d.-.a; Beukelman & Mirenda, 2013).

Symbols

Symbols can be graphic (e.g., photographs, text), auditory (e.g., spoken words), gestural, or tactile (e.g., textures, objects) and can be unaided, such as facial gestures, or aided, such as pictures (ASHA, n.d.-a). The concept of symbols is multifaceted and can be described given their visual relationship to an actual concept (also known as iconicity); their level of stability or transience; and their acquisition hierarchy (ASHA, n.d.-a; Beukelman & Mirenda, 2013).

Iconicity can be thought of as how guessable the symbol is, without assistance (ASHA, n.d.-a). Symbol iconicity ranges from transparent, where the symbol demonstrates a clear relationship to the concept (e.g., a drawing of a house that represents *home*; Figure 18–4A), to opaque, where the symbol does not demonstrate a clear relationship to the concept without an established meaning (e.g., the ASL sign for *home*; Figure 18–4B) (Drager & Light, 2010; Drager et al., 2003).

Symbol stability refers to how dynamic or static a symbol is. Spoken symbols (i.e., words) and manual signs are very dynamic and transient, whereas graphic symbols are considered static or permanent (Beukelman & Mirenda, 2013). Symbols that are more static and permanent place lower cognitive demands on both the sender and the receiver than do dynamic or transient symbols. Dynamic symbols require sustained attention, memory, and sequencing abilities, which can sometimes exceed developing or preserved skills (Fager, Hux, Beukelman, & Karantounis, 2006).

Table 18–3. Common Myths and Truths About Augmentative and Alternative Communication (AAC)

Myth	Truth
There are prerequisite skills, cognition levels, and communicative abilities required for AAC assessment and intervention.	Although language and cognition are interrelated, it remains unclear which force drives the other, and without a method of communication, cognition cannot be demonstrated or assessed definitively.
	AAC access has been demonstrated to support the early cognitive and linguistic skills necessary for the development of language.
There is a minimum age for AAC assessment and intervention.	The earliest AAC intervention can apply to a child's behaviors, gestures, cooperative actions, and sounds.
	AAC use benefits infants and toddlers, based on evidence suggesting that a child's early learning experiences in the first 3 years of life are foundational to subsequent brain development.
Language acquisition follows a symbolic representational hierarchy that flows from objects to written words.	During the early phases of language development, symbol type (i.e., iconic or abstract) may not be a significant factor in intervention since, ultimately, all symbols function similarly.
AAC use will interfere with a child's speech or vocal development.	AAC use does not impede vocalizations or oral language. AAC has been shown to encourage vocalizations and oral language by increasing communication opportunities.
	Children typically use the most efficient method of communicating, and with the inherent advantages that speech offers over AAC, children will move to speech when possible.
AAC implementation should be delayed until a consistent verbal communication delay is confirmed over time.	Communication across all modes in the early childhood years should be made available to the child.
	Delaying AAC implementation, when behaviors and physical limitations suggest a risk for impaired speech, can have a negative effect on the long-term development of speech and language.
The introduction of AAC decreases the users' need to work on speech.	Natural speech improvements often correlate with the introduction of AAC.
	AAC users typically use multiple communication modes, including technology, gestures, and natural speech.
Speech, regardless of how limited it is, should be the primary mode of communication.	Children and adults who are left without a reliable means to communicate even their basic wants and needs have the potential to demonstrate behavior problems, social failure, academic challenges, and learned helplessness.
The use of AAC makes individuals look different from their peers.	Rather than inhibiting language production, the implementation of AAC has the potential to inhibit challenging communicative behavior and build more socially acceptable behaviors.
	Ultimately, individuals look more atypical when they are unable to express themselves.
AAC use represents the last resort in speech-language intervention.	Early introduction of AAC fosters communication and language skills, and diminishes communication failure for both beginning communicators and those with acquired disabilities.
	AAC intervention is holistic in that it addresses improving communication skills across all modes, including verbal skills.

Table 18–3. *continued*

Myth	Truth
AAC, if unsuccessful, can be considered a failure after the implementation of only a limited set of AAC strategies or techniques.	Because AAC is a continuum that may involve a variety of strategies and support levels, multiple attempts may be necessary to find the right combination of strategies, aids, support, and techniques.

Sources: ASHA, n.d.-a Beukelman & Mirenda, 2013; Beukelman, Fager, Ball, & Dietz, 2007; Branson & Demchak, 2009; Cress & Marvin, 2003; Light & Drager, 2007; National Scientific Council on the Developing Child, 2007; Romski & Sevcik, 2005; Augmentative and Alternative Communication Connecting Young Kids (YAACK), n.d.

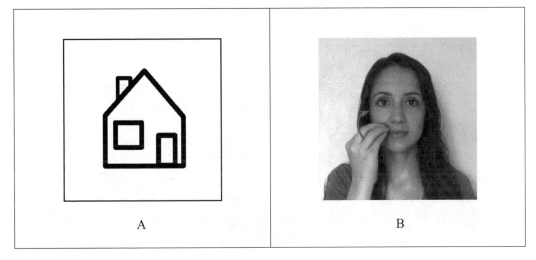

Figure 18–4. Example of transparent versus opaque symbol iconicity. **A.** Black and white icon of *home. Boardmaker.* Copyright 2018. Tobii Dynavox, Pittsburgh, PA All rights reserved. Used with permission. **B.** American Sign Language (ASL) sign for *home.*

As to acquisition hierarchy, symbols can be arranged in order, given their visual relationship to the actual concept, progressing from real objects (i.e., realia) to a signed representation of a concept (e.g., ASL; ASHA, 2004). Symbols that are more concrete, such as a juice box representing *juice*, are easier to comprehend than more abstract representations, such as the signed Amerind symbol for *more* (Figure 18–5; Fried-Oken, Beukelman, & Hux, 2012). Abstract symbols typically require training to use and understand.

Box 18–1 contains a generally accepted symbol hierarchy with respect to ease of acquisition, starting more easily acquired symbols (i.e., objects) and progressing to symbols requiring more effort to acquire (i.e., traditional orthography). Research conducted on symbol use for people with acquired communication impairments suggests that including contextually rich photographs (Figure 18–6) may lead to more successful expressive and receptive symbol use (Fried-Oken et al., 2012).

Figure 18–5. Amerind Symbol for *more*. *Board-maker.* Copyright 2018. Tobii Dynavox, Pittsburgh, PA. All rights reserved. Used with permission.

Box 18–1. Symbol Acquisition Hierarchy

1. Objects
2. Color photographs
3. Black and white photographs
4. Miniature objects

5. Black and white line drawings
6. Blissymbols
7. Traditional orthography

Sources: Beukelman & Mirenda, 2013; Glennen & DeCoste, 1997.

Figure 18–6. Example of a contextually rich photograph.

On AAC systems, symbols can be arranged in multiple ways, such as alphabet-based methods that use traditional spelling as a means of generating messages. A second way that symbols can be arranged is through single-meaning message generation, where a single graphic icon represents a single word or message, such as when touching an image with a school indicates it is time to go to school. A final method of symbol arrangement is the use of semantic compaction, which is based on iconic encoding with multiple meanings. This concept will be explained more fully in the discussion of vocabulary arrangement (ASHA, n.d.-a).

Aids

Aids, or devices, are used to convey or receive the actual message, such as switch-activated devices or a series of symbols that convey meaning (ASHA, n.d.-a). Augmentative and alternative communication aids can be either aided or unaided, although most people who are nonverbal use multiple communication modalities that incorporate both aided and unaided systems (ASHA, n.d.-a).

Unaided Communication. Unaided communication methods involve solely the individual's body (Beukelman & Mirenda, 2013). Unaided communication methods offer an efficient communication method without the need for external devices. Successful unaided communication requires a shared understanding between communication partners of the meaning or situational context represented by a nod, gesture, vocalization, or symbol. This makes communication with unfamiliar partners more difficult, unless the communicative act is transparent (i.e., guess-able) enough to establish a clear meaning. Box 18–2 lists examples of unaided communication. Unaided communication strategies require at least a minimal level of motoric ability. Typical users include people with dysarthria or people who have experienced a stroke or a traumatic brain injury, who are able at least partially to use their preserved cognitive, linguistic, visual, and motoric abilities to convey their messages (ASHA, n.d.-a; Beukelman & Mirenda, 2013).

Aided Communication. Aided communication methods involve the use of tools, equipment, or devices in addition to an individual's body (ASHA, n.d.-a). Aided AAC systems offer increased message length, complexity, speed, and comprehensibility to the communication partner. Aided communication strategies also require at least a minimal level of motoric ability and cognition. It is important to note that there is an inverse relationship between AAC system complexity and the complexity of an individual's communication needs. There is also a direct relationship between reliance on an interlocutor, or communication partner and the complexity of an individual's communication needs, as seen in Figure 18–7.

> ### Box 18–2. Examples of Unaided Communication
>
> - Speech
> - Eye movements
> - Head nods
> - Gestures
> - Vocalizations
> - Sign language
> - Facial expressions

Figure 18–7. Factors influencing augmentative and alternative communication (AAC) intervention and use.

People with a variety of disorders (e.g., childhood apraxia of speech, apraxia of speech, amyotrophic lateral sclerosis) who are able to use preserved cognitive, linguistic, visual, or motoric abilities to communicate are typical users of aided AAC (Beukelman & Mirenda, 2013; Glennen & DeCoste, 1997).

The class of aided systems can be further broken down into the categories of low-tech and high-tech (Loncke, 2014). Low-tech AAC systems are typically hand-made and not computer based. Box 18–3 lists examples of low-tech, aided communication and Appendices 18–A to 18–D describes some of them.

An additional set of aided low-tech communication devices are those that use

---

Box 18–3. Examples of Low-Tech Aided Communication

- Paper and pencil (e.g., for use in writing and drawing)
- Communication books (Appendix 18–A)
- Eye-gaze boards (Appendix 18–B)
- Alphabet boards (Appendix 18–C)
- Choice boards (Appendix 18–D)
- Real objects
- Remnant books (e.g., movie tickets, concert programs, menus from recent life events)

an electronic component, but are limited in their output (Loncke, 2014). Examples of these include:

- Tactile communicators (Appendix 18–E)
- Switch and button communicators (Appendix 18–F)

High-tech AAC systems typically contain microcomputer chips and can be dedicated solely to AAC use or can be a program or app on a non-dedicated mobile device or a computer (Beukelman & Mirenda, 2013). They might offer message retrieval and storage, stored or synthetic speech, prediction features, and complex vocabulary (Beukelman & Mirenda, 2013). A significant benefit of AAC systems with speech-generating devices, or voice output, is their ability to enhance communicative interaction between people (Cress & Marvin, 2003). Voice output can be accomplished through stored speech, also called digitized speech, which is similar to a tape recording, and synthesized speech, which

is computer generated. The quality of synthesized speech varies based on the system utilized. Stephen Hawking, the British physicist, was probably the most well known user of a synthetic voice (Figure 18–8). Although Hawking was British, his voice used an American accent and in 2006 Hawking stated, "I have kept it [the voice] because I have not heard a voice I like better and because I have identified with it (Reuters, 2018).

AAC users identify the voice quality of AAC systems as being highly important and consider them extensions of the self. Improvements in this technology can have a profound impact on overall quality of life (Mills, Bunnell, & Patel, 2014). Although options for speech output remain limited, recent advances in synthesized speech include voice conversion (Mills et al., 2013), which works by extracting data from a speech corpus and generating a unique synthetic voice for each individual. Although still a relatively new technology, as voice conversion techniques continue to develop there will be more and better choices for AAC users

Figure 18–8. Stephen Hawking with his high-tech augmentative and alternative communication (AAC) system. Courtesy of Bing Images, free to share and use commercially.

that including natural-sounding and intelligible speech. Typically, AAC systems offer a narrow selection of pre-stored voices, which can be customized by altering loudness, rate, and pitch. Some synthesized voices are very intelligible listeners and others can be robot-like, requiring careful listening. An example of digitized speech is when a classmate or peer pre-records a short phrase (e.g., "Let's go to recess") with an AAC device, which can then be selected and played by the AAC user in a communicative context. Recent advances in technology also allow AAC users, such as those diagnosed with a progressive disease (e.g., amyotrophic lateral sclerosis, multiple sclerosis), to preserve samples of their speech within a computer system to be retrieved at a later date, when they are no longer able to communicate vocally (Mills et al., 2013).

Box 18–4 lists examples of high-tech, aided communication that you can find samples of in Appendices 18–G to 18–J. These are but a few examples of the many high-tech communication devices available to AAC users. As you grow in your skills and experience with AAC, you will no doubt learn about many more options.

Strategies

Because AAC users typically communicate at a fraction of the rate of natural speakers (2 to 15 words per minute versus 200 words per minute), *strategies*, which are used to improve and refine messages and increase the rate of communication, are of high value to AAC users and their communication partners (ASHA, n.d.-a; Beukelman & Mirenda, 2013). Strategies can be used across aided and unaided communication and low- and high-tech devices, and may decrease the cognitive and motoric demands on users. Although a complete review of all available strategies is beyond the scope of this chapter, Table 18–4 lists a few examples. Additional methods of refining and improving messages and enhancing the rate of communication are topic identification and partner-focused questions (Beukelman & Mirenda, 2013).

Techniques

Techniques are either direct or indirect selection methods available to users of AAC communication to transmit the message itself (ASHA, n.d.-a; Beukelman & Mirenda, 2013).

Direct selection involves an interaction between the motoric abilities of the AAC user and the manual, mechanical, or technological options offered by the communication device. It can be low-tech or high-tech, and allows users to make a direct communication choice via voice, a body

---

Box 18–4. Examples of High–Tech Aided Communication Devices

- Speech-generating devices (SGD) and voice output communication aids (VOCAs) (Appendix 18–G)
- Text-to-speech devices (Appendix 18–H)
- Computers, iPads, and tablets, with software or apps for communication purposes (Appendices 18–I and 18–J)

Table 18–4. Examples of Augmentative and Alternative Communication Strategies

Strategy	Definition	Example
Encoding	The use of prestored, shortened code to represent a longer message	The use of the letters GG to represent the phrase "Please get my glasses."
Prediction	A dynamic interaction between the AAC user and the AAC device or communication partner that allows for prediction of the balance of a partially formulated message at the letter, word, or phrase level,	Letter: Based on rules of spelling and letter patterns. Word: Based on context and rules of syntax. Phrase: Based on context and topic and sophisticated computer algorithms that incorporate natural language constructs.
Sequencing	Combining symbols to create spontaneous, novel utterances for communication and that moves beyond the single-symbol level.	An example of a sequenced phrase can be seen in Figure 18–9.

Figure 18–9. Example of symbol sequencing. *Boardmaker.* Copyright 2018. Tobii Dynavox, Pittsburgh, PA. All rights reserved. Used with permission.

part, such as a hand or the head, or some form of technical aid, such as a light pointer, adapted mouse, or a switch. Examples of direct selection techniques are highlighted in Box 18–5 (Beukelman & Mirenda, 2013).

Recent advances in computer technology allow an additional method of direct selection using the eyes, referred to as eye tracking. High-tech devices can track the movements of the eye and register

Box 18–5. Examples of Direct Selection Methods

- Eye-gaze
- Physical contact
  - Manual touch or pressure on keyboard or switch
- Pointing (no contact)
- Voice recognition activation

a location on the screen where an AAC user gazes. If the user holds her gaze in that position or blinks, the system registers that as a selection (e.g., activation of a symbol on the screen; Fager, Bardach, Russell, & Higginbotham, 2012).

For those individuals without sufficient motoric abilities to make direct selections, *indirect selections* compensate for these limitations. With indirect selection, also called scanning, users make a communication choice through intermediary steps facilitated by their communication partner or the device (Beukelman & Mirenda, 2013). To use indirect selection, the AAC user may make a selection from a series of symbols. For example, symbols can be presented auditorily, as when a communication partner calls out individual letters of the alphabet and waits for confirmation or rejection of a specific letter choice. Symbols can also be presented visually, as when a communication partner points to symbols on a communication board or when a high-tech system highlights a symbol by changing its background color, placing a dark outline around the symbol, and so forth. The AAC user selects a desired symbol using some form of physical confirmation to the listener, such as a head nod or eye-blink, or a tap of the finger, wrist, or head on a switch (Appendix 18–F), which then triggers the AAC device. The speed and timing of the auditory or visual scanning can be individualized to reflect the cognitive, linguistic, visual, auditory, and motoric abilities of the user.

AAC Intervention Guidelines

AAC intervention occurs within the context of a team of stakeholders that includes the AAC users and their families (ASHA, n.d.-a). In addition to you and your supervising SLPs, this team of related professionals can also include general and special education teachers, physical therapists, occupational therapists, and rehabilitation engineers (Beukelman & Mirenda, 2013). As with all other speech-language intervention, AAC intervention revolves around the individualized goals written by a speech-language pathologist (SLP). For your reference, Chapter 7 (Lesson Plans and Goals) contains sample AAC objectives. Augmentative and alternative communication intervention looks much like other speech-language intervention except that input and output can be mediated through alternative means, such as vocalizations, signs, objects, or a low- or high-tech device. Best practices suggest focusing on the goal of the intervention rather than modality of production. One of the basic premises of AAC intervention, which mirrors a basic premise of all speech-language intervention, is that it should be functional, take place in naturalistic contexts and situations (Beck, Stoner, & Dennis, 2009), and be led by the AAC user's interests, innate curiosities, actions, and behaviors (Cress & Marvin, 2003; Hourcade, Everhart Pilotte, West, & Parette, 2004; Romski & Sevcik, 2005).

Best practices suggest that the clinician overlay targeted language or provide a verbal model in parallel with symbol manipulation or referencing (Beck, Stoner, & Dennis, 2009; Dada & Alant, 2009). This method of evidence-based intervention, called *augmented input strategies*, has the potential to enhance expressive and receptive language skills. Modeling language allows users to learn, restore, and use language. An example of this method is when a clinician points to an icon for baby and crib and comments to the child, "Oh look, the baby is sleeping," or when working with adults, asking an individual.

"How many grandchildren do you have?" while pointing to icons representing *two* and *three* (Figure 18–10; Beck, Stoner, & Dennis, 2009). When implementing AAC intervention with adults who have cognitive or communication impairments and may have difficulty with symbolic representation (e.g., aphasia), augmented input strategies increase the likelihood of symbol comprehension and communication.

The dynamic aspect of AAC means that users may need to use multiple AAC systems, based on their audience and communication partners. For example, individuals may use vocalizations and signs with familiar communication partners (i.e., at home), and may use a picture-based system with unfamiliar communication partners (i.e., community members; ASHA, 2010). Similarly, because AAC is dynamic and multi-modal, modifications to the AAC system will likely be needed over the course of intervention. These modifications can involve all com-

ponents of the AAC system, such as the symbols used and the strategies and techniques employed. For children developing their speech, language, and communication abilities, the AAC components may increase in complexity and the messages increase in length. For adults with acquired CCNs, AAC modifications may be required due to speech, language, and communication improvements or due to diminishing capabilities that may accompany degenerative conditions (Beukelman & Ball, 2002).

As discussed in greater detail in Chapter 5 (Cultural and Linguistic Diversity), individuals' cultural experiences and background also influence intervention. While much of the research on AAC use has focused on Anglo-European culture, ideals and values, SLPAs must be aware of the values, ideals, and considerations of other cultures, ethnicities, and languages (ASHA, n.d.-b; Beukelman & Mirenda, 2013;) as cultural norms have a significant effect on the implicit and explicit rules of communication and language (Hetzroni & Harris, 1996). The concepts of collectivism, cooperation, interdependency, family hierarchies, respect, politeness, and levels of directness within the communication cycle vary across cultures, social communities, customs, and languages and must be considered by SLPAs involved in the implementation of AAC systems. Best practices in AAC implementation allow users to code-switch, which means to adjust the content and complexity of their communication based on their communication partner/partners, whether they be peers, family members, or health care or educational professionals (ASHA, n.d.-a). Additional factors to consider include user and family attitudes toward technology and the possible stigmatization of disabilities,

Figure 18–10. *Boardmaker* choice icons. *Boardmaker.* Copyright 2018. Tobii Dynavox, Pittsburgh, PA. All rights reserved. Used with permission.

rehabilitation services, and education (ASHA, n.d.-a; Beukelman & Mirenda, 2013; Parette & Scherer, 2004). These factors should be carefully considered, especially given the fact that stigmatization is closely associated with abandonment of AT (Parette & Scherer, 2004).

Lastly, vocabulary selection and organization play a key role in AAC intervention. It is generally accepted that both adults and children with CCNs benefit when a meaningful, functional, individualized, and motivating vocabulary is available to them. Vocabulary selection is an ongoing process and is typically accomplished with the participation of AAC users and people significant to them, including family, friends, and related professionals such as SLPAs. Assessing vocabulary needs can involve ecological inventories or questionnaires (Fallon, Light, & Paige, 2001), communication diaries, and standardized vocabulary lists (Beukelman & Mirenda, 2013; Van Tatenhove, 2009). Vocabulary selections may depend on where the vocabulary is being used (e.g., home versus school), age, gender, disease progression, stage of language development, and literacy level (Beukelman & Mirenda, 2013).

Once established, the vocabulary should be broken down into the categories of core and fringe vocabulary for purposes of organization with the AAC device. *Core vocabulary* refers to words or messages that are highly functional, occur frequently across individuals, and relate to basic functional needs and social exchanges. *Fringe vocabulary* refers to words or messages that are specific to an individual or context (Beukelman & Mirenda, 2013; Van Tatenhove, 2009). As mentioned earlier, it is important to consider individual factors when creating a vocabulary for individuals with CCNs.

Two significant factors are the individual's level of language of development and literacy (Davidoff, 2017). Table 18–5 contains examples of core vocabulary for toddlers and adults, although it is not exhaustive. Just as individuals who use AAC to communicate present with unique profiles, their vocabularies too should be individualized.

Once the vocabulary has been defined, it must be organized physically and linguistically to promote efficient and effective communication. Whether creating a communication book or installing software, the vocabulary must be organized based on users' cognitive, communicative, and motoric abilities, their communication partners' knowledge and experience level, the communicative context, and frequency of use (Beukelman & Mirenda, 2013; Glennen & DeCoste, 1997). Vocabulary can be organized by semantic categories (e.g., people, locations, actions, activities) and syntax (e.g., parts of speech). Box 18–6 (Van Tatenhove, 2007) contains some basic tenants for vocabulary organization.

Table 18–5. Examples of Core Vocabulary for Toddlers and Adults

Toddler	Adult
All done	Go
Different	Eat
Help	Yes
Mine	No
More	Stop
Not/don't	Home
Stop	Restroom
That	
What	

Sources: Glennen & DeCoste, 1997; Van Tatenhove, 2007.

Box 18–6. Vocabulary Organization

■ Place core vocabulary with broad language functions in prominent positions that can be accessed quickly and easily, and place extended vocabulary in secondary positions that may be accessed through multiple steps or on subsequent pages.
■ Words or phrases that regulate activities or behaviors (e.g., more, again, help, all gone, all done) should hold prominent positions.
■ Words used to comment and relate to others (e.g., fun, good, bad, like) can hold secondary positions.
■ The words *yes* and *no* do not need to be in prominent positions if the user has an alternative and reliable method to communicate these ideas.

Helpful Tips

Chapter 5 includes tips for communicating with individuals with disabilities. These recommendations are applicable to AAC users as well. In addition, it is important to keep in mind that AAC users expend a considerable amount of energy and cognitive resources on communication, and they must adapt their communicative choices based on their available resources (Fried-Oken, Beukelman, & Hux, 2012). Best practices suggest the following (Accessible Technology Coalition, 2011):

■ Face the person.
■ Treat AAC users with the same manners and level of respect you use with others.
■ Speak directly to the AAC user; never talk about them with someone else when they are present.
■ Communication with the use of AAC takes additional time and energy—allow the AAC user time to compose and communicate their message.
■ Do not limit your questions to a simple *yes/no* format.
■ Do not be afraid to ask for clarification.
■ Always ask permission to provide assistance or touch their AAC device.
■ Be patient when experiencing technological glitches.
■ Avoid condescension.
■ Remember at all times that a person's silence does not necessarily reflect their desire to communicate.

SUMMARY

We end by reflecting on the words used in the introduction. Having read this chapter, you are now more familiar with the challenges and complexities of AAC. But you are now also more familiar with the ways AAC supports communicative competence, self-expression, and individual agency. While you may still conceive of yourself as a novice in the world of AAC, you have a theoretical foundation from which to approach your work with individuals with CCNs. Over time, this theoretical foundation will develop into sound clinical judgment and practice. After that, it is up to you to bridge any remaining gaps that stand between you and the individuals with CCNs you serve. And I wish you the best of luck in this very important work.

REFERENCES

Accessible Technology Coalition. (2011). *Etiquette in communicating with AAC users*. Retrieved from http://www.access-to-justice.org/pdfs/5_Etiquette_tips.pdf

American Speech-Language-Hearing Association (ASHA). (n.d.-a). *Augmentative and alternative communication*. Retrieved from http://www.asha.org/Practice-Portal/Professional-Issues/Augmentative-and-Alternative-Communication/

American Speech-Language-Hearing Association. (n.d.-b). *Cultural competence*. Retrieved from https://www.asha.org/Practice-Portal/Professional-Issues/Cultural-Competence//

American Speech-Language-Hearing Association. (n.d.-c). *International Classification of Functioning, Disability, and Health (ICF)*. Retrieved from https://www.asha.org/slp/icf/

American Speech-Language-Hearing Association. (2001). *Scope of practice in speech-language pathology*. Rockville, MD: Author.

American Speech-Language-Hearing Association. (2002). *2002 Omnibus survey caseload report: SLP*. Rockville, MD: Author.

American Speech-Language-Hearing Association [ASHA]. (2004). *Roles and responsibilities of speech-language pathologists with respect to augmentative and alternative communication: technical report* [Technical report]. Available from http://www.asha.org/policy

American Speech-Language-Hearing Association. (2010). *Communication services and supports for individuals with severe disabilities: FAQs*. Retrieved from http://www.asha.org/uploadedFiles/Communication-Services-Severe-Disabilities.pdf

American Speech-Language-Hearing Association. (2013). *Speech-language pathology assistant scope of practice*. Available from http:// www.asha.org/policy

American Speech-Language-Hearing Association. (2016). *Schools survey report: SLP caseload characteristics trends* 1995–2016. Rockville, MD: Author. Retrieved from https://www.asha.org/uploadedFiles/2016-Schools-Survey-SLP-Caseload-Characteristics-Trends.pdf

American Speech-Language-Hearing Association. (2017). *SLP health care survey report: Caseload characteristics and trends 2005–2017*. Rockville, MD: Author. Retrieved from https://www.asha.org/uploadedFiles/2017-SLP-Health-Care-Survey-Caseload-Characteristics-and-Trends-2005–2017.pdf

Augmentative and Alternative Communication (AAC) for Connecting Young Kids (YAACK). (n.d.). *Does AAC impede natural speech?—And other fears*. Retrieved from https://communicationmatrix.org/uploads/5346/YAACK%20posting%20AAC%20does%20not%20impeded%20speech.pdf

Barker, R. M., Akapa, S., Brady, N. C., & Thiemann-Bourque, K. (2013). Support for AAC use in preschool, and growth in language skills, for young children with developmental disabilities. *Augmentative and Alternative Communication, 29*(4), 334–346. doi:10.3109/07434618.2013.848933

Beck, A. R., Stoner, J. B., & Dennis, M. L. (2009). An investigation of aided language stimulation: Does it increase AAC use with adults with developmental disabilities and complex communication needs? *Augmentative and Alternative Communication, 25*(1), 42–54. doi:10.1080/07434610802131059

Beukelman, D. R., & Ball, L. J. (2002). Improving AAC use for persons with acquired neurogenic disorders: Understanding human and engineering factors. *Assistive Technology, 14*, 33–44. doi:10.1080.10400435.2002.10132053

Beukelman, D. R., Ball, L. J., & Fager, S. (2008). An AAC personnel framework: Adults with acquired complex communication needs. *Augmentative and Alternative Communications, 24*(3), 255–267. doi:10.1080/07434610802388477

Beukelman, D. R., Fager, S., Ball, L., & Dietz, A. (2007). AAC for adults with acquired neurological conditions: A review. *Augmentative and Alternative Communications, 23*(3), 230–242. doi:10.1080/07434610701553668

Beukelman, D. R., & Mirenda, P. (2013). *Augmentative and alternative communication: Supporting children and adults with complex communication needs.* Baltimore, MD: Paul H. Brookes.

Blackstone S., Williams M., & Wilkins D. (2007). Key principles underlying research and practice in AAC. *Augmentative and Alternative Communication, 23*(3), 191–203. doi:10.1080/07434610701553684

Brady, N., Bruce, S., Goldman, A., Erickson, K., Mineo, B., Ogletree, B., . . . Wilkinson, K. (2016). Communication services and supports for individuals with severe disabilities: Guidance for assessment and intervention. *American Journal on Intellectual and Developmental Disabilities, 121,* 121–138. doi:10.1352/1944-7558-121.2.121

Branson, D., & Demchak, M. (2009). The use of augmentative and alternative communication methods with infants and toddlers with disabilities: A research review. *Augmentative and Alternative Communications, 25*(4), 274–286. doi:10.3109/07434610903384529

Bugaj, C. R., & Norton-Darr, S. (2010). *The practical and fun guide to assistive technology in public schools: Building or improving your district's AT team.* Washington, DC: International Society for Technology in Education.

Calculator, S. N., & Black, T. (2009). Validation of an inventory of best practices in the provision of augmentative and alternative communication services to students with severe disabilities in general education classrooms. *American Journal of Speech-Language Pathology, 18,* 329–342. doi:10.1044/1058-0360(2009/08-0065)

Cress, C. J. (2004). Augmentative and alternative communication and language: Understanding and responding to parent's perspectives. *Topics in Language Disorders, 24*(1), 51–61.

Cress, C. J. & Marvin, C. (2003). Common questions about AAC services in early intervention. *Augmentative and Alternative Communication, 19*(4), 254–272. doi:10.1080/07434610310001598242

Dada, S., & Alant, E. (2009). The effect of aided language stimulation on vocabulary acquisition in children with little or not functional speech. *American Journal of Speech-Language Pathology, 18,* 50–64. doi:10.1044/1058-0360(2008/07-0018)

Davidoff, B. E. (2017). AAC with energy—Earlier. *The ASHA Leader, 22,* 48–53. doi:10.1044/leader.FTR2.22012017.48

Fager, S., Bardach, L., Russell, S., & Higginbotham, J. (2012). Access to augmentative and alternative communication: New technologies and clinical decision-making. *Journal of Pediatric Rehabilitation Medicine, 5,* 53–61. doi:10.3233/PRM-2012-0196

Fager, S., Hux, K., Beukelman, D. R., & Karantounis, R. (2006). Augmentative and alternative communication use and acceptance by adults with traumatic brain injury. *Augmentative and Alternative Communications, 22*(1), 37–47. doi:10.1080/07434610500243990

Fallon, K. A., Light, J. C., & Paige, T. K. (2001). Enhancing vocabulary selection for preschoolers who require augmentative and alternative communication (AAC). *American Journal of Speech-Language Pathology, 10*(1), 81–94. doi:10.1044/1058-0360(2001/010)

Fried-Oken, M., Beukelman, D. R., & Hux, K. (2012). Current and future AAC research considerations for adults with acquired cognitive and communication impairments. *Assistive Technology, 25,* 56–66. doi:10.1080/10400435.2011.648713

Glennen, S. L., & DeCoste, D. C. (1997). *Handbook of augmentative and alternative communication.* New York, NY: Delmar Cengage Learning.

Hetzroni, O. E., & Harris, O. L. (1996). Cultural aspects in the development of AAC users. *Augmentative and Alternative Communication, 12*(1), 52–58. doi:10.1080/07434619612331277488

Hourcade, J., Everhart Pilotte, T., West, E., & Parette, P. (2004). A history of augmentative and alternative communication for individuals with severe and profound disabilities. *Focus on Autism and other Developmental Disabilities, 19*(4), 235–244. doi:10.1177/10883576040190040501

Hux, K., Weissling, K., & Wallace, S. (2008). Communication-based interventions: Augmentative and alternative communication for people with aphasia. In R. Chapey (Ed.), *Language intervention strategies in aphasia and related neurogenic communication disorders* (pp. 813–836). Baltimore, MD: Lippincott Williams & Wilkins.

Light, J. (1988). Interaction involving individuals using augmentative and alternative communication systems: State of the art and future directions. *Augmentative and Alternative Communication, 4*(2), 66–82. doi:10.1080/07434618812331274657

Light, J. C., & Drager, K. (2007). AAC technologies for young children with complex communication needs: State of the science and future research directions. *Augmentative and Alternative Communication, 23*(3), 204–216. doi:10.1080/07434610701553635

Light, J., & McNaughton, D. (2012). The changing face of augmentative and alternative communication: Past, present, and future challenges. *Augmentative and Alternative Communication, 28*(4), 197–204. doi:10.3109/07434618.2012.737024

Light, J. C., Parsons, A. R., & Drager, K. D. R. (2002). "There's more to life than cookies": Developing interactions for social closeness with beginning communicators who require augmentative and alternative communication. In J. Reichle, D. Beukelman, & J. Light (Eds.), *Exemplary practices for beginning communicators: Implications for AAC* (pp. 187–218). Baltimore, MD: Paul H. Brookes.

Loncke, F. (2014). *Augmentative and alternative communication: Models and applications for educators, speech-language pathologists, psychologists, caregivers, and users.* San Diego, CA: Plural.

Mills, T., Bunnell, H. T., & Patel, R. (2014). Toward personalized speech synthesis for augmentative and alternative communication. *Augmentative and Alternative Communication, 30*(3), 226–236. doi:10.3109/07434618.2014.924026

National Scientific Council on the Developing Child. (2007). *The timing and quality of early experiences combine to shape brain architecture: Working paper No. 5.* Retrieved from: http://developingchild.harvard.edu

Parette, P., & Sherer, M. (2004). Assistive technology use and stigma. *Education and Training in Developmental Disabilities, 39*(3), 271–226.

Pinker, S. (1994). *The language instinct.* New York, NY: William Morris and Company.

Romski, M., & Sevcik, R. A. (2005). Augmentative communication and early intervention: Myths and realities. *Infants & Young Children, 18*(3), 174–185. doi:10.1097/00001163-200507000-0002

Sandle, P. (2018, March 14). Stephen Hawking's voice was his trademark. *Reuters.* Retrieved from https://www.reuters.com/article/people-hawking-voice/stephen-hawkings-voice-was-his-trademark-idUSL8N1QW6U2

Sigafoos, J., Schlosser, R. W., & Sutherland, D. (2013). Augmentative and alternative communication. In J. H. Stone & M. Blouin (Eds.), *International encyclopedia of rehabilitation.* Retrieved from https://www.researchgate.net/profile/David_Beukelman2/publication/230852920_Augmentative_and_Alternative_Communication/links/54871c4d0cf268d28f070dbc/Augmentative-and-Alternative-Communication.pdf

Staehely, J. (2000). Prologue: The communication dance. In M. Fried-Oken & H. A. Bersani, Jr. (Eds.), *Speaking up and spelling it out: Personal essays on augmentative and alternative communication* (pp. 1–12). Baltimore, MD: Paul H. Brookes.

Van Tatenhove, G. M. (2007). *Normal language development, generative language & AAC.* Retrieved from http://www.texasat.net/Assets/1--normal-language--aac.pdf

Van Tatenhove, G. (2009). Building language competence with students using AAC devices: Six challenges. *Perspectives on Augmentative and Alternative Communication, 18*(2), 38–47.

World Health Organization. (2014). *International Classification of Functioning, Disability and Health.* Geneva, Switzerland: Author. Retrieved from http://www.who.int/classifications/icf/en/

Wu, Y. & Voda, J. A. (1985). User-friendly communication board for nonverbal, severely physically disabled individuals. *Archives of Physical Medicine & Rehabilitation, 66,* 827–828.

APPENDIX 18–A
Example of Communication Book

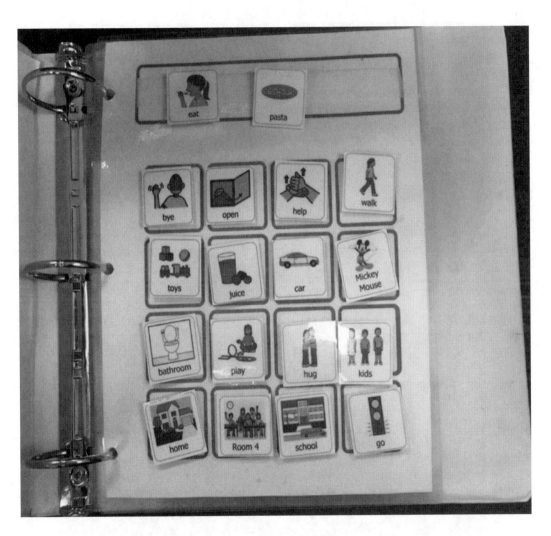

Note. Users point to symbols on the page to communicate.

Source: Boardmaker. Copyright 2018 Tobii Dynavox. All rights reserved. Used with permission.

APPENDIX 18–B
Example of Eye-Gaze Board

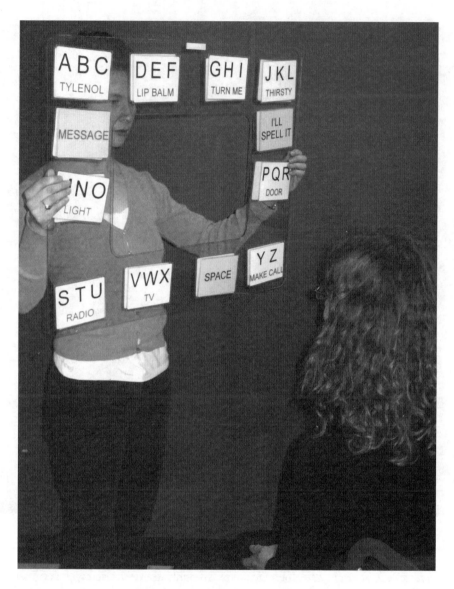

Note. The eye-gaze board is held up between the AAC user and the communication partner. The communication partner places his or her face within the boundaries of the hole in the center of the board and locks gaze with the AAC user before posing a question. The AAC user indicates his or her communication choice by gazing at the desired box and the communication partner confirms the choice verbally.

Source: Courtesy of Bing Images, free to share and use commercially.

APPENDIX 18–C
Example of Alphabet Boards

Traditional Alphabet Board

A	B	C	D	E	F
G	H	I	J	K	L
M	N	O	P	Q	R
S	T	U	V	W	X
Y	Z				
0	1	2	3	4	5
6	7	8	9		

Vowel-Based Alphabet Board (Wu & Voda, 1985)

A	B	C	D		
E	F	G	H		
I	J	K	L	M	N
O	P	Q	R	S	T
U	V	W	X	Y	Z

Note. AAC users communicate messages via alphabet boards by pointing to each letter to form words and phrases or by indicating their choice of auditorily presented letters with an agreed-upon method (e.g., blinking, finger raising, nodding).

APPENDIX 18–D
Example of Choice Board

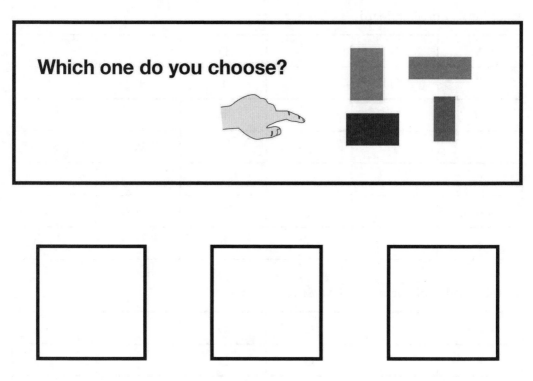

Note. Blank boxes can contain words or visual icons representing items or activities; users indicate a specific choice by pointing to a box(es).

APPENDIX 18-E
Totally Tactile Communicator

Note. Designed especially for visually impaired users, this communicator features brightly colored plates with raised designs and adjustable activation time (1–12 seconds) that gives users time to feel the plates (i.e., pre-recorded message choices) before activating their message. Features six levels for a total of 36 messages and a total record time of 300 seconds, 7 seconds per message.

Source: Totally Tactile Communicator. Enabling Devices, Hawthrone, NY. Used with express permission: Information available at http://www.enablingdevices.com

APPENDIX 18–F
Example of Switch Communicator
(Big-Talk Triple–Play Sequencer)

Note. A message is recorded using digitized speech (i.e., recorded human speech). AAC users press a button to play a message in a communicative context. Can also be used as a switch, when attached with a wire to a switch-enabled device. Switch-enabled devices systematically present options to AAC users. When the desired option is highlighted, pressing the switch activates a corresponding symbol on the switch-enabled system. This process is also known as scanning.

Source: Enabling Devices, Hawthorne, NY. Used with express permission. Information available at http://www.enablingdevices.com

APPENDIX 18–G
Speech Generating Device: *GoTalk Express 32*

Note. Users select an icon that makes the system play a pre-recorded message (also known as digitized speech).

Source: *GoTalk Express* 32. Attainment Company, Verona, WI. Used with express permission. Information can be found at http://www.attainmentcompany.com/gotalk-express-32

APPENDIX 18-H
Text-to-Speech Device: *LightwriterSL50TM*

Note. Users type words and the device converts written text into voice output.

Source: LightwriterSL50-Connect. Copyright. Abilia Ltd., Cambridge, England. Used with permission.

APPENDIX 18–I

Visual Scene Display: *Speaking Dynamically Pro* Software

Note. The user selects a "hot spot," and the software is programmed to speak out an associated phrase, such as "T.V." or "I want to play a game," using either digitized or synthesized speech.

Source: Boardmaker. Copyright 2018, Tobii Dynavox, Pittsburgh, PA. All rights reserved. Used with permission.

APPENDIX 18–J
Words For Life Application on an iPad Tablet

Note. User generate voice output by selecting icon(s).

CHAPTER 19

Adults with Acquired Neurologic Disorders

The brain is more than an assemblage of autonomous modules, each crucial for a specific mental function. Every one of these functionally specialized areas must interact with dozens or hundreds of others, their total integration creating something like a vastly complicated orchestra with thousands of instruments, an orchestra that conducts itself, with an ever-changing score and repertoire.

—Oliver Sacks

The topic of this chapter is acquired neurologic disorders and specifically those that occur in adults. This chapter will first cover some foundational knowledge, including important terms and definitions and a general description of the brain and its functions. Key principles helpful to understanding the settings where services are provided for adults with neurologic disorders are discussed. This is followed by a discussion of the nature, scope, and general treatment principles of several

507

common acquired neurologic disorders in adults.

It is important to first highlight that this chapter is by no means exhaustive in providing the critical information you need to effectively serve as a speech-language pathologist assistant (SLPA) for adults with acquired neurologic disorders (and their families). An entire textbook could be written on that topic alone and there are many such books available. Rather, this chapter serves as a review and reminder of several key principles. Your training as an SLPA has likely been more limited in this topic area, due in part to the very broad scope of the speech-language pathology field. It is impossible to cover every possible disorder, population, and setting where SLPAs are present within the limited scope of training required of SLPAs. In addition, SLPAs are less likely to provide services to adults with neurologic disorders in medical settings, than they are to provide services to children in school settings. This is due to differences in the nature and scope of services for adults and also the fee structures and billing options available in each setting.

This chapter is only devoted to adults with acquired neurologic disorders. This is not because children do not acquire neurologic disorders. To the contrary, children also experience acquired neurologic disorders, but the research evidence for children and adults in this area is distinctly different. In children, neurologic disorders impact a developing brain that is acquiring language, cognitive, and motor skill, whereas in adults, acquired neurologic disorders impact language, cognitive, and motor skills that have already developed. As such, the impacts, outcomes, and intervention approaches are different between adults and children

with acquired neurologic disorders. If you are working with a child with an acquired neurologic disorder, you should seek assistance from your supervising speech-language pathologist (SLP) as to the nature of the specific disorder, its impacts, and best practices for intervention. Do not assume that the details discussed in this chapter, specific to adults, are transferable to children, as that is likely not the case given the reasons already stated above.

FOUNDATIONAL KNOWLEDGE

Neurologic disorders are "diseases of the brain, spine and the nerves that connect them. There are more than 600 diseases of the nervous system, such as brain tumors, epilepsy, Parkinson's disease and stroke as well as less familiar ones such as frontotemporal dementia . . . " (University of California San Francisco [UCSF] Health, n.d., Neurological Disorders, para. 1). Often diseases of this nature are also described using the related terms *neurogenic* (originating in nervous tissue) or *neurological* (of or relating to neurology). Neurologic disorders in adults can be parsed into three categories: developmental (also called congenital), progressive, and acquired (Toronto Acquired Brain Injury Network, 2005). This chapter focuses on the latter, acquired neurologic disorders. Box 19–1 contains a brief description of each type of neurologic disorder.

As might be expected given the essential function of the brain to all human behavior, neurologic disorders can cause a wide range of impairments to physical, cognitive and psychological functioning (BIAA, 2012). The quote at the start of this chapter underscores this point, as does

Box 19–1. Categories of Neurologic Disorders

Developmental or Congenital Neurologic Disorders

A neurologic disorder that an individual is born with, such as cerebral palsy, muscular dystrophy, autism

Progressive Neurologic Disorders

A neurologic disease with a continuous gradual deterioration of brain function, such as dementia, Alzheimer's disease, and Parkinson's disease.

Acquired Neurologic Disorders

A neurologic disorder resulting from damage to the brain that occurs after birth, and is neither developmental nor progressive. Acquired neurologic disorders, also known as acquired brain injury (ABI), encompass both traumatic and non-traumatic brain injuries (Teasdale, Cullen, Marshall, Janzen, & Bayley, M. 2017). Traumatic ABI (sometimes referred to as traumatic brain injury, TBI) occurs as a result of an external force on the brain, such as with a car accident, fall, assault, or sports-related injury. Non-traumatic ABI occurs are alterations in brain function or caused by an internal force (Brain Injury Association of America (BIAA), 2012). which means those due to a medical problem or diseases such as stroke, brain tumors, and infection. Table 19–1 list additional examples of acquired brain injuries.

Table 19–1. Examples of Acquired Brain Injury (Traumatic and Non-Traumatic)

Traumatic Brain Injury Causes	Non-Traumatic Brain Injury Causes
• Falls	• Strokes (hemorrhage, blood clot)
• Assaults	• Infectious diseases (meningitis, encephalitis)
• Motor vehicle accidents	• Seizures
• Sports and recreation injuries	• Electric shocks
• Abusive head trauma (shaken baby syndrome, child, spousal, and elder abuse)	• Tumors
	• Metabolic disorders
• Gunshot wounds	• Neurotoxic poisoning (carbon monoxide, lead exposure)
• Workplace injuries	
• Military actions (blast injury)	• Lack of oxygen (drowning, choking, hypoxic and anoxic injuries)
	• Drug overdoses

Source: Brain Injury Association of America, 2012, Brain Injury Overview para. 5.

the following quote about the brain and its functions (BIAA, 2012):

> The human brain is magnificent and complex. The brain is made up of many parts, each with a specific and important function. It controls our ability to balance, walk, talk, and eat. It coordinates and regulates our breathing, blood circulation, and heart rate. It is responsible for our ability to speak, to process and remember information, make decisions, and feel emotions. Every brain is unique, ever-changing, and extremely sensitive to its environment. (Functions of the Brain, para. 1)

Always remember that a person with a brain injury is a person first. No two people are exactly the same and neither are their neurologic disorders. The effects of an acquired brain injury depends on factors unique to each person and the nature of their injury (BIAA, 2012). Although a detailed discussion of the brain and its function is beyond the scope of this chapter, a brief review of the general makeup of the brain is worthwhile as you consider your role in service as an SLPA for adults with acquired neurologic disorders.

The brain is comprised of roughly equal-size halves (also known as hemispheres of the brain): a left and a right hemisphere (Figure 19–1). Although they are roughly equal in size, they are not identical and they differ in terms of their functions (BIAA, 2012). The right side of the brain controls the left side of the body,

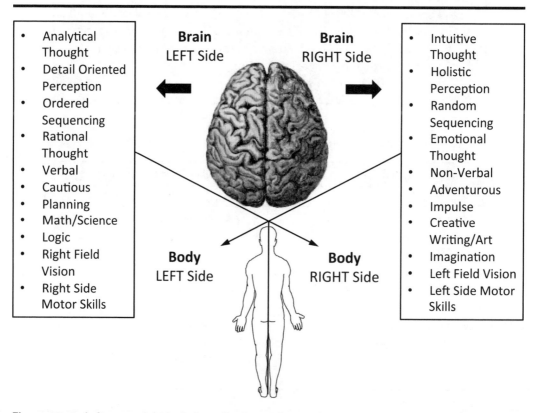

Brain LEFT Side
- Analytical Thought
- Detail Oriented Perception
- Ordered Sequencing
- Rational Thought
- Verbal
- Cautious
- Planning
- Math/Science
- Logic
- Right Field Vision
- Right Side Motor Skills

Brain RIGHT Side
- Intuitive Thought
- Holistic Perception
- Random Sequencing
- Emotional Thought
- Non-Verbal
- Adventurous
- Impulse
- Creative Writing/Art
- Imagination
- Left Field Vision
- Left Side Motor Skills

Body LEFT Side

Body RIGHT Side

Figure 19–1. Left versus right brain lateralization and control.

while the left side of the brain controls the right side of the body (see Figure 19–1). Common functions associated more with the left hemisphere than the right include analytical, logical, precise, organized, detached, and literal thinking (BIAA, 2012, Functions of the Brain). Common functions ascribed more to the right hemisphere than the left include creative, imaginative, intuitive, conceptual, empathetic, figurative thinking. These are perhaps false distinctions, however, as the two hemispheres of the brain are highly integrated and collaborate with one another to varying degrees in every important skill and life function. But because certain functions rely more on one hemisphere than the other, different patterns of impairment can result depending on the side of the brain impacted. Table 19–2 summarizes potential impairments as a result of injuries to a specific side of the brain.

Specific structures and regions of the brain affected by acquired neurologic disorders include the brainstem, cerebellum, and the four lobes of the brain (frontal, temporal, parietal, and occipital lobes;

Figure 19–2). Certain functions rely more on some of these structures and regions than others. As a result, general patterns of impairment arise when damage occurs in specific areas (BIAA, 2012, Functions of the Brain):

- Frontal lobe damage can impact speaking, motor functions, recall and control of emotions, impulses, and behavior.
- Temporal lobe damage may lead to difficulty with language production and comprehension, memory, social cognition, and complex visual processing.
- Parietal lobe damage can lead to difficulty integrating information from the five primary senses (sight, hearing, taste, smell, and touch), attention, proprioception (sensing where your own body parts are in space), and spatial cognition.
- Occipital lobe damage causes vision problems, like perceiving the size and shape of objects, and color and motion perception.

Table 19–2. Common Characteristics of Injuries to the Right Versus Left Hemispheres of the Brain

Left-Hemisphere Brain Injuries	Right-Hemisphere Brain Injuries
• Difficulties understanding language (receptive language)	• Visual-spatial impairments
• Difficulties signing, speaking and verbal output (expressive language)	• Visual memory deficits
• Catastrophic emotional reactions (depression, anxiety)	• Left-side neglect (inattention to the left side of the body)
• Right-side neglect (inattention to the left side of the body)	• Decreased awareness of deficits
• Impaired logic	• Altered creativity and music perception
• Sequencing difficulties	• Loss of "the big picture" type of thinking
• Decreased control over right-sided body movements	• Decreased control over left-sided body movements

Source: Brain Injury Association of America, 2012.

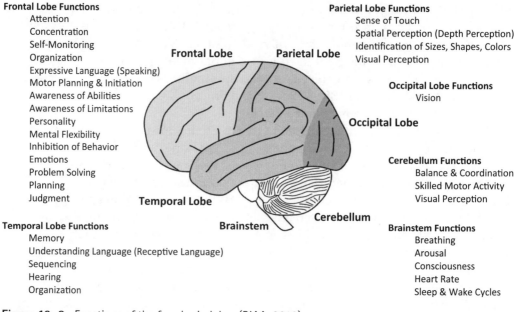

Frontal Lobe Functions
  Attention
  Concentration
  Self-Monitoring
  Organization
  Expressive Language (Speaking)
  Motor Planning & Initiation
  Awareness of Abilities
  Awareness of Limitations
  Personality
  Mental Flexibility
  Inhibition of Behavior
  Emotions
  Problem Solving
  Planning
  Judgment

Parietal Lobe Functions
  Sense of Touch
  Spatial Perception (Depth Perception)
  Identification of Sizes, Shapes, Colors
  Visual Perception

Occipital Lobe Functions
  Vision

Cerebellum Functions
  Balance & Coordination
  Skilled Motor Activity
  Visual Perception

Temporal Lobe Functions
  Memory
  Understanding Language (Receptive Language)
  Sequencing
  Hearing
  Organization

Brainstem Functions
  Breathing
  Arousal
  Consciousness
  Heart Rate
  Sleep & Wake Cycles

Figure 19–2. Functions of the four brain lobes (BIAA, 2012).

- Cerebellar damage may lead to difficulty with coordination of balance and movement.
- Brainstem damage can affect the body's involuntary functions, such as breathing, heart rate, and other functions critical to survival.

SERVICE PROVISION FOR ADULTS WITH NEUROLOGIC DISORDERS

The majority of services provided to adults with acquired neurologic disorders occurs within health care settings, especially in the early stages of recovery, but services are also provided in non-school private practice settings. Table 19–3 provides a brief description of settings of this nature. Although the exact numbers are not known, a smaller percentage of SLPAs are employed in health care settings, as compared to school and other non-health care settings, in part because there are fewer speech-language pathologists (SLPs) in health care settings. A 2011 American Speech-Language-Hearing Association (ASHA) membership count found that only 38% of certified SLPs were employed in health care settings (ASHA, 2011). In 2002, a survey of ASHA members in health care settings revealed the rarity of SLPA employment in these settings, with 98% of SLP respondents indicating SLPAs were *not* used in their departments (ASHA, n.d.-a, n.d.-b). This number may be increasing, however, given that a 2009 ASHA membership survey found that 32% of SLPs in health care settings reported employing one or more SLP support personnel in their department (ASHA, n.d.-b). Other reasons for a smaller numbers of SLPAs in health care

Table 19–3. Health Care and Non-School Private Practice Settings

Health Care Settings	
Acute Care Hospital	Inpatient care provided in an acute care medical facility
Inpatient Rehab	Free standing rehabilitation hospitals or rehabilitation units in acute care hospitals designed to support intensive, interdisciplinary rehabilitation of disabling conditions.
Outpatient	Outpatient services provided in a hospital
Skilled Nursing Facility	Skilled nursing units are usually either hospital-based or in a long-term care facility with skilled nursing care 24 hours a day. Rehab therapy services may be provided. Intermediate or extended care settings have 24-hour medical supervision, but skilled nursing services are not required.
Non-School Private Practice Settings	
Office Based	Any free-standing speech and hearing clinic or office-based private practice clinic providing speech-language services.
Home Health	Speech and language services provided in the home.

Source: American Speech-Language-Hearing Association, 2017.

settings could be the nature of services provided, the population served, or billing regulations for health care settings. Presently, Medicare policy precludes reimbursement for SLPA services. Private insurance reimbursement for SLPA services is variable based on the insurer (ASHA, n.d.-a).

Some cardinal features of speech-language pathology in healthcare settings include the use of a World Health Organization (WHO) International Classification framework, patient-centered care, interdisciplinary teams, and use of adult learning principles. Each of these are briefly discussed below.

World Health Organization International Classification Framework

The World Health Organization's (WHO) International Classification of Function-

ing, Disability and Health (ICF) is integral to understanding the recovery, outcome, and services associated with neurologic disorders. The ICF is *biopsychosocial*, as it integrates medical, psychological, and social perspectives of disability and function (WHO, 2002, pp. 9, 19). It addresses the concept of *disability* as something every human being may experience in their life, through a change in health or environment. Figure 19–3 is one representation of the WHO ICF model. As can be seen, disability and functioning are outcomes of the interactions between health conditions (diseases, disorders, and injuries) and contextual factors (personal and environmental; Ostergren, 2017). Personal contextual factors, such as gender, race, education, and coping strategies are independent of the health condition, but may influence how a person functions. Environmental contextual factors are factors outside of the person's control, such as family,

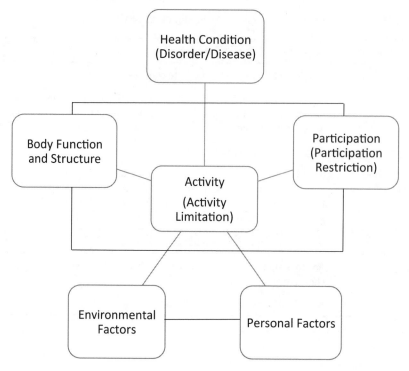

Figure 19–3. World Health Organization (WHO) International Classification of Functioning, Disability and Health (ICF).

work, laws, and cultural norms. There is a synergistic relationship among all three levels of human functioning: functioning of the body or body part(s) (body structure and function), executing tasks or actions (activity), and involvement in life situations (participation). Note that the first of those need not involve the whole person (e.g., a specific body part could be impaired), but the latter two occur at the level of the whole person (e.g., limited activity, restricted participation). As an SLPA you should be familiar with this framework and its related terminology. It is discussed clinically in health care settings and may be frequently referenced in the resources materials your supervising SLP asks you to read and research on the topic of acquired neurologic disorders.

Patient-Centered Care

Patient-centered care is another key feature of services for adults with acquired neurologic disorders, regardless of the setting where services are provided (Cott, 2004; Ostergren, 2017). Several long-standing principles of patient-centered care include (Picker Institute, n.d.):

- Respect for patients' values, preferences, and expressed needs,
- Coordination and integration of care,
- Information, communication, and education,
- Physical comfort,

- Emotional support and alleviation of fear and anxiety,
- Involvement of family and friends,
- Continuity and transition, and
- Access to care

In addition, patient-centered principles also include those listed in Table 19–4. These are each important factors to consider when providing services to adults with neurologic disorders. Take a moment to consider how these factors might influence the services you provide for adults with acquired neurologic disorders.

Interdisciplinary Teams

The third foundational feature of most rehabilitation settings for adults with neurologic disorders is interdisciplinary teams (Brasure et al. 2013; Ostergren, 2017). The most critical member of any interdisciplinary team are the individu-

Table 19–4. Client-Centered Rehabilitation Principles from the Client Perspective

Individualization of programs to the needs of each client in order to prepare them for life in the real world
Mutual participation with health care professionals in decision-making and goal setting
Outcomes that are meaningful to the client
Sharing appropriate and timely information and education according to clients' wishes
Emotional support
Family and peer involvement throughout the rehabilitation process
Coordination and continuity across multiple service sectors

Source: Cott (2004, pp. 1418-1419); Ostergren (2017).

als with neurologic disorders (and their family members). The composition of additional team members varies based on the age of the individual, the nature of impairments, the stage of recovery, and specialized training of particular team members. The team works together to provide integrated services and identify ways to optimize environmental and personal factors impacting daily function (Ostergren, 2017). Examples of potential team members are listed in Table 19–5. The table includes you, as a paraprofessional team member.

Adult Learner Principles

It is helpful to consider core tenants of adult learning pertaining to the services

Table 19–5. Interdisciplinary Team Members

Primary care physician
Psychologist
Speech-language pathologist
Audiologist
Rehabilitation psychologist
Behavioral specialist
Dietitian
Educator
Occupational therapist
Physical therapist
Psychiatrist
Social worker
Case manager
Therapeutic recreation specialist
Vocational rehabilitation counselor
Paraprofessionals

Source: Joint Committee on Interprofessional Relations Between the American Speech-Language-Hearing Association and Division 40 (Clinical Neuropsychology) of the American Psychological Association.

you provide to this population. An adult learner (Knowles, 1984a, 1984b)

- Has an independent self-concept and can direct his or her own learning,
- Has accumulated a reservoir of life experiences that is a rich resource for learning,
- Has learning needs closely related to changing social roles,
- Is problem-centered and interested in immediate application of knowledge, and
- Is motivated to learn by internal rather than external factors

Additional aspects of service provision for adults include are listed below (Knowles, 1984a; 1984b):

- Adults should be involved in the planning and evaluation of their instruction.
- Adults' experience (including mistakes) provides a basis for learning activities.
- Adults are most interested in learning about subjects that have immediate relevance to their life.
- Adult learning is problem-centered rather than content-oriented.

Take a moment to consider how these principles shape the services you provide as an SLPA working with adults with acquired neurologic disorders (as compared to services for children). Do these principles change specific aspects of your approach? They should, as many of them necessitate that your methods allow for more independence, self-direction, and self-determination. They also require that you work closely with your supervising SLP to make the function, purpose,

and rationale of the services you provide very clear to the adult you are working with. I encourage you to revisit this list frequently as an SLPA who is providing services to adults (not just those with neurologic disorders). Adherence to these principles will mean the difference between successful and unsuccessful treatment services for adult learners.

TREATMENT FOUNDATIONS

Before we discuss treatment approaches specific to given neurologic disorders, it is helpful to first take a 360 degree bird's-eye view of the foundations of treatment of neurologic disorders. Many treatment approaches have common core features and aims. There is a framework I adapted from various descriptions of treatment foundations in this area, including the Institute of Medicine's (IOM) descriptions for cognitive rehabilitation therapy (CRT) for TBI (IOM, 2011). It categorizes treatment approaches as either restoration, calibration, or compensation (Figure 19–4). *Restoration* approaches seek to improve, strengthen, or normalize an impaired function (IOM, 2011). Restoration approaches commonly involve repetition and drills or exercise-like activities, gradually increasing in difficulty and demand, to target an impaired process (IOM, 2011). Treatment in this frame is thought to act as restorative in overcoming damage related to a brain injury. *Compensation* approaches seek to provide alternative strategies for completing everyday activities, despite residual deficits (IOM, 2011). Compensation approaches are commonly divided into internal and external strategy compensation (IOM, 2011). External strategies uti-

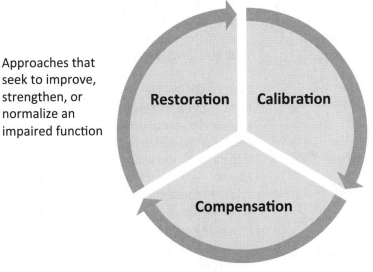

Figure 19–4. Framework of Treatment Approaches for Neurologic Disorders. Ostergren, J. (2017). *Cognitive Rehabilitation Therapy for Traumatic Brain Injury: A Guide for Speech-Language Pathologists.* Copyright 2017. San Diego, CA: Plural Publishing, Inc. All rights reserved. Reprinted with permission.

lize items external to the individual, such as augmentative and alternative communication (AAC), alarms, notebooks, notes, and calendars,. Internal strategies utilize internal processes such as word finding strategies, mnemonics, visualization, and word association. Lastly, *calibration* approaches seek to refine awareness, understanding, and self-measurements of performance (e.g., thinking about thinking) and use that information to shape performance. As you learn more about specific approaches in the sections that follow, I encourage you to reflect on these descriptions and identify aspects of specific techniques that appear to align with one, two, or more of these approaches.

Seeing these connections and the underlying themes will increase your understanding of any specific technique.

COMMON NEUROLOGIC DISORDERS

The acquired neurologic disorders discussed in this section are aphasia, right hemisphere brain dysfunction (RHBD), cognitive-communicative disorders associated with TBI, apraxia of speech, and dysarthria. Dysphagia, a disorder of swallowing, is also common, but ASHA's Scope of Practice for SLPAs has specific limitations on services provided by SLPAs for dysphagia. Specifically it states that, SLPAs may not (ASHA, 2013, Responsibilities Outside the Scope for Speech-Language Pathology Assistants, para. 2):

- Screen or diagnose patients or clients for feeding or swallowing disorders,
- Use a checklist or tabulate results of feeding or swallowing evaluations, or
- Demonstrate swallowing strategies or precautions to patients, family, or staff.

Some state regulations also limit provisions of services for dysphagia by SLPAs. As such, this chapter does not discuss dysphagia and its treatment. However, as with any personnel providing services to individuals potentially at risk of dysphagia, SLPAs should know the common signs and symptoms of dysphagia and the related topics of aspiration and tube feeding, as discussed in Chapter 6.

Aphasia

Aphasia is defined as an "impairment of language, affecting the production or comprehension of speech and the ability to read and write" (The Stroke Foundation, 2017, Glossary, para. 4). ASHA adds that aphasia is "an acquired neurogenic language disorder resulting from an injury to the brain—most typically, the left hemisphere" (ASHA, n.d.-c, para. 1). While impairments in cognitive skills can co-occur with aphasia, individuals with aphasia generally have intact nonlinguistic cognitive skills, such as memory and executive function. Aphasia involves varying degrees of impairment in four primary areas:(ASHA, n.d.-c):

- Spoken language expression
- Spoken language comprehension
- Written expression
- Reading comprehension

Box 19–2 (ASHA, n.d.-c) describes common signs and symptoms of aphasia for each of these impairments. Aphasia is also classified into different types (Table 19–6). Figure 19–5 depicts a decision flowchart about specific presenting features as they relate to these classifications.

The most frequent cause of aphasia is a stroke (National Institute on Deafness and Other Communication Disorders [NIDCD], 2015). Chapter 6 describes in more detail the origins of stroke and its common signs and symptoms. Other causes of aphasia are severe blows to the head, brain tumors, gunshot wounds, brain infections, and progressive neurological disorders, such as Alzheimer's disease (NIDCD, 2015). NIDCD (2015) estimated that there are 180,000 new cases of aphasia per year in the United States and that approximately 1 million people in the United States are living with aphasia. This translates to 1 in 250 people in the United States today (ASHA, n.d.-c).

Research has shown that individuals who receive treatment designed to reduce language impairments associated with aphasia improve to a greater extent than individuals who do not receive treatment (Simmons-Mackie & Kagan, 2007). Treatment is generally provided as early as tolerated (Brady et al., 2016; The Stroke Foundation, 2017). Table 19–7 contains a description of common treatment approaches for aphasia. Technology is increasingly advancing the treatment of aphasia, including computer-based software and a variety of low and high-technology approaches to AAC.

Box 19–2. Common Signs and Symptoms of Aphasia
(ASHA, n.d.–c, Signs and Symptoms)

Impairments in Spoken Language Expression

- Having difficulty finding words (anomia)
- Speaking haltingly or with effort
- Speaking in single words (e.g., names of objects)
- Speaking in short, fragmented phrases
- Omitting small words like *the, of,* and *was* (i.e., telegraphic speech)
- Making grammatical errors
- Putting words in the wrong order
- Substituting sounds or words (e.g., *table* for *bed; wishdasher* for *dishwasher*)
- Making up words (e.g., jargon)
- Fluently stringing together nonsense words and real words, but leaving out or including an insufficient amount of relevant content

Impairments in Spoken Language Comprehension

- Having difficulty understanding spoken utterances
- Requiring extra time to understand spoken messages
- Providing unreliable answers to "yes/no" questions
- Failing to understand complex grammar (e.g., "The dog was chased by the cat.")
- Finding it very hard to follow fast speech (e.g., radio or television news)
- Misinterpreting subtleties of language (e.g., taking the literal meaning of figurative speech such as "It's raining cats and dogs.")
- Lacking awareness of errors

Impairments in Written Expression (Agraphia)

- Having difficulty writing or copying letters, words, and sentences
- Writing single words only
- Substituting incorrect letters or words
- Spelling or writing nonsense syllables or words
- Writing run-on sentences that don't make sense
- Writing sentences with incorrect grammar

> ### *Impairments in Reading Comprehension (Alexia)*
>
> - Having difficulty comprehending written material
> - Having difficulty recognizing some words by sight
> - Having the inability to sound out words
> - Substituting associated words for a word (e.g., *chair* for *couch*)
> - Having difficulty reading non-content words (e.g., function words such as *to, from, the*)

Table 19–6. Types of Aphasia

Aphasia Type	Characteristics
Nonfluent Aphasias	
Broca's	Anomia, short phrase length, agrammatism, impaired prosody and intonation, relatively poor ability to repeat words and phrase, relatively good auditory comprehension, usually associated with right hemiparesis (one-sided weakness) or hemiplegia (one-sided paralysis), and may co-occur with dysarthria and apraxia of speech.
Transcortical Motor	Anomia, impaired initiation of spontaneous speech, short phrase length, preserved ability to repeat words and phrases (unlike in Broca's aphasia), relatively good auditory comprehension, and may co-occur with hemiparesis.
Mixed Nonfluent	Severe anomia, short phrase length, verbal output may be limited to stereotypic utterances, poor ability to repeat words and phrases, relatively poor auditory comprehension, with modality deficits less severe than with global aphasia but more severe than with Broca's aphasia.
Global	Severe deficits in all areas of language comprehension and production; profound anomia with virtually no speech output (may be restricted to stereotypic utterances), very poor auditory comprehension, often associated with right hemiplegia, and may co-occur with severe dysarthria, oral apraxia, apraxia of speech, and dysphagia.
Fluent Aphasias	
Wernicke's	Marked anomia, fluent but often meaningless speech (jargon), well-articulated and prosodic speech consisting of many error types (e.g., phonemic, semantic, and neologistic paraphasias), significant impairment in auditory comprehension, and poor repetition ability.
Transcortical Sensory	Severe anomia, fluent and in many cases meaningless speech (jargon), poor auditory comprehension, persevered ability to repeat words and phrases (unlike in Wernicke's aphasia), with prosodic features relatively preserved.
Conduction	Anomia, fluent output that may be interrupted by word-finding pauses or attempts to self-correct, frequent phonemic paraphasias, significant difficulty with repetition (disproportionate to other impairments), and good auditory comprehension.
Anomic	Significant word-finding difficulties in presence of otherwise fluent and grammatical speech, and relatively or entirely intact auditory comprehension and repetition.

Sources: Brookshire, 2015; Helm-Estabrooks, Albert, & Nicholas, 2014.

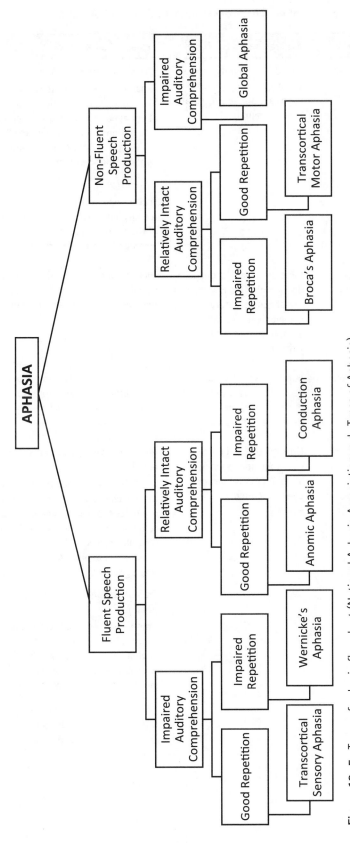

Figure 19–5. Types of aphasia flowchart (National Aphasia Association, n.d., Types of Aphasia).

Table 19–7. Common Treatment Approaches for Individuals with Aphasia

Treatment Type	General Treatment Goals	Example Approaches
Community Support and Integration	Provide community support and help individuals with aphasia more fully integrate into community life.	*Community Aphasia Groups* Expand "opportunities to socialize, converse, share ideas and feelings, receive support, and learn more about aphasia and aphasia resources" (ASHA, n.d.-b., Community Support and Integration, para. 10) via group treatment with individuals with aphasia (and their family members). *Life Participation Approach to Aphasia (LPAA)* Focuses on long-term management of aphasia and reengaging individuals with aphasia in activities of their choosing by implementing home and community based treatment.
Constraint-Induced Language Therapy (CILT)	Increase spoken language by discouraging (constraining) use of compensatory communication strategies, such as gestures and writing.	Focus on verbal production without the concurrent use of other communication modalities, via massed practice (multiple trials) and high-intensity training.
Melodic Intonation Therapy (MIT)	Improve expressive language using the prosodic elements of speech (i.e., melody, rhythm, and stress)	Engage undamaged areas of the right hemisphere to facilitate language expression using the intact function of singing (and other visual and tactile cues)
Multimodal Treatment	Use effective and efficient communication strategies as an alternative means of communication.	*Augmentative and Alternative Communication (AAC)* Use aided and unaided communication techniques to supplement or replace spoken language. Examples of aided techniques include picture communication symbols, line drawings, Blissymbols, tangible objects, and speech-generating devices. Examples of unaided techniques include manual signs, gestures, and finger spelling. *Promoting Aphasics' Communication Effectiveness (PACE)* Train individuals and their partners to improve conversation by using any and multiple modes of communication (spoken language, gestures, drawing, writing, partner support) to convey a meaningful and personally relevant message. *Visual Action Therapy (VAT)* Trains individuals with aphasia (commonly global aphasia) to use hand gestures to communicate wants and needs.

Table 19–7. *continued*

Treatment Type	General Treatment Goals	Example Approaches
Partner Approaches	Engage the communication partner in facilitating improved communication.	*Conversational Coaching* Teach verbal and nonverbal communication strategies to individuals with aphasia and their primary communication partners. The SLP serves as a coach, helping the communication partner select and deploy effective communication techniques. *Supported Communication Intervention (SCI)* Teach multimodal communication strategies to communication partners to support the dynamic and social process of communication for the individuals with aphasia.
Script Training	Use intact knowledge of scripts (understanding, remembering, and recalling event sequences of an activity) to facilitate participation in personally relevant activities.	Help the individuals with aphasia create, learn, and automatically use scripted monologues or dialogues during activities of interest.
Syntax Treatments	Improve the grammatical structure for sentence-level deficits.	*Sentence Production Program for Aphasia (SPPA)* Focus on sequential and structured practice of eight specific sentence types. *Treatment of Underlying Forms (TUF)* Treat sentence-level deficits by starting with more complex sentence structures that generalize to less complex sentences that share similar properties.
Word-Finding Treatments	Improve word finding deficit (anomia) in spontaneous utterances.	*Gestural Facilitation of Naming (GES)* Pair verbal expressions with intact gestural abilities to activate word retrieval. *Response Elaboration Training (RET)* Sequentially shape and elaborate on verbal responses using shaping, reinforcement, modeling, and structured cuing. *Semantic Feature Analysis Treatment* Train persons with aphasia in identifying the important semantic features thought to activate the needed semantic network for successful word retrieval. *Verb Network Strengthening Treatment (VNeST)* Improve the production of basic syntactic structures in sentences by targeting retrieval of verbs and their related semantic networks and associations. *Word Retrieval Cuing Strategies* Use structured phonological (beginning sound of a word) and semantic (contextual) cues to prompt word recall.

Source: ASHA, n.d.-b, Treatment Options.

Right Hemisphere Brain Damage

Right hemisphere brain damage (RHBD), also referred to as right hemisphere brain dysfunction or right hemisphere damage, is "an acquired brain injury—usually secondary to stroke or TBI—that causes impairments in language and other cognitive domains that affect communication." (ASHA, n.d.-d). Estimates indicate that 50% to 78% of individuals with RHBD exhibit one or more communication impairments (Lehman Blake, Frymark, & Venedictov, 2013) due to cognitive or language deficits.

In the realm of cognition, RHBD can impact attention, memory, and executive control (Lehman Blake, Frymark, & Venedictov, 2013). Examples of difficulties stemming from RHBD include the following (ASHA, n.d.-d., Signs and Symptoms, para. 11):

- Reduced sustained attention,
- Reduced selective attention (easily distracted),
- Reduced attention to detail,
- Unilateral visual neglect—typically, the left side,
- Decreased or no awareness of deficits (anosognosia),
- Reduced reasoning and judgment,
- Difficulty with sequencing and problem solving,
- Impaired executive functioning,
- Reduced inhibition, and
- Reduced recognition of facial expression.

In relation to language, RHBD can affect semantic processing of words, discourse processing (including narratives), prosody, and pragmatics. Generally syntax, grammar, phonological processing, and word retrieval are preserved in RHBD (ASHA, n.d.-h.). Box 19–3 contains a list of language deficits common to RHBD. Individuals with RHBD may also present with aprosodia, which is reduced (or absence of) normal variations in pitch, loudness, intonation, and rhythm of speech (Blake, 2018). Aprosody combined with reduced emotional expressiveness and diminished facial expressions may also lead to an appearance of flat affect in RHBD.

RHBD results from etiologies similar (causes) to those of aphasia, including stroke, TBI, brain tumors, and other neurological illnesses and injuries (Lehman Blake, Frymark, & Venedictov, 2013). Many individuals with RHBD may go untreated, making the exact incidence and prevalence of RHBD unknown. Following stroke, damage to the right hemisphere of the brain occurs in 42% to 49% of patients (ASHA, n.d.-h.).

The most commonly reported treatment areas reported for people with RHBD are difficulties with swallowing and the cognitive functions of memory and problem solving (ASHA, 2017). Disorders of expression, comprehension and pragmatics are also reported, but to a lesser degree than other cognitive symptoms (ASHA, 2017). Table 19–8 provides a summary of treatment approaches for RHBD.

Cognitive–Communicative Disorders Following Traumatic Brain Injury

Traumatic brain injury, also referred to as neurotrauma, is defined as "a disruption in the normal function of the brain that can be caused by a bump, blow, or jolt to the head or a penetrating head injury"

Box 19–3. Language Deficits Common to RHBD
(ASHA, n.d.-d., Language)

Discourse Comprehension Deficits

- Difficulty understanding abstract language, figurative language, lexical ambiguities, or information that can be interpreted in multiple ways
- Difficulty making inferences and understanding the global meanings of discourse such as topic, gist, and big picture
- Difficulty understanding jokes, irony, and sarcasm
- Difficulty understanding others' emotions

Discourse Production Deficits

- Verbosity (using more words than needed)
- Egocentric (self-centered) and tangential (peripheral or erratic) comments that digress from the topic
- Focus on irrelevant details
- Disorganized thoughts
- Impulsive and poorly organized responses

Pragmatic Communication Deficits

- Reduced eye contact
- Poor turn taking
- Decreased conversation initiation

Semantic Processing Deficits

- Understanding the metaphorical meaning of words (e.g., "a sea of grief" and "roller coaster of emotions")

(Centers for Disease Control [CDC], 2015, p. 15). An explosive blast can also cause a TBI (CDC, 2015). TBI can result when the head suddenly and violently hits an object, or when an object pierces the skull and enters brain tissue (National Institute of Neurologic Disorders and Stroke [NINDS], n.d.). TBI can range in severity (from mild to severe). The presence of any of the following clinical signs is considered a disruption in normal brain function after a TBI (Menon, Schwab, Wright, & Maas, Demographics and Clinical Assessments Working Group, 2010):

- Any period of loss of or decreased consciousness
- Any loss of memory for events immediately before (retrograde amnesia) or after the injury (post-traumatic, or anterograde amnesia);

Table 19–8. Treatment Approaches for RHBD

Treatment Type	General Treatment Goals	Example Approaches
Language Treatment	Improve: • Narrative and conversational discourse • Understanding and managing alternate meanings • Pragmatics	*Narrative and Conversational Discourse Training* Develop skills in making inferences and understanding the topic, gist, and big picture of conversation through either • Guided inference-generating that requires the individual to label, identify, and explain the relationship among items • Macrostructure tasks that require the individual to identify the "big picture" of news stories, picture scenes, or conversations and/or organize information into a logical sequence to support a main idea *Understanding and Managing Alternate Meanings Treatment* Improve the ability to understand lexical ambiguities, generate alternate meanings, and understand nonliteral language through tasks that require the individual to • Group words according to their positive or negative associations • Provide multiple and alternative meanings • Interpret figurative language *Treatment for Pragmatic Deficits* Improve social communication skills through coaching, visual and verbal feedback, video modeling, rehearsal, role-play, and individual and group practice, targeting • Use of appropriate and social and cultural conversational conventions, such as nonverbal cues, turn-taking, organized and on-topic conversation, and social boundaries. • Understanding other peoples' beliefs, attitudes, and emotions and using that understanding to navigate social situations
Prosody	Improve expression and/or interpretation of prosody, such as varying pitch, loudness, and rhythm	*Direct Treatment Approaches for Prosody* Improve conscious control in expression of prosody by using production drills and practice. *Compensatory Treatment Approaches for Prosody* Focus on techniques to compensate for difficulties in expression or interpretation of prosody, such as • Teaching the individual to use cues from the speaker that convey emotions other than prosody, such as word choice, facial expression, and body language • Asking communication partners and the person with RHBD to explicitly state emotions to avoid misunderstanding in expression or interpretation of prosody

Table 19–8. *continued*

Treatment Type	General Treatment Goals	Example Approaches
Attention, Memory, and Executive Function Treatment	Improve attention, memory, and executive functioning deficits	*Attention Treatment* Direct Treatment Approaches for Attention Target sustained, selective, alternating, and/or divided attention deficits, using • Computerized attention training programs • Practice engaging in structured or real-world tasks that require a specific level of attention, gradually increasing the complexity of tasks and type of attention as treatment progresses Metacognitive and Compensatory Strategy Approaches for Attention Help the person understand the nature, scope, and impact of attention deficits through a series of guided exercises with clinician feedback, followed by training in individualized strategies and techniques the person can use to mitigate or minimize the negative impacts of attention deficits on daily tasks. Environmental Modification Approaches for Attention Mitigate and minimize attention deficits by eliminating threats to attention in the environment, such as turning off or moving away from the TV, choosing the best time of day to complete important tasks, or organizing work space and removing distracting items. *Memory Treatment* Provide training and practice in compensating for memory impairments through the use of external and internal strategies, including the following (ASHA, n.d.-h, Attention, Memory, and Executive Function). External Strategies • To-do lists • Notes • Calendars • Alarms and timers • Medication reminders • Journals • Labels Internal Strategies • Mnemonics, such as assigning an abbreviation for information to be recalled (e.g., B.A.D. for bread, aspirin, and detergent to be purchased at the store) • Visualization, repetition, and rehearsal of information to be recalled • Semantic elaboration, such as identifying and describing as many salient features as possible of the information to be remembered or linking the information with preexisting knowledge.

continues

Table 19–8. *continued*

Treatment Type	General Treatment Goals	Example Approaches
Attention, Memory, and Executive Function Treatment *continued*	Improve attention, memory, and executive functioning deficits	*Executive Function* Develop skills for solving problems, thinking flexibly, setting and completing goals, staying on task, and staying organized, including Metacognitive and Compensatory Strategy Approaches for Executive Function Help the person understand the nature, scope, and impact of executive function deficits through a series of guided exercises with clinician feedback, followed by training in individualized strategies and techniques the person can use to mitigate or minimize the negative impacts of deficits in executive function on daily tasks. Environmental Modification Approaches for Executive Function Mitigate and minimize executive function deficits by eliminating threats to them in the environment, such as making sure that items and materials are stored near where they will be used, labeling boxes, drawers, and cabinets to indicate content, color-coding tabs in a file drawer to identify categories (e.g., medical records or bills) to optimize organization and problem solving.

Source: ASHA, n.d.-h. Treatment Options.

- Muscle weakness, loss of balance and coordination, disruption of vision, change in speech and language, or sensory loss;
- Any alternation in mental state at the time of the injury such as confusion, disorientation, slowed thinking, or difficulty concentrating.

It is important to note that concussion, defined as follows (McCrory, Meeuwisse, Aubry et al., 2013, pp. 1–2), is also considered TBI:

1. Caused either by a direct blow to the head, face, neck, or elsewhere on the body by an "impulsive" force (i.e., the brief force produced when two objects collide).

2. Typically results in the rapid onset of short-lived impairment of neurological function that resolves spontaneously. However, in some cases, symptoms and signs may evolve over a number of minutes to hours.

3. May result in neuropathological changes, but the acute clinical symptoms largely reflect a functional disturbance rather than a structural injury and as such, no abnormality is seen on standard structural neuroimaging studies.

4. Results in a graded set of clinical symptoms that may or may not involve loss of consciousness.

TBI is classified by the mechanism of primary injury (Ostergren, 2017). Table 19–9 has brief descriptions of primary injuries and their sub-classifications related to TBI. Not included in the table are blast or explosive injuries to the brain, which are thought to be a unique form of primary injury (Magnuson, Leonessa, & Ling, 2012).

Traumatic brain injury is a major cause of death, especially among young people, and a significant source of lifelong disability (CDC, 2017). So much so that it is often described as a silent epidemic and unfortunately, the incidence of TBI is on the rise globally (CDC, 2017). Each year in the United States, 2.5 million people sustain a TBI, either as an isolated injury or along with other injuries (CDC, 2017). Every day, 153 people die from injuries related to TBI (CDC, 2017). Falls are the most prevalent cause of TBI in the United States (CDC, 2017); other common sources include motor vehicle accidents and violence.

Individuals with TBI can experience a wide variety of symptoms including physical, visual, auditory and vestibular, neurobehavioral, swallowing, and communication impairments (ASHA, n.d.-e). Communication impairments after TBI are common and enduring in nature (Larkins, 2007). They are often attributed to disruptions of attention, memory, executive function, or social cognition (McDonald, Togher, & Code, 2014; Murdoch, 2010).

Table 19–9. Injury Classifications in Traumatic Brain Injury (TBI)

Primary Brain Injury	
Resulting from initial mechanical forces of the trauma (Greve & Zink, 2009)	
Penetrating/Open-Head Injury: A penetrating brain injury (also known as an open-head injury) occurs when the skull is pierced by an object (NINDS, n.d.)	*High-Velocity Penetrating Brain Injury* Resulting from high-velocity objects, such as rifle bullets, artillery shells, and shell fragments, traveling at a high speed penetrating the skull (Kazim et al, 2011; Young et al., 2015). *Low-Velocity Penetrating Brain Injury* Results from a penetrating object traveling at a lower rate of speed (as compared to high-velocity projectiles), such as clubs, baseball bats, and knives (Kazim et al., 2011; Young et al., 2015).
Nonpenetrating/Closed-Head Injury: A nonpenetrating brain injury (also known as closed-head injury) occurs as a result of an external force that produces rapid rotation or shaking of the brain within the skull (an impact to the skull; NINDS, n.d.).	*Nonacceleration Head Injuries* Resulting from damage to brain tissue primarily from a moving object striking the skull when the head is restrained, causing deformation of the skull at the point of impact (McLean & Anderson, 1997).If the force and nature of the object create a fracture to the skull and rupture of the meninges, this is referred to as a penetrating head injury (as above).The skull is slightly elastic, however, and can press inward to some degree, without being penetrated. *Acceleration and Deceleration Head Injuries* Resulting from damage due to movement of the brain within the skull when the head is not restrained, such as the moving head striking a stationary or moving object, or when the head is shaken violently.

Source: Ostergren, 2017.

As such, they are described as *cognitive-communication* disorders, which "encompasses difficulty with any aspect of communication that is affected by disruption of cognition." (ASHA, 2005, para. 1). They are defined as,

> A set of communication features that result from underlying deficits in cognition. Communication difficulties can include issues with hearing, listening, understanding, speaking, reading, writing, conversational interaction and social communication. These disorders may occur as a result of underlying deficits with cognition, that is: attention, orientation, memory,

organization, information processing, reasoning, problem solving, executive functions, or self-regulation. (College of Audiologists and Speech-Language Pathologists of Ontario, CASLPO, 2015, p. 2)

This interconnected relationship between communication and cognition is reflected in Figure 19–6, which shows communication at the center of the processes of attention, memory, executive function, and social cognition (Ostergren, 2017; Strutchen, n.d.). Table 19–10 provides additional examples of communication deficits associated with attention, memory, and executive function following TBI.

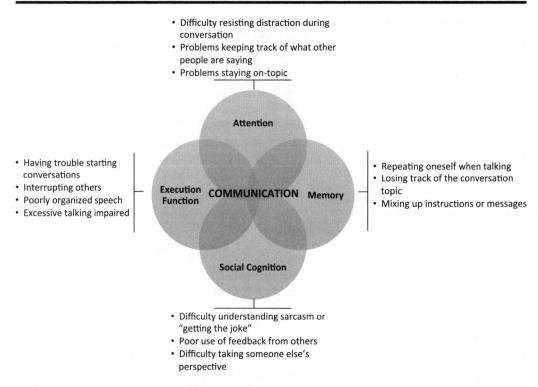

Figure 19–6. Communication at the intersection of attention, executive function, memory, and social communication. Ostergren, J. (2017). *Cognitive Rehabilitation Therapy for Traumatic Brain Injury: A Guide for Speech-Language Pathologists.* Copyright 2017. San Diego: Plural Publishing, Inc. All rights reserved. Reprinted with permission.

Table 19–10. Communication Deficits Associated with Cognitive Functions Commonly Impaired in TBI

Attention
Difficulty responding appropriately to incoming information
Difficulty learning new information
Difficulty filtering out irrelevant stimuli
Difficulty conversing in situations with distractions, background noise, and multiple participants
Difficulty managing the demands of high-level activity
Difficulty sustaining attention when reading complex or lengthy material
Difficulty shifting attention as needed
Difficulty maintaining or changing topics in conversation
Tangential discourse
Social avoidance to compensate for sense of overstimulation

Memory
Difficulty recalling instructions or messages
Difficulty learning new information
Difficulty remembering names of individuals, appointments, directions, or location of personal effects
Difficulty recalling details when reading complex or lengthy material
Difficulty maintaining topic or remembering purpose of conversation
Repetition of ideas, statements, questions, conversations, or stories
Failure to use compensatory strategies to improve performance on everyday tasks

Executive Function
Lack of coherence in discourse
Lack of organization in planning daily activities
Difficulty implementing plans and actions
Difficulty initiating conversations
Problems recognizing and repairing conversational breakdowns
Inability to determine the needs of communication partners
Difficulty making inferences or drawing conclusions
Difficulty assuming another person's perspective
Difficulty interpreting the behavior of others
Difficulty evaluating validity of information
Verbose; lack of conciseness in verbal expression
Decreased comprehension of abstract language, humor, or indirect requests
Difficulty meeting deadlines
Difficulty formulating realistic goals
Difficulty recognizing complexity of tasks and need for simplification
Difficulty anticipating consequences of actions
Inappropriate comments

Source: Cornis-Pop et al., 2012, Traumatic Brain Injury.

One type of treatment for cognitive-communication disorders following TBI is cognitive rehabilitation therapy (CRT). CRT is "a systematic, functionally oriented service of therapeutic cognitive activities, based on an assessment and understanding of the person's brain-behavior deficits. Services are directed to achieve functional changes by (1) reinforcing, strengthening, or reestablishing previously learned patterns of behavior, or (2) establishing new patterns of cognitive activity or compensatory mechanisms for impaired neurological systems." (Harley et al., 1992, p. 63) CRT is provided in either individual or group format. It is expected to (ASHA, n.d.-e., Treatment Options):

- Capitalize on strengths and address weaknesses related to underlying structures and functions that affect communication,
- Facilitate the individual's activities and participation by assisting the person in acquiring new skills and strategies, and

- Modify contextual factors that serve as barriers and enhance facilitators of successful communication and participation, including development and use of appropriate accommodations.

Table 19–11 summarizes CRT approaches for cognitive-communication disorders. A prominent element of CRT is training in the use of assistive technology for cognition (ATC; Leopold, Lourie, Petras, & Elias, 2015). ATC is designed to, "increase, maintain, or improve functional capabilities for individuals whose cognitive changes limit their performance of daily activities" (Scherer, 2012, p. 159). ATC can be divided into low technology, medium technology, and high technology (Sohlberg, 2011). High technology includes the use of increasingly popular mainstream technology such as smartphones and tablet computers. Table 19–12 lists examples of ATC categorized by their level of technology and function (task specific or multifunction).

Table 19–11. Treatment Approaches for Cognitive-Communication Disorders After Traumatic Brain Injury (TBI)

Treatment Type	General Treatment Goals	Example Approaches
Compensatory Strategy Training	Maximize the performance and capitalize on intact skills through either modifying the environment or providing internal and external supports.	Support communication and cognition by identifying, training, and generalizing external and/or internal compensatory strategies. Examples of external strategies are the assistive technology for cognition (ATC) devices and supports listed in Table 19–12. Internal strategies include • Mnemonics, such as assigning an abbreviation for information to be recalled (e.g., B.A.D. for bread, aspirin, and detergent to be purchased at the store) • Visualization, repetition, and rehearsal of information to be recalled • Semantic elaboration, such as identifying and describing as many salient features as possible of the information to be remembered or associating the information with preexisting knowledge.

Table 19–11. *continued*

Treatment Type	General Treatment Goals	Example Approaches
Computer Assisted Technology (CAT)	Target cognitive processing using commercial software and mobile applications.	Provide consistent feedback to individuals on their performance during cognitive tasks using software or mobile applications that administer repeated trials targeting specific skills or functional tasks, adapted to the individual's performance.
Drill and Practice Training	Establish new networks or stimulate damaged neural networks to restore them using practice and drills for specific skills.	Use repetition of target behaviors to develop new or lost skills and abilities.
Dual Task Training	Improve task complexity by targeting the ability to carry out two competing tasks (typically requiring equal amounts of attention).	Systematic practice and feedback on a combination of two cognitive tasks—a cognitive and motor task, or two motor tasks.
Errorless Learning	Develop new skills or relearn previously developed skills by practicing them without error.	Treatment tasks structure opportunities for repeated practice with a target skill, that • Breaks down the target task into small, discrete steps or units • Provides models before the client is asked to perform the target task • Encourages the client to avoid guessing • Immediately corrects errors and carefully fades prompts once a behavior is established
Metacognitive Skills Training	Improve awareness and self-monitoring of cognitive and communication deficits.	Treatment tasks engage individuals in structured and guided self-reflection and self-regulation in order to facilitate better recognition of problem situations and identification of functional strategies that facilitate success in achieving everyday goals after a TBI.
Social Communication Training	Improve functional conversational skills and success in navigating social situations.	Important components of social communication treatment includes (ASHA, n.d.-a., Treatment Options) • Sharing knowledge with and training everyday communication partners • Selecting highly specific and personal goals and incorporating extensive practice of social behaviors in the situations in which they are required • Situational coaching prior to challenging situations • Situational training to improve social perception and interpretation of others' behaviors to improve self-monitoring of stress • Focusing on social success • Counseling to help an individual identify a sense of self that includes positive social interaction strategies

Source: ASHA, n.d.-a., Treatment Options.

Table 19–12. Sample Assistive Technologies for Cognition Aids Categorized by Function and Level

Task specific	Multifunctional
Low technology	
Calculator	Sticky notes
Pillbox with reminder	Voice mail, answering machine
Phone dialer	Checklists
Alarm clock	Appointment calendars
Electronic speller, thesaurus, dictionary	Memo pads for the car
Oven timer	
Watch, clock	
Labeler	
Key finder	
Mail sorter baskets	
Map, posted directional signs	
Financial planner	
Posted instructions	
Mid technology	
Camera	Voice recorder/digital recorder
	Cell phone
	Pager
	Data watches
High technology	
Global positioning system (GPS) device	Specialized task guidance systems
Specialized software programs for facilitated writing, reading, or email	Smartphones
	Personal digital assistants

Source: Sohlberg, 2011.

Dysarthria

Dysarthria is broadly defined as "an impaired ability to produce clear speech due to the impaired function of the speech muscles" (The Stroke Foundation, 2017, Glossary, para 15). More specifically, dysarthria describes a group of neurologic speech disorders with "abnormalities in the strength, speed, range, steadiness, tone, or accuracy of movements required for breathing, phonatory, resonatory, articulatory, or prosodic aspects of speech production" (Duffy, 2013, p. 4). This can be related to sensorimotor problems, such as weakness (paresis), paralysis, incoordination, involuntary movements, or excessive, reduced, or variable muscle tone (Duffy,

2013). Impairments due to dysarthria range from speech that has mild articulatory imprecision to speech that is totally unintelligible. Box 19–4 lists several common signs of dysarthria (ASHA, n.d.-f). Dysarthria can be one of several types based on the perceptual features of the speaker (Table 19–13).

Anything that causes brain damage can cause dysarthria, including stroke, TBI, and tumors (ASHA, n.d.-f) and a variety of progressive neurologic disorders such as Parkinson's disease, amyotrophic lateral sclerosis (ALS), cerebral palsy, and dementia. The true incidence and prevalence of dysarthria is not known and will vary based on the cause. Research suggests that 8% to 60% of individuals with stroke and 10% to 65% of individuals with TBI present with dysarthria (ASHA, n.d.-f).

Treatment for dysarthria focuses on "facilitating the efficiency, effectiveness, and naturalness of communication" (ASHA, n.d.-f, Treatment). Restoration approaches target the speech production subsystems and compensatory approaches target communication strategies, environmental modifications, and AAC. Medical or surgical interventions are also used to treat dysarthria

(ASHA, n.d.-f). Table 19–14 summarizes of treatment approaches for dysarthria.

Apraxia of Speech

Apraxia is defined as "impaired planning and sequencing of movement that is not due to weakness, incoordination or sensory loss" (The Stroke Foundation, 2017, Glossary, para. 5). There are different forms of apraxia, including limb apraxia, oral apraxia, apraxia of gait, apraxia of swallowing, and apraxia of speech (ASHA, n.d.-g). Often these forms co-occur (ASHA, n.d.-g). Apraxia of speech (AOS) refers to impaired planning and sequencing of speech, including difficulty initiating and executing movements for speech in the absence of weakness in the speech muscles (National Clinical Guideline Centre, 2013). There are two forms of AOS: *acquired* AOS, caused by damage to the parts of the brain responsible for speaking, and *childhood* AOS (also known as developmental apraxia of speech, developmental verbal apraxia, or articulatory apraxia), which is present from birth. Consistent with the theme of this chapter, the sections that follow describe acquired AOS.

Box 19–4. Common Signs of Dysarthria

- Slurred or mumbled speech that can be hard to understand
- Slow speech
- Rapid speech
- Quiet speech
- Inability to easily move tongue, lips, and jaw properly
- Robotic or choppy speech
- Changes in voice quality (e.g., hoarseness, breathiness, stuffiness, hypernasality)

Table 19–13. Common Types of Dysarthria and their Perceptual Characteristics

Dysarthria Type	Perceptual Speech Characteristics
Flaccid	• Continuous breathiness • Diplophonia • Audible inspiration or stridor • Nasal emission • Short phrases • Hypernasality • Rapid deterioration and recovery with rest • Imprecise alternating motion rates (AMRs)
Spastic	• Slow rate • Strained or harsh voice quality • Pitch breaks • Slow and regular AMRs
Ataxic	• Irregular articulatory breakdowns • Excess and equal stress • Distorted vowels • Excessive loudness variation • Irregular AMRs
Hypokinetic	• Monopitch • Monoloudness • Reduced loudness and stress • Tendency for rapid or accelerated rate • Inappropriate silences • Rapidly repeated phonemes • Palilalia • Rapid, "blurred" AMRs
Hyperkinetic	• Prolonged intervals • Sudden forced inspiration or expiration • Transient breathiness • Transient vocal strain or harshness • Voice stoppages/arrests • Voice tremor • Myoclonic vowel prolongation • Intermittent hypernasality • Marked deterioration with increased rate • Inappropriate vocal noises • Intermittent breathy or aphonic segments • Distorted vowels • Excessive loudness variation • Slow and irregular AMRs
Unilateral Upper Motor Neuron	• Slow rate • Imprecise articulation • Irregular articulatory breakdowns • Strained voice quality • Reduced loudness

Source: Duffy, 2013, as cited by ASHA, n.d.-g, Distinguishing Perceptual Characteristics and Physiologic Findings by Dysarthria Type.

Table 19–14. Treatment Approaches for Dysarthria

Treatment Type	General Treatment Goals	Example Approaches
Speech Production Subsystem Treatment	Target the speech-production subsystems of • Respiration, • Phonation, • Articulation, and • Resonance	Use drills, practice, strength, and conditioning training for impacted muscles; postural adjustments; and facilitative techniques to directly target the impacted subsystems of speech.
Communication Strategies	Target a variety of strategies used by individuals with dysarthria and their communication partners to enhance speech intelligibility and comprehensibility.	Identify, train, and generalize the following strategies: Speaker Strategies: • Maintain eye contact • Gain listeners' attention and introduce topics before speaking • Use pointing and gesturing to help convey meaning • Look for signs that communication partners have not understood the message • Use conversational repair strategies Communication-Partner Strategies: • Use active listening and make efforts to understand the speaker's message • Ask for clarification information • Provide feedback and encouragement • Optimize ability to hear the speaker and to see the speaker's visual communication cues, such as wearing prescribed hearing aids and glasses during conversations
Environmental Modification	Identify and modify the environment to optimize speech intelligibility and comprehensibility.	Optimize speech by eliminating environmental threats to intelligibility and comprehensibility, such as reducing background noise, ensuring that the environment has good lighting, improving proximity between the speaker and his or her communication partner, and using face-to-face seating for conversations.
Augmentative and Alternative Communication (AAC)	Instruct speakers in strategies to supplement or replace speech.	Train in the use of aided and unaided communication techniques to supplement or replace spoken language. Examples of aided techniques include picture communication symbols, and line drawings. Examples of unaided techniques include manual signs, gestures, and finger spelling. Other AAC approaches for dysarthria include voice amplifiers, artificial phonation devices (e.g., electrolarynx and intraoral devices), and oral prosthetics to reduce hypernasality.

Source: ASHA, n.d.-h., Treatment Options.

Acquired forms of AOS often co-occur with dysarthria and aphasia (National Clinical Guideline Centre, 2013). Because of this, and challenges in distinguishing among certain types of errors, there is no reliable data on the incidence and prevalence of acquired AOS in adults (ASHA, n.d.-g; Duffy, Strand, & Josephs, 2014). When AOS is documented as the primary, but not the only communication disorder present, estimates suggest it comprises approximately 7% of all motor speech disorders (Duffy, 2013 as cited in ASHA, n.d.-g).

Treatment approaches for AOS focus on facilitating the efficiency, effectiveness, and naturalness of communication (ASHA, n.d.-g) by either improving speech production or using AAC to enhance communication effectiveness. Treatment for AOS also focuses on minimizing barriers to successful communication, such as (ASHA, n.d.-g, Treatment, para. 5):

■ Modifying the environment (e.g., reducing background noise, maintaining eye contact, and decreasing the distance between speaker and listener);
■ Informing listeners about the individual's communication needs and his or her preferred method of communication; and
■ Encouraging speakers to use strategies for repairing breakdowns in communication (e.g., repeating, rephrasing, gesturing, writing).

Table 19–15 summarizes common treatment approaches for AOS.

Table 19–15. Common Treatment Approaches for Apraxia of Speech (AOS)

Treatment Type	General Treatment Goals	Example Approaches
Articulatory–Kinematic	Address the symptoms of AOS using the principles of motor programming and planning.	Approaches include elements of the following: • Provide frequent and intensive practice of speech targets • Focus on accurate speech movement • Include external sensory input for speech production (e.g., auditory, visual, tactile, cognitive cues) • Consider practice schedules, such as random versus blocked practice • Provide appropriate types and schedules of feedback regarding performance
Sensory Cueing	Teach movement sequences for speech by incorporating sensory input (e.g., visual, auditory, proprioceptive, and tactile cues).	Provide a variety of sensory feedback (either separately or in combination) on important aspect of motor learning and planning.
Rate and Rhythm Control	Improve speech production by addressing rate and rhythm control (also known as prosodic facilitation).	Increase the length of utterances, decrease dependence on the clinician, and decrease reliance on prosodic patterns by guiding individuals through a gradual progression of steps.
Augmentative and Alternative Communication (AAC)	Supplement or replace speech by instruct individuals in strategies.	Supplement or replace spoken language with training in the use of aided and unaided communication techniques. Aided techniques include picture communication symbols and line drawings. Unaided techniques include manual signs, gestures, and finger spelling.
Script Training	Facilitate participation in personally relevant activities using intact knowledge of scripts (understanding, remembering, and recalling event sequences of an activity).	Help individuals to create, learn, and automatically use scripted monologue or dialogue during activities of interest.

Source: ASHA, n.d.-c.

REFERENCES

American Psychiatric Association. (2013). *Diagnostic and statistical manual of mental disorders* (5th ed.). Arlington, VA: Author.

American Speech-Language-Hearing Association (ASHA). (n.d.-a). *Frequently asked questions: Speech-Language Pathology Assistants.* Retrieved from https://www.asha.org/associates/SLPA-FAQs/

American Speech-Language-Hearing Association (ASHA). (n.d.-b). *Executive summary: SLP health care survey 2002.* Retrieved from https://www.asha.org/research/memberdata/exec_sum/

American Speech-Language-Hearing Association (ASHA). (n.d.-c). *Aphasia.* Retrieved from https://www.asha.org/Practice-Portal/Clinical-Topics/Aphasia/

American Speech-Language-Hearing Association. (n.d.-d). *Right hemisphere damage.* Retrieved from https://www.asha.org/Practice-Portal/Clinical-Topics/Right-Hemisphere-Damage/

American Speech-Language-Hearing Association. (n.d.-e). *Traumatic brain injury in adults.* Retrieved from https://www.asha.org/Practice-Portal/Clinical-Topics/Traumatic-Brain-Injury-in-Adults/

American Speech-Language-Hearing Association. (n.d.-f). *Dysarthria in adults.* Retrieved from https://www.asha.org/PRPSpecificTopic.aspx?folderid=8589943481&section=Treatment

American Speech-Language-Hearing Association. (n.d.-g). *Acquired apraxia of speech.* Retrieved from https://www.asha.org/Practice-Portal/Clinical-Topics/Acquired-Apraxia-of-Speech/

American Speech-Language-Hearing Association. (2005). *Roles of speech-language pathologists in the identification, diagnosis, and treatment of individuals with cognitive-communication disorders: Position statement* [Position statement]. Retrieved from https://www.asha.org/policy/ps2005-00110.htm

American Speech-Language-Hearing Association (ASHA). (2011). *Current status of SLP employment in health care settings.* Retrieved from https://www.asha.org/careers/recruitment/healthcare/recruit_current/

American Speech-Language-Hearing Association (ASHA). (2013). *Speech-language pathology assistant scope of practice.* Retrieved from https://www.asha.org/policy/sp2013-00337/

American Speech-Language-Hearing Association. (2017). *National Outcomes Measurement System: Adults in healthcare–acute hospital national data report 2017.* Rockville, MD: National Center for Evidence-Based Practice in Communication Disorders.

Blake, M. L. (2018). *The right hemisphere and disorders of cognition and communication: Theory and clinical practice.* San Diego, CA: Plural.

Brain Injury Association of America (BIAA). (2012). *Brain injury basics.* Retrieved from https://www.biausa.org/brain-injury

Brasure, M., Lamberty, G. J., Sayer, N. A., Nelson, N. W., Macdonald, R., Ouellette, J., & Wilt. T. J. (2013). Participation after multidisciplinary rehabilitation for moderate to severe traumatic brain injury in adults: A systematic review. *Archives of Physical Medicine and Rehabilitation, 94*(7), 1398–1420.

Brookshire, R. (2015). *Introduction to neurogenic communication disorders.* St. Louis. MO: Mosby.

Centers for Disease Control and Prevention (CDC). (2015). *Report to Congress on traumatic brain injury in the United States: Epidemiology and rehabilitation.* National Center for Injury Prevention and Control; Division of Unintentional Injury Prevention. Atlanta, GA. Retrieved from http://www.cdc.gov/traumaticbraininjury/pdf/tbi_report_to_congress_epi_and_rehab-a.pdf

Centers for Disease Control and Prevention (CDC). (2017). *TBI: Get the facts.* Retrieved from https://www.cdc.gov/traumaticbraininjury/get_the_facts.html

College of Audiologists and Speech-Language Pathologists of Ontario. (2015). *Practice standards and guidelines for acquired cognitive communication disorders.* Toronto, Canada: Author. Retrieved from http://www.caslpo.com/sites/default/uploads/files/PSG_EN_Acquired_Cognitive_Communication_Disorders.pdf

Cornis-Pop, M., Mashima, P.A., Roth, C.A., MacLennan, D.L., Picon, L.M., Smith Hammond, C., . . . Frank, E.M. (2012). Cognitive-communication rehabilitation for combat-related mild traumatic brain injury. *Journal of Rehabilitation Research & Development, 49*(7), xi–xxxi.

Cott, C. A. (2004). Client-centered rehabilitation: Client perspectives. *Disability & Rehabilitation, 26*(24), 1411–1422.

Duffy, J. R. (2013). *Motor speech disorders: Substrates, differential diagnosis, and management.* **St. Louis, MO: Elsevier.**

Duffy, J. R., Strand, E. A., & Josephs, K. A. (2014). Motor speech disorders associated with primary progressive aphasia. *Aphasiology, 28,* **1004–1017.**

Harley, J. P., Allen, C. Braciszewski, T. L., Cicerone, K. D., Dahlberg, C., Evans, S., . . . Smigelski, J.S. (1992). Guidelines for cognitive rehabilitation. *NeuroRehabilitation, 2,* 62–67.

Helm-Estabrooks, N. Albert, M., & Nicholas, N. (2014). *Manual of aphasia and aphasia therapy.* Austin, TX: Pro-Ed.

Institute of Medicine. (2011). *Cognitive rehabilitation therapy for traumatic brain injury: Evaluating the evidence.* Washington, DC: The National Academies Press. doi:10.17226/13220

Kazim, S. F., Shamim, M. S., Tahir, M. Z., Enam, S. A., & Waheed, S. (2011). Management of penetrating brain injury. *Journal of Emergencies, Trauma, and Shock, 4*(3), 395–402.

Knowles, M. (1984a). *The adult learner: A neglected species* (3rd ed.). Houston, TX: Gulf.

Knowles, M. (1984b) *Andragogy in action.* San Francisco, CA: Jossey-Bass.

Larkins, B. (2007). The application of the ICF in cognitive-communication disorders following traumatic brain injury. *Seminars in Speech and Language, 28*(4), 334–342.

Lehman Blake, M., Frymark, T., & Venedictov, R. (2013). An evidence-based systematic review on communication treatments for individuals with right hemisphere brain damage. *American Journal of Speech-Language Pathology, 22,* 146–160.

Leopold, A., Lourie, A., Petras, H., & Elias, E. (2015). The use of assistive technology for cognition to support the performance of daily activities for individuals with cognitive disabilities due to traumatic brain injury: The current state of the research. *NeuroRehabilitation, 37*(3), 359–378.

Magnuson, J., Leonessa, F., & Ling, G. (2012). Neuropathology of explosive blast traumatic brain injury. *Current Neurology and Neuroscience Reports, 12*(5), 570–579.

McCrory P., Meeuwisse, W. H., Aubry, M., Cantu, B., Dvořák, J., Echemendia, R. J., . . . Turner, M. (2013). Consensus statement on concussion in sport: The 4th international conference on concussion in sport held in Zurich, November 2012. *British Journal of Sports Medicine, 47,* 250–258.

McDonald, S., Togher, L., & Code, C. (2014). *Social and communication disorders following traumatic brain injury.* New York, NY: Psychology Press.

McLean, A. J., & Anderson, R. W. G., (1997). Biomechanics of closed head injury. In P. Reilly & R. Bullock (Eds.), *Head injury: Pathophysiology and management of severe closed head injury.* New York, NY: Chapman & Hall.

Menon, D. K., Schwab, K., Wright, D. W., Maas, A. I., and Demographics and Clinical Assessment Working Group of the International and Interagency Initiative toward Common Data Elements for Research on Traumatic Brain Injury and Psychological Health. (2010). Position statement: Definition of traumatic brain injury. *Archives of Physical Medicine and Rehabilitation, 91*(11), 1637–1640.

Merriam, S. B. (2001). Andragogy and self-directed learning: Pillars of adult learning theory. *New Directions for Adult & Continuing Education, 2001*(89), 3–14.

Murdoch, B. E. (2010). Speech-language disorders associated with traumatic brain injury. In B. E. Murdoch (Ed.), *Acquired speech and language disorders: A neuroanatomical and functional neurological approach* (2nd ed., pp. 118–152). Oxford, UK: Wiley-Blackwell.

National Aphasia Association. (n.d.). *Aphasia definitions.* Retrieved from https://www.aphasia.org/aphasia-definitions/

National Clinical Guideline Centre. (2013). *Stroke rehabilitation: Long-term rehabilitation after stroke.* London, UK: National Institute for Health and Care Excellence, (Clinical Guideline 162), 4–591.

National Institute of Neurologic Disorders and Stroke. (2015). *Traumatic brain injury: Hope through research* (NIH Publication No. 15-2478). Retrieved from https://www.ninds.nih.gov/Disorders/Patient-Caregiver-Education/Hope-Through-Research/Traumatic-Brain-Injury-Hope-Through

National Institute on Deafness and Other Communication Disorders. (2015). *NIDCD fact sheet: Aphasia* (NIH Pub. No. 97-4257). Retrieved from https://www.nidcd.nih.gov/sites/default/files/Documents/health/voice/Aphasia6-1-16.pdf

Ostergren, J. (2017). *Cognitive rehabilitation therapy for traumatic brain injury: A guide for speech-language pathologists.* San Diego, CA: Plural.

Picker Institute. (n.d.). *Principles of patient-centered care.* Retrieved from: http://cgp.pickerinstitute.org/?page_id=1319

Scherer, M. J. (2012). *Assistive technologies and other supports for people with brain impairment.* New York, NY: Springer.

Simmons-Mackie, N., & Kagan, A. (2007). Application of the ICF in aphasia. *Seminars of Speech and Language, 28*(4), 244–253.

Sohlberg, M. (2011). Assistive technology for cognition. *ASHA Leader, 16*(2), 14.

Strutchen, M.A. (n.d.) *Social communication and traumatic brain injury (TBI): A guide for professionals.* Houston, TX: Traumatic Brain Injury Model System at TIRR Memorial Hermann Brain Injury Research Center. Retrieved from http://www.tbicommunity.org/resources/publications/professional_education_social_comm.pdf

Sohlberg, M. (2011). Assistive technology for cognition. *ASHA Leader*, *16*(2), 14.

Teasdale, R., Cullen, N., Marshall, S., Janzen, S., & Bayley, M. (2017). *Evidence-based review of moderate to severe acquired brain injury: Introduction and methodology.* Retrieved from https://www.abiebr.com/sites/default/files/modules/Module%201_V12_Intro.pdf

The Stroke Foundation. (2017). *Clinical guidelines for stroke management 2017.* Melbourne, Australia: The Stroke Foundation. Retrieved from https://informme.org.au/Guidelines/Clinical-Guidelines-for-Stroke-Management-2017

Toronto Acquired Brain Injury Network. (2005). *Definition of acquired brain injury.* Retrieved from http://www.abinetwork.ca/definition

University of California San Francisco Health. (n.d.). *Neurological disorders.* Retrieved from https://www.ucsfhealth.org/conditions/neurological_disorders/

World Health Organization (WHO). (2002). *Towards a common language for functioning, disability and health: ICF.* Geneva, Switzerland: Author. Retrieved from http://www.who.int/classifications/icf/training/icfbeginnersguide.pdf

Young, L., Rule, G. T., Bocchieri, R. T., Walilko, T. J., Burns, J. M., & Ling, G. (2015). When physics meets biology: Low and high-velocity penetration, blunt impact, and blast injuries to the brain. *Frontiers in Neurology, 6*(89), 1–19.

Index

Note: Page numbers in **bold** reference non-text material

confidentiality of, 196
data collection section of, **198**, 201, 204. *See also* Data collection
educational field use of, 196
goals
 defining of, 197
 sample, **198**, 243–247
materials/equipment section of, **198**, 202
objectives
 components of, 199, **199**
 condition statement of, **200**, 200–201
 criterion of, **200**, 201
 deciphering of, **200**, 200–201
 definition of, 197, 199
 example of, **198**
 performance statement of, 200, **200**
 sample, 243–247
origins of, 196
prompts and modifications section of, **198**, 202–204
sample, **198**
Liability insurance, 9–10, 24–25
Life Participation Approach to Aphasia, **522**
LightwriterSL50, 504
Linguistic facilitation, **431**
Liquid gliding, 362, 374
Liquid oxygen systems, 183
Listening, 79, 132, 135, 140
Literacy development, 295
Literature-based units, 430–432
LLD. *See* Language learning disorders
Long-term goals, 197
Low-road processing, 290
Low-tech aided communication, **486**, 486–487
Lung abscess, 184

M

Mainstream culture, 159
Mainstream Euro-Americans, 159
Malpractice insurance, 9
Materials/equipment section, of lesson plans, **198**, 202
Maximal oppositions contrast, 375–376
Mean length of utterance, 264, **265**, 269
Mechanical corrective feedback, **310**
Medical abbreviations, 133, 143–144

Medical conditions. *See also* Acquired neurologic disorders; Neurologic disorders
 airway obstruction, 180, **180**
 allergic reactions, 180–181
 heart attack, 179, **179**
 overview of, 177–178
 seizures, 180, **181**
 stroke, **178**, 178–179
 traumatic brain injury, 179–180
Medical setting
 direct observation of skills checklist for, 72
 job description for, 60–61
 reports in, sample, 228–242
 self-evaluation of intervention sessions in, 155–156
Medically fragile, 28
Melodic intonation therapy, **522**
Mentee, 82, **83**
Mentor
 finding of, 82
 how to find, 82, 84
 roles of, **83**
 supervisor and, differences between, 82
Mentoring
 definition of, 82
 goal setting for, 84
 guidelines for, **85**
 mentee, 82, **83**
 mentor. *See* Mentor
 relationship, 82, 84
Metacognitive skills training, **533**
Metaskills, 426
Methicillin-resistant Staphylococcus aureus, **173**
Minimal oppositions, 374–375, **375**
Minimal pairs, 374–375. **375**
Minority groups, 157
Misspelled words, 152
Mistakes, learning from, 133
MIT. *See* Melodic intonation therapy
Mixed nonfluent aphasia, **520**
MLU. *See* Mean length of utterance
Modeling of tasks, 301, **302**, 429
Morals, laws versus, 91
Morphemes, 264, **265**, 377, 415, 463
Morphological acquisition, **391**